The Art of EKG Interpretation

A Self-Instructional Text

Sixth Edition

with Special Sections on

➤ Hemodynamic Monitoring

➤ Diagnosis and Treatment of Acute Coronary Syndromes

➤ Pacemaker Basics

➤ Advanced Pacemaker Features and Interventions

➤ Antiarrhythmic, Thrombolytic and Platelet Inhibitor Agents

➤ Pediatric EKG Interpretation

➤ Advanced Practice

Karen S. Ehrat, Ph.D.

KENDALL/HUNT PUBLISHING COI
4050 Westmark Drive   Dubuque, Iowa

Book Team

Chairman and Chief Executive Officer Mark C. Falb
Senior Vice President, College Division Thomas W. Gantz
Director of National Book Program Paul B. Carty
Editorial Development Manager Georgia Botsford
Developmental Editor Lynne Rogers
Vice President, Production and Manufacturing Alfred C. Grisanti
Assistant Vice President, Production Services Christine E. O'Brien
Prepress Editor Amanda Smith
Permissions Editor Corrina Vohl
Designer Jenifer Chapman

THIS BOOK IS DEDICATED

TO MEMBERS OF

THE HEALTH CARE COMMUNITY

. . . PROFESSIONALS AND STUDENTS . . .

WHO ARE STRIVING TO LEARN THE

COMPLEXITIES OF EKG INTERPRETATION

AND RELATED TOPICS

AS PAINLESSLY AS POSSIBLE!

CONTRIBUTING AUTHORS

Stephanie L. Woods, Ph.D., R.N.
Victoria A. Paparelli, M.S.N., R.N., CCNS-AC
Mike Lucey, Pharm. D.

ACKNOWLEDGMENTS

Every writer attempts to recognize individuals who support or contribute to a publication. This author shares that motivation, but humbly acknowledges the magnitude of that effort. I especially wish to thank past learners (professionals and students) and faculty whose comments and suggestions have supported the evolution of this text and the intergenerational transfer of knowledge.

Special geographic acknowledgments are also in order! From the *Cactus Belt,* Tucson Medical Center and the University of Arizona are credited with supporting the genesis of this text. The *Rust Belt,* St. Joseph's Mercy Hospital Centers, Mt. Clemens, Michigan, supplied contributing authors and they, in turn, supplied expanded content. Later in *River City*, Cincinnati, Mercy Hospital Anderson furnished unique and challenging monitor tracings to further challenge the reader. The *Outer Banks* of North Carolina unknowingly contributed sea shells later discovered on the cover of the fourth edition, and, the *Alamo City* and Baptist Health System birthed the millennium edition. This sixth edition calls for special acknowledgments noted below.

A special thank you is extended to the following persons, facilities and staff for collecting challenging rhythm strips for this edition!

Virginia Dempsey, President/CEO Marymount Medical Center, London, Kentucky

Chris Dumas, Chief Nursing Officer, St. Luke's Baptist Hospital, San Antonio, Texas

Pam Flentge, Chief Nursing Officer, Southwest General Hospital, San Antonio, Texas

Payton Flynn, RN Nurse Manager Adult Medical/Surgical Specialty, Christus Santa Rosa Hospital, San Antonio, Texas

Lea Martinez, RN Director Critical Care, North Central Baptist Hospital, San Antonio, Texas

Brooks Sutton, Chief Operating Officer, St. Clare Hospital, Lakewood, Washington.

Alphabetically, Mike Lucey, Victoria Paparelli and Stephanie Woods win *best supporting author awards* for their respective contributions to this text. I gratefully acknowledge their work and the past contributions of Deanna Culberson, Delores Schultz and Jane Werth.

Finally, I must thank Margaret Reihner who has provided editorial assistance. Absent her able support, this text would be a mere collection of monitor tracings and meaningless diagrams!

For the many other supporters I have failed to mention, I trust a *sincere* thank you will be accepted!!

ABOUT THE AUTHOR

The author is a self-described "non-traditional educator" who promotes the lighter side of learning. Dr. Ehrat is a prolific writer and public speaker. Her work experiences span the health care spectrum, from Indian Health Services, Critical Care, Education and Research, to Executive Management. Dr. Ehrat's educational memorabilia includes a diploma from St. Luke's, St. Louis, a Master's of Science degree in Nursing and a Doctor of Philosophy degree in Higher Education from the University of Arizona.

Dr. Ehrat is well-respected by professional colleagues and is described by students (medical, nursing, para-professional and everyday, ordinary non-medical variety) as a dynamic instructor!

A LONG-WINDED INTRODUCTION
WORTH READING

Cardiac rhythms can be *relatively* straight forward or *amazingly* confounding. **Not to worry**! The purpose of this text is to provide the reader with an excellent baseline understanding of both the simple and more complex rhythms, imparting terminology along the way. Importantly, a consistent methodology for evaluating and describing rhythms is emphasized throughout. Numerous illustrations and analogies serve to aid learning and demystify complex concepts. Sufficient structure has been incorporated to prevent even the novice learner from floundering! At the conclusion of the text, the reader will be *comfortable* describing simple and complex rhythm disorders and determining when action is warranted. Several *Advanced Study* ( ) discussions are included for the more adventurous student.

This sixth edition of *The Art of EKG Interpretation* considers rapidly expanding diagnostic and therapeutic interventions and provides additional rhythm interpretation practice exercises. Faculty and student suggestions have been incorporated into the content. The author's undergirding assumptions remain unchanged: complex material can be easily learned when it is broken into its simplest, component parts; learning technical material can be both *fun* and *painless*; and, humor aids adult learning!

One introductory point deserves *special* attention. Professionals in cardiac monitoring areas excel in the everyday use of complex, technical terminology. The new learner should consider that the use of highly technical terminology is simply a means for distinguishing one's practice specialty . . . similar to surgeons wearing green, surgical nurses displaying Kelly clamps, ICU nurses draping stethoscopes over their shoulders, etc. Rest assured, comfort with terminology will follow as a *natural* consequence of rhythm description!!

This text has been structured to allow for *self-paced learning* and utilizes a self-instructional format. Information and encouragement are provided under headings labeled **Input**. **Practice Exercises** follow Input sections. Practice Exercise answers are provided under **Feedback** headings. Practice rhythm strips are included throughout.

As a final *important* word, please be advised that diagnostic and therapeutic interventions change at rates *faster than speeding bullets*! Both technologic and pharmacologic developments, in concert with clinical research, continue to evolve the efficacy of both diagnosis and treatment of rhythm disorders and related pathology. The reader is always advised to consult the most current version of the American Heart Association's **Advanced Life Support** for treatment updates.

CONTENTS

(Participant Objectives Precede Each Section 👓)

LEADing into Section 1,   1

The Standard Limb Leads, 4

The Augmented Leads, 6

The Precordial Leads, 7

Bedside Monitoring, 9

Section 1: The Conduction System and Related Matters,   15

Input Section 1.1:   The Conduction System, 16

Input Section 1.2:   The P Wave and P-R Interval, 17

Input Section 1.3:   The QRS Complex, 19

Input Section 1.4:   The ST Segment, the T Wave and U wave . . . (followed by a word about the QT
                       interval and QRS interval and QRS-ST segment), 22

Input Section 1.5:   Paper Time, 24

Input Section 1.6:   Measuring P, P-R, and QRS Intervals, 26

Input Section 1.7:   Calculating Heart Rate, 29

Input Section 1.8:   Sinus Rhythm, 34

Input Section 1.9:   Interpreting Dysrhythmias, 35

Section 2: Sinus and Atrial Dysrhythmias,   45

Input Section 2.1:   Steps for Interpreting Dysrhythmias, 46

Input Section 2.2:   Sinus Arrhythmia, 47

Input Section 2.3:   Sinus Bradycardia, 50

Input Section 2.4:   Sinus Tachycardia, 53

Input Section 2.5:   Wandering Atrial Pacemaker (W.A.P.), 55

Input Section 2.6:   Premature Atrial Contractions, 56

Input Section 2.7:   Atrial Tachycardia and Re-entry Mechanisms, 61

                       Multifocal Atrial Tachycardia (MAT), 62

                       🎓 Atrial Re-entry Mechanisms (Advanced Study), 63

Input Section 2.8:   Atrial Flutter, 69

Input Section 2.9:   Atrial Fibrillation, 73

Input Section 2.10:   Atrial Flutter-Fibrillation ("flutter-fib"), 76

Input Section 2.11:   Sick Sinus Syndrome (Brady-Tachy Syndrome), 77

Input Section 2.12:   Bypass Re-Entry Mechanisms (Wolff-Parkinson-White Syndrome)
                                  Advanced Study, 78

                                  Wolff-Parkinson-White Syndrome, 78

Section 3: Junctional Escape and Ectopic Rhythms,   89

Input Section 3.1:   Junctional Escape Rhythm, 90

                              Retrograde P Wave, 92

                              The Hidden P Wave, 94

Input Section 3.2:   Premature Junctional Beats, 98

Input Section 3.3:   Junctional Tachycardia, 100

Section 4: Ventricular Ectopic and Escape Rhythms,   107

Input Section 4.1:   Premature Ventricular Contractions, 108

                              P Wave Buried in QRS Complex, 109

                              Retrograde P Wave, 109

                              R on T Phenomenon, 112

                              Multiformed or Multifocal P.V.C.s, 112

                              Interpolated P.V.C.s, 114

Input Section 4.2:   Fusion (Dressler) Beats, 116

Input Section 4.3:   Ventricular Tachycardia, 119

                              Capture Beats, 122

Input Section 4.4:   Ventricular Re-Entry Mechanisms (Advanced Study), 124

Input Section 4.5:   Torsades de Pointes (TdP) (Advanced Study), 126

                              Calculating the QTc Interval, 127

Input Section 4.6:   Ventricular Flutter, 127

Input Section 4.7:   Ventricular Fibrillation, 128

Input Section 4.8:   Pulseless Electrical Activity (PEA), 130

Input Section 4.9:   Ventricular Escape Beats and Rhythms, 131

                              Atrial Kick, 133

Section 5: Conduction Disturbances and Heart Block,   141

Input Section 5.1:   Sinus Arrest (Sinus Pause) and Sinus Block, 142

Input Section 5.2:   Atrial Tachycardia with Block, 144

Input Section 5.3:   Early Studies and Relevant History, 145

Table of Heart Blocks, 146

Input Section 5.4:   First Degree AV Block, 147

Input Section 5.5:   Second Degree AV Block, 150

—Mobitz Type I—Wenckebach, 150

—Mobitz Type II, 152

2:1 AV Conduction, 154

Input Section 5.6:   Complete Heart Block (CHB), 157

Input Section 5.7:   Bundle Branch Block, 162

Right Bundle Branch Block (RBBB), 163

Rate Dependent Bundle Branch Block, 165

Left Bundle Branch Block (LBBB), 165

Section 6: Artifact . . . To Be, or Not To Be . . . by Delores D. Schultz,   177

Input Section 6.1:   Introduction to Artifact, 178

Input Section 6.2:   Sixty-Cycle Interference, 180

Input Section 6.3:   Motion Artifact, 182

Input Section 6.4:   Artifact Produced by Electrical Devices, 189

Input Section 6.5:   "Off the Monitor", 190

Input Section 6.6:   Concerns Associated with Artifact, 193

Clues for Identifying Artifact, 193

Section 7: Cardioversion and Defibrillation,   199

Input Section 7.1:   Refractory and Vulnerable Phases of the Cardiac Cycle, 200

Synchronized Cardioversion, 201

Defibrillation (nonsynchronized shock), 201

Automatic External Defibrillator (AED) functioning, 203

Section 8: Pacemaker Basics,   209

Input Section 8.1:   Pacemaker Fundamentals, 210

Types of Pacemakers, 210

Temporary Pacemakers, 210

Transcutaneous Pacing, 211

Epicardial Pacing, 211

Permanent Pacemakers, 211

Anatomy of a Pacemaker, 213

Indications for Pacing: Short-Term and Long-Term, 213

Recognizing Pacemaker Rhythms, 213

A Demand Ventricular Pacemaker, 214

Dual Lead AV Sequential Pacing, 214

Input Section 8.2:   Determining Pacemaker Rate, 216

Input Section 8.3:   More about Capture, 217

Input Section 8.4:   Failure to Sense, 219

Input Section 8.5:   The Pacemaker Rhythm, 220

NASPE Programming Sequences, 220

Pacer Interrogation, 221

Section 9: Advanced Pacemaker Features and Interventions by Victoria A. Paparelli (The *Not so Basics* of Pacemaker Function!),   227

Input Section 9.1:   Rate Responsive or Rate Modulated Pacing, 229

NBG Pacemaker Code, 230

Sensors, 231

Markers, 233

Atrial and Ventricular Electrograms, 234

Input Section 9.2:   Hysteresis, Mode-Switch and Auto Capture, 236

Hysteresis, 236

Lag Behind Function, 236

Mode Switch or Atrial Tachycardia Response (ATR), 237

Auto Capture, 238

Input Section 9.3:   Atrial Arrhythmia Suppression/Atrial Rate Stabilization (AKA Atrial Overdrive Pacing for Atrial Dysrhythmias), 240

Atrial Fibrillation, 240

Atrial Flutter, 240

Rapid Atrial Pacing, 241

Overdrive Suppression, 241

Input Section 9.4:   Pacemaker Mediated Tachycardia (PMT), 242

Re-entry Circuits, 242

Lack of Atrial Capture, 243

Input Section 9.5:   Implantable Devices for Overdrive Pacing and Defibrillation, 245

AICD, PCD, ICD, 245

NBG and NBD Pacemaker Codes, 245, 246

Comparison of Older/Newer Pacing Devices, 246

Anti-Tachycardia (Overdrive) Pacing, 247

Implantable Defibrillators (ICDS), 247

Counters, 248

Supraventricular Discriminator Options, 254

Input Section 9.6:   Bi-Ventricular Pacing, 255

Coronary Sinus Lead, 255

LBBB Patterns, 256

Re-synchronization Therapy, 257

Section 10: Electrolyte Changes,   261

Input Section 10.1:   Ions, Electrolytes, and Potassium, 262

Anions and cations, 262

Serum Potassium, 263

Hypokalemia, 263

QT Interval Measurement, 263

Dysrhythmias Associated with Hypokalemia, 265

Hyperkalemia, 266

Dysrhythmias Associated with Hyperkalemia, 267

Input Section 10.2:   Serum Calcium, 268

Hypocalcemia, 269

Hypercalcemia, 269

Input Section 10.3:   Magnesium, 272

Calculating a QTc interval, 272, 273

Section 11: The Identification of Ischemia, Injury, and Infarct,   277

A Brief Introduction, 278

The Classification Scheme for Myocardial Insult, 279

The Standard 12 Lead Electrocardiogram, 280

Orientation of Leads to the Left Ventricular Surfaces, 281

Myocardial Blood Supply, 282

Input Section 11.1:   Myocardial Ischemia, 283

Input Section 11.2:   Myocardial Injury and Infarction, 288

Muscle Layers of the Heart, 288

Diagnosis of Myocardial Infarction or ACS, 289

Injury (ST Segment Elevation), 289

Reciprocal ST Depression, 290

The Pathologic Q Wave, 291

Loss of R Wave, 291

Normal and Altered Depolarization of the Ventricles, 291

Infarct Resolution, 299

Lateral Wall Myocardial Infarction, 300

Inferior Wall Myocardial Infarction, 300

Anteroseptal Wall Myocardial Infarction, 300

Low Lateral Wall (Apical) Myocardial Infarction, 300

Ventricular Dysrhythmias, 304

Input Section 11.3:   Posterior Wall Myocardial Infarction, 312

Input Section 11.4:   Serum Markers, 313

Ck-Mb (Creatine Kinase-Myocardial Band), 313

Myoglobin, 313

Cardiac Troponins (T and I), 313

Summary of Coronary Artery Compromise, 318

Section 12: The Diagnosis and Treatment of Acute Coronary Syndromes by Stephanie L. Woods,   321

Input Section 12.1:   Coronary Artery Disease and Progression to Acute Coronary Syndrome, 322

Input Section 12.2:   Non-Emergent Diagnosis and Treatment of Coronary Artery Disease, 322

Minimally Invasive Diagnostic Tests, 323

Invasive Diagnostic Tests, 323

Elective Treatment Options, 324

Medical Management Options, 324

Interventional Options, 324

Surgical Options, 324

Algorithm for Diagnosis and Treatment
of Non-Emergent CAD, 325

Input Section 12.3:   Diagnosis and Treatment of Acute Coronary Syndrome (ACS), 326

Ask-Assess-Treat, 326

Classifying Patients According To 12-Lead EKG Evidence, 327

Treatment Plans, 328

Algorithm for Diagnosis and Treatment of ACS, 329

Section 13: The Fundamentals of Hemodynamic Monitoring by Stephanie L. Woods,   333

Input Section 13.1:   Hemodynamic Monitoring and Cardiac Output, 334

Non-Invasive and Invasive Hemodynamic Parameters, 334

Blood Flow through the Heart, 334

Diastole and Systole, 335

The Effects of Pressure, Vessel Characteristics, Viscosity,
Resistance and Volume, 337

Preload, Contractility, Afterload and Heart Rate (The Components
of Cardiac Output), 339

Starling's Law, 339

Measuring Left Heart Pressures, 341

Input Section 13.2:   The Pulmonary Artery Catheter (Swan-Ganz), 343

Cardiac Output, 344

Input Section 13.3:   Pressures and Wave Forms, 344

Right Atrial (RA) Pressure Waveform, 346

Right Ventricular (RV) Pressure Waveform, 348

Pulmonary Artery (PA) Pressure Waveform, 351

Pulmonary Capillary Wedge Pressure (PCWP) vs. Left Atrial Pressure, 353

Pulmonary Capillary Wedge Pressure (PCWP) vs. Left Ventricular End
Diastolic Pressure (LVEDP), 355

Non-Invasive Indicators for Assessing Cardiac Output, 356

Section 14: Antiarrhythmic, Thrombolytic and Platelet Inhibitor Agents by Mike Lucey, 365

Input Section 14.1:   Pharmacologic Processes and Therapeutic Ranges, 366

        The Body's Four Processes for Drug Handling, 366

        Absorption, 367

        Distribution, 367

        Metabolism, 368

        Excretion, 368

        Serum Drug Concentrations and the
          "Therapeutic Range", 369

Input Section 14.2:   Control of Heart Rate by Autonomic Nerves, 370

Input Section 14.3:   Antiarrhythmic Drugs: Actions at Receptor Sites, 371

Input Section 14.4:   The Classification of Antiarrhythmic Drugs, 372

        Class I Drugs, 373

        Class II Drugs: Beta-Blockers, 374

        Class III Drugs, 375

        Class IV Drugs (Calcium Channel Blocker), 375

        Important Antiarrhythmics without "Class", 376

        Digoxin, 376

        Magnesium, 378

Input Section 14.5:   Treatment of Specific Rhythm Disorders, 379

        Atrial Fibrillation and Atrial Flutter, 379

        Ventricular Ectopy: PVCs, 379

        Sustained Ventricular Tachycardia, 380

        Ventricular Fibrillation and Pulseless
          Ventricular Tachycardia, 381

Input Section 14.6:   Platelet Inhibitor and Thrombolytic Drug Treatment for Acute
Myocardial Infarction, 381

        Reperfusion Arrhythmias, 382

        Mechanism of Action—Thrombolytic Agents, 382

        Mechanism of Action—GPIIB/IIIA Inhibitors, 383

Input Section 14.7:   The Use of Drug-Eluting Stents in Percutaneous
Coronary Interventions, 385

Section 15: Kidstuff by Jane D. Werth,   391

Input Section 15.1:   Genral Rules and Concepts, 393

Heart Rate Norms, 394

The P Wave, 394

The P-R Interval, 395

QRS Duration, 396

QT Interval, 396

The ST Segment, 396

The T Wave, 397

Input Section 15.2:   Sinus Anomalies, 398

Sinus Arrhythmia, 399

Sinus Bradycardia, 400

Sinus Tachycardia, 401

Sinus Arrest, 402

Sick Sinus Syndrome, 403

Input Section 15.3:   Atrial Dysrhythmias, 404

Premature Atrial Contractions (P.A.C.), 404

Atrial Tachycardia, 405

Paroxysmal Supraventricular Tachycardia
    (P.S.V.T.), 407

Atrial Flutter, 408

Atrial Fibrillation, 409

Wandering Atrial Pacemaker (W.A.P.), 410

Input Section 15.4:   Junctional Dysrhythmias and Rhythms, 412

Junctional Escape Rhythm, 412

Junctional Escape Beats, 413

Premature Junctional Contractions (P.J.C.s), 413

Junctional Tachycardia, 414

Input Section 15.5:   Ventricular Dysrhythmias, 415

Premature Ventricular Contractions (P.V.C.s), 415

Ventricular Tachycardia, 417

Ventricular Flutter, 418

Ventricular Fibrillation, 418

Input Section 15.6:   Complex Dysrhythmias, 420

                        Pulseless Electrical Activity (PEA), 420

                        Inherited Long QT Syndrome (LQTS), 420

Input Section 15.7:   Conduction Disturbances, 421

                        First Degree Heart Block, 422

                        Second Degree Heart Block, 422

                        Mobitz Type I Second Degree Heart Block, 422

                        2:1 AV Conduction, 423

                        Mobitz Type II Second Degree Heart Block, 424

                        Third Degree Heart Block (AKA Complete Heart Block), 424

                        Bundle Branch Block, 426

                        Right Bundle Branch Block, 426

                        Left Bundle Branch Block, 427

Input Section 15.8:   Drug and Electrolyte Induced Dysrhythmias, 428

                        Hypokalemia, 429

                        Hyperkalemia, 429

                        Digitalis Toxicity, 430

Input Section 15.9:   Kids' Artifact, 432

Section 16: Test Your Skill, 439

Section 17: The Final Analysis: Advanced Arrhythmia Interpretation Practice, 459

Index, 527

Important note from the management: "LEADS" may be confusing to the novice learner. Later in the text, you will be directed to reread this section!

Welcome to this book! You're probably wondering who I am . . . Right? Well, this is me.

Actually, this is the back of my head. If you think it would be difficult to recognize me in a crowd . . . I'll help you out by showing you my best side. . . .

 (Cute, huh?)

If you're still uncertain about my identity, you can view me from any angle that you choose.

Sometimes, if one has a common face, it's necessary to look closely to determine identity!
The same thing holds true when looking at monitors tracings or electrocardiograms. Sometimes all those "peculiar" waves and bumps are *almost* **impossible** to identify. However, by looking at the various wave forms and patterns from different views or angles, identity becomes more clear.

Before you start through this book, there are several things you should know. For instance, all cell membranes in the body are charged . . .

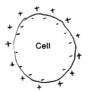

. . . and *charged* means that the cell membranes have *electrical potentials*.

When cells are in a **resting** or **polarized** state, the cell membranes carry a net positive charge.

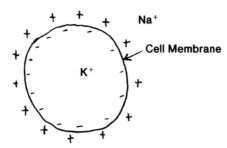

This charge or electrical potential results from the difference of intra and extracellular electrolyte concentrations. Technically speaking, the development of energy or electrical potential is dependent upon the dissipation or restitution of the ionic gradient across the cell membrane. The electrical potentials created by this charge can be measured on EKG.

When the cells are electrically stimulated, the cells depolarize and contract. The cell membrane which is usually only slightly permeable to sodium (Na⁺), allows Na⁺ ions to rush into the cell while potassium (K⁺) moves out of the cell.

This shift in electrolyte concentrations reverses the charge on the cell membrane and is known as **depolarization**.

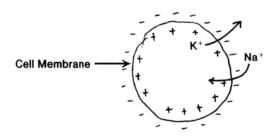

Once depolarization occurs, the cell activity transports Na⁺ back to the cell membrane surface, and K⁺ diffuses back into the cell.

That brings us back to where we started. This returning to the resting state is called **repolarization**.

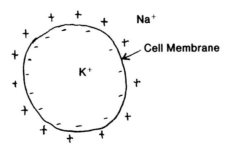

It is this process of **depolarization** and **repolarization** of the myocardial cells that produces the various wave forms observed on the EKG or cardiac monitor. The EKG or monitoring unit *measures and displays (or records) electrical potential . . . it tells one nothing about muscle contraction.*

It is well worth remembering that electrical depolarization occurs *before* cardiac muscle contraction . . . and that electrical repolarization *follows* cardiac muscle contraction!

Rather than tackling the history of electrical potential measurement, we will just accept the fact that the standard EKG machine has the capability of measuring electrical potential using a 12 lead system.

If you think of leads as simply providing different views or angles from which to view the heart's electrical activity, the subject is less confounding.

The standard 12 lead EKG system has 5 electrodes. One electrode is placed on each extremity, while the 5th electrode is used as a **floating electrode** . . . or used for recording from the chest wall.

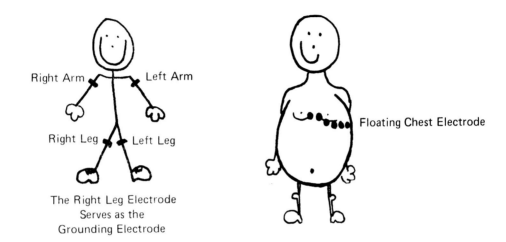

Right Arm   Left Arm

Right Leg   Left Leg

The Right Leg Electrode
Serves as the
Grounding Electrode

Floating Chest Electrode

There are actually three different types of leads . . . **standard limb leads**, **augmented leads**, and **precordial** or **chest leads**. Each lead is made up of a negative ⊖ and a positive ⊕ electrode. These electrodes sense both the magnitude and the direction of the electrical forces and record surface information from the heart borders. Because that sounds a bit confusing, each type of lead will be discussed separately. Whew!

First, however, there are a few critical points to consider. Though these points will be discussed later in the text, they will assist you in understanding the EKG presentations associated with the various leads.

LV

First, the major (net) direction of ventricular electrical activation is leftward (moving right to left), through the free wall of the left ventricle (LV) as noted by the arrow in the above diagram.

Secondly, ventricular depolarization or activation is recorded on the EKG as a QRS complex. QRS complexes are either positive (upright) or negative (directed downward) depending upon the placement of the electrodes and the movement of the depolarization force toward, or away from, those electrodes. Study the diagram at the top of the next page.

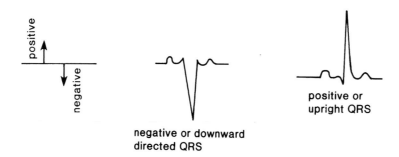

negative or downward
directed QRS

positive or
upright QRS

The QRS (usually the most easily identified wave formation) represents ventricular depolarization or activation. When the major (net) direction of ventricular depolarization spreads through the left ventricular (LV) muscle moving toward a positive ⊕ electrode, the QRS deflection on the EKG will appear upright or positive.

depolarization

When the major (net) direction of ventricular depolarization spreads through the LV heart muscle moving *away from* a positive ⊕ electrode or *toward* a negative ⊖ electrode, the QRS deflection will appear negative or directed downward.

depolarization

Sounds *fairly simple* . . . right?!

As we move forward, you will notice that various electrodes change their *polarity* . . . in other words, sometimes a given electrode is positive ⊕, and sometimes that same electrode is negative ⊖. ***Not to worry!*** The EKG recording machine is programmed to change the polarity when the various lead channels are selected ***Whew!***

Now . . . more about the 12 leads. . . .

The Standard Limb Leads

The **standard limb leads** are leads I, II, and III and they record frontal plane activity. These leads are *bipolar leads* . . . which means that each of these leads has two electrodes which record the electrical potential of the heart flowing toward two extremities. In other words, each lead records the difference of electrical potential between two selected electrode sites.

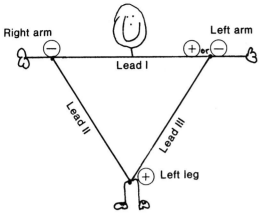

Leads I, II, and III are all electrically equidistant from the myocardial activity. The right arm is always the negative ⊖ pole, while the left leg is always the positive ⊕ pole. The left arm electrode is positive ⊕ in Lead I and negative ⊖ in Lead III.

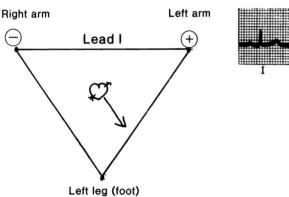

Lead I records the difference of potential between the left arm and the right arm. Specifically, in Lead I, the positive electrode is on the left arm and the negative electrode is on the right arm. The important thing to observe is that the direction of depolarization (see arrow) moves more generally toward the positive ⊕ electrode. Thus, the QRS (which represents ventricular depolarization) is predominantly positive or upright in Lead I.

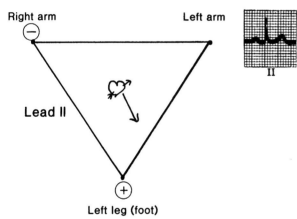

Lead II records the difference of potential between the left leg and the right arm. In Lead II, the left leg electrode is positive and the right arm electrode is negative. Notice the direction of depolarization (see arrow) moves generally toward the positive ⊕ electrode. Therefore, the QRS in Lead II is positive or upright.

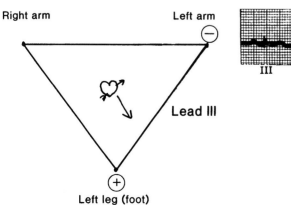

Lead III records the difference of potential between the left leg and the left arm. In Lead III, the left leg electrode is positive and the left arm electrode becomes negative. Once again, you will see that the direction of depolarization (see arrow) moves between the positive ⊕ and the negative ⊖ electrodes. Thus, we can expect that the QRS in Lead III will appear partly positive and partly negative. *Neat, huh!*

The Augmented Leads

The **augmented leads**, leads aVR, aVL, and aVF are designed to increase the amplitude of the deflections by 50% over those recorded by the standard limb leads. The augmented leads are unipolar in nature (one electrode on the body) and record electrical potential from both the right and left arms and the left leg.

P.S. aVR stands for augmented voltage right arm
aVL stands for augmented voltage left arm
aVF stands for augmented voltage foot

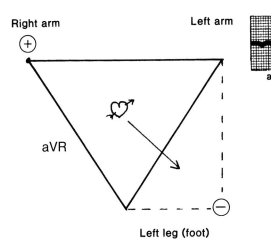

Lead aVR faces the heart from the right shoulder and is oriented to the cavity of the heart. In lead aVR, the right arm electrode extends in an imaginary direction between the left arm and left leg electrodes. The *important* thing to notice is that the direction of depolarization (see arrow) moves toward the negative ⊖ electrode. Thus, the QRS is directed negatively in lead aVR.

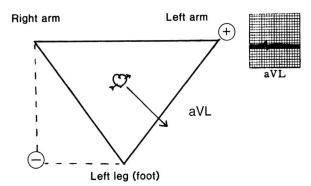

Lead aVL faces the heart from the left shoulder and is oriented to the left ventricle. In lead aVL, the left arm electrode is positive. The negative electrode extends in an imaginary direction between the right arm and left leg electrodes. The *important* thing to notice is that the direction of depolarization (see arrow) moves more or less perpendicular to the positive and negative electrodes. Thus, the QRS complex viewed from lead aVL is neither extremely positive nor negative.

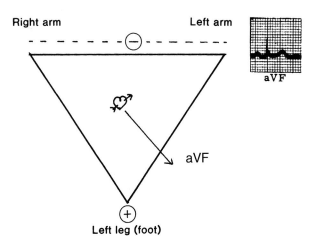

Lead aVF faces the heart from the hip and is oriented to the inferior surface of the left ventricle. In lead aVF, the left leg electrode is positive. The negative electrode extends in an imaginary direction between the right arm and left arm electrodes. The *important* point to notice here is that the direction of depolarization (see arrow) moves principally toward the positive ⊕ electrode. Thus, the QRS complex viewed from lead aVF is positive.

The Precordial Leads

There are six **chest** or **precordial leads** that are identified by the letters V, V_1, V_2, V_3, V_4, V_5, and V_6. The V leads record electrical potential in the *horizontal plane* and provide six views of the heart's activity! There is a single positive electrode which is moved to all six positions on the chest wall.

Lead V_1 is located over the 4th intercostal space to the right of the sternal border.
Lead V_2 is located over the 4th intercostal space to the left of the sternal border.
Lead V_3 is located between V_2 and V_4.
Lead V_4 is located at the 5th intercostal space on the mid-clavicular line.
Lead V_5 is located at the 5th intercostal space on the anterior axillary line.
Lead V_6 is located at the 5th intercostal space on the midaxillary line.

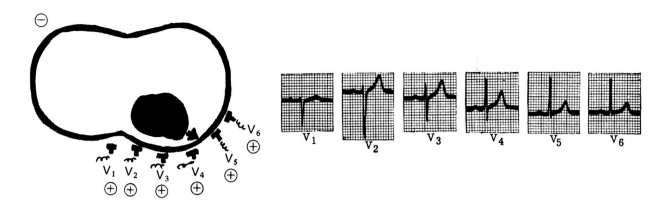

You are probably wondering where the negative electrodes are if the V leads are all positive! (You will remember that each lead is made up of both a positive ⊕ and a negative ⊖ electrode . . . remember? Well, in the precordial leads (V leads), the negative electrode extends backwards or posteriorly toward an imaginary point created by the limb leads.

Normally the *major* (net) direction of ventricular depolarization moves from *right to left* (see arrow above). Thus, the QRS deflections in the right precordial leads (V_1 and V_2) are mostly negative (the wave of depolarization is moving away from the positive chest electrode). As the positive ⊕ chest electrode is moved further left, the QRS deflections become positive (the wave of depolarization is moving toward the positive electrodes).

Now that you are no doubt **thoroughly** perplexed, let me reinforce the important points to remember about leads. . . .

When the major (net) direction of depolarization (electrical activity) spreads through the heart muscle toward a positive pole (electrode), the QRS deflection on the EKG will appear upright or positive.

When the major (net) direction of depolarization (electrical activity) spreads through the heart muscle moving away from a positive pole (electrode) or toward a negative pole (electrode), the deflections will be inverted or negative.

In the absence of electrical activity, there will be no wave forms to record.

Electrical inactivity or electrical silence is recorded as a straight line called an **isoelectric line**. So here's an isoelectric line _____ representing electrical silence.

If you think all this is confusing, you're right! It also means that you're progressing in a *normal* fashion. **Honest!** "LEADing into Section 1" is *purely* introductory! The content will be reviewed later in the text.

Whew!

Probably the *most* important thing to remember is that the 12 EKG leads allow one to look at the various surfaces of the left ventricle . . . or simply look at the electrical activity from different views or angles.

Since the left ventricle (***the pump***) is the most important heart chamber, recording leads are designed to capture electrical activity on the various left ventricular surfaces.

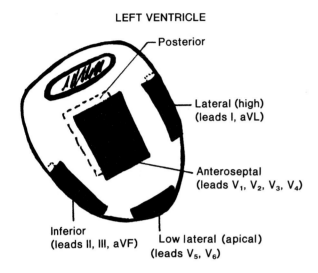

LEFT VENTRICLE
- Posterior
- Lateral (high) (leads I, aVL)
- Anteroseptal (leads V₁, V₂, V₃, V₄)
- Inferior (leads II, III, aVF)
- Low lateral (apical) (leads V₅, V₆)

Leads I and aVL view the lateral surface of the left ventricle (high lateral).

Leads II, III, and aVF view the inferior surface of the left ventricle.

Leads V_1, V_2, V_3, and V_4 view the anteroseptal surface of the left ventricle.

Leads V_5 and V_6 view the low lateral or apical surface of the left ventricle.

There are no leads that directly view the posterior region of the left ventricle.

So, with the introduction now *under your belt*, you can proceed on to Section 1.

P.S. If the content is not securely under your belt, *don't worry!* "LEADing into Section 1" comes at the beginning of the text because history and tradition so dictates! It makes much more sense when you reread this section later in the text. So progress ahead without a care!

Bedside Monitoring

Besides monitoring systems provide for the ongoing observation of cardiac rhythms. It is important to recognize that monitoring technology is ever expanding. Wireless EKG monitoring is now available using Bluetooth technology. This technology provides for continuous monitoring without antennas, thus allowing both patients and staff greater degrees of freedom! The wireless system, made up of disposable cables and a small transceiver, communicates via radio waves to a transceiver attached to the monitoring system. To date, however, most hospitals employ traditional five lead monitoring systems.

5 Lead Monitoring Systems

Most beside monitoring systems utilize a five lead arrangement which allows for the monitoring of all leads within the capability of the system. In a five lead system, four electrodes are placed in stationary positions as indicated in the diagram at the top of the page 10. The fifth electrode (labeled Ⓥ) can be placed in any of the $V_1 - V_6$ positions as shown on page 7. (To monitor on a specific V lead, the V electrode will need to be moved to that position.)

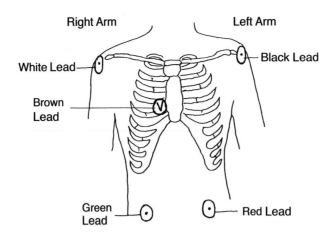

The Ⓥ lead electrode has been placed in the V_1 position.
The Ⓥ lead electrode can be repositioned to any of the precordial lead positions (V_1-V_6).

You will notice the WHITE lead attaches to the electrode positioned on the upper outer part of the right arm; the BLACK lead attaches to the electrode located in the same position on the upper outer left arm; the GREEN lead attaches to the electrode positioned on the right hip, just outside the nipple line; the RED lead attaches to the electrode placed in that same position on the left hip. **(Electrode placement at points where the limbs attach to the torso assists in eliminating motion artifact and keeps the field (chest area) clear in the event that emergency procedures are necessary.)**

Expect *lead clinicians* remember correct lead placement locations by the following.

> **White on right,**
> **Black (smoke) over fire (Red). . . .**

. . . then all one has to remember is that the GREEN lead attaches to the electrode placed opposite the RED lead, and the Brown lead connects to the chest (precordial) electrode!

The five lead system allows one to select (using the lead selector) the preferred lead(s) to be monitored. Most five lead monitoring systems allow two leads to be simultaneously monitored.

3 Lead Monitoring Systems

Owing to the cost of monitoring systems and equipment, some health care institutions utilize a three lead bedside monitoring system. A three lead monitoring system is made up of a positive ⊕ electrode, a negative ⊖ electrode, and a ground Ⓖ electrode. Depending on how these three electrodes are positioned on the chest surface, the resulting monitor picture will closely resemble the standard, bipolar limb leads I, II and III.

A three lead monitoring system has lesser capabilities than a five lead system, requiring the electrodes to be repositioned in order to monitor the specific limb leads. Using a three lead system, it is not possible to obtain true V (or chest) leads; instead, the electrodes can be repositioned to obtain Modified Chest Lead (MCL) positions. A three lead system affords a single channel for EKG monitoring (only one EKG lead can be viewed on the monitor).

The following diagrams demonstrate electrode placement for obtaining leads I, II, and III and MCL_1 and MCL_6, modified chest leads.

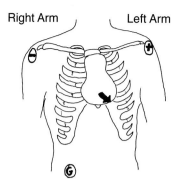

Lead I

In the bedside version of lead I, the general (net) direction of ventricular depolarization (see arrow) is moving more toward the positive $\oplus$ electrode. Thus, the QRS in lead I will be positively deflected or directed.

Notice that the left arm electrode is positive $\oplus$; the right arm electrode is negative $\ominus$; the right leg (name, not location) electrode serves as the ground.

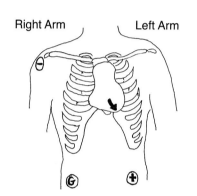

Lead II

In the bedside version of lead II, the net direction of ventricular depolarization (see arrow) is moving toward the positive $\oplus$ electrode. Thus, the QRS in lead II is positively deflected or directed.

Notice that the left leg (name, not location) electrode is positive $\oplus$; the right arm electrode is negative $\ominus$; the right leg (name, not location) electrode serves as the ground.

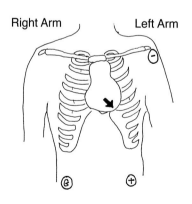

Lead III

In the bedside version of lead III, the net direction of ventricular depolarization (see arrow) flows between the positive $\oplus$ and negative $\ominus$ electrodes. Thus, the QRS observed in lead III is partly positive and partly negative.

Observe that the left leg electrode (name, not location) is positive $\oplus$; the left arm electrode is negative $\ominus$; the right leg (name, not location) serves as the ground.

It is also possible to arrange the three bedside monitoring electrodes to mimic certain precordial leads, specifically leads V_1 and V_6. However, since the precordial leads are unipolar in nature (using a positive electrode on the chest wall with an imaginary negative electrode), and our bedside monitoring system is bipolar, certain modifications must be made. Thus, these leads are referred to as **modified chest leads (MCL)**!

Modified Chest Leads

As will be discussed later in the text, certain rhythm abnormalities are best viewed from leads approximating right (V_1) or left (V_6) precordial leads. By adjusting the bedside monitoring lead placement, one can achieve modified versions of these two leads.

Lead MCL$_1$ (modified V_1)   **Lead MCL$_6$** (modified V_6)

    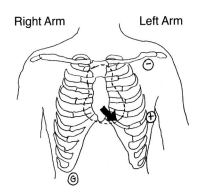

The positive $\oplus$ electrode is positioned as V_1 at the 4th intercostal space to the right of the sternum. The negative $\ominus$ electrode is placed on the left arm. The ground electrode can be placed anywhere.

Remember ... V_1 is a right chest lead ... so, MCL$_1$ is a modified right chest lead.

Because the net direction of ventricular depolarization (see arrow) moves between the positive $\oplus$ and negative $\ominus$ electrodes, the QRS in lead MCL$_1$ will be partly positive and partly negative.

The positive $\oplus$ electrode is positioned as V_6 at the 5th intercostal space on the left mid-axillary line. The negative electrode $\ominus$ is placed on the left arm. The ground electrode can be placed anywhere.

Remember ... V_6 is a left chest lead ... so, MCL$_6$ is a modified left chest lead.

You will notice that the net direction of ventricular depolarization (see arrow) moves toward the positive $\oplus$ electrode. Thus, the QRS observed in lead MCL$_6$ will be positive or upright.

In both of the above modified systems (MCL$_1$ and MCL$_6$), the left arm electrode is the negative $\ominus$ electrode. The positive electrode is placed in the appropriate V lead position. If you need review, please turn back to page 7.

Note: MCL stands for "modified chest—left arm" lead.

Let me **reassure** you once again! If you are uncertain or confused, please understand that this is a **normal** state. It will all begin to fall into place as we move along. **Trust me!** And, be assured that manufacturers of monitoring equipment include diagrams for lead placement.

Notes

_____

_____

_____

_____

_____

_____

_____

_____

_____

_____

_____

_____

_____

_____

_____

_____

_____

_____

_____

_____

_____

Notes

The Conduction System and Related Matters

Objectives

When you have completed Section 1, you will be able to describe, identify or calculate

1. normal electric impulse transmission across the myocardium

2. P, Q, R, S, T cardiac cycle

3. heart rate

4. paper time

5. sinus rhythm

6. the conduction system

7. a method for interpreting dysrhythmias

Input Section 1.1: The Conduction System

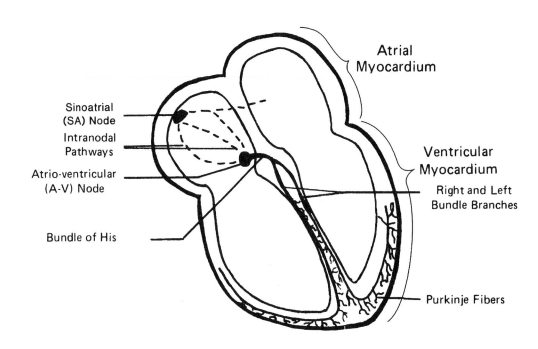

   Each normal heart beat is the result of an electrical impulse that originates in the sinoatrial (SA) node. The SA node lies at the junction of the superior vena cava and the right atrium. *The SA node is the normal heart's physiologic pacemaker, initiating impulses at a rate between 60–100 times per minute. From the SA node, the impulse travels across intranodal pathways activating the atria. The activation (or depolarization) of the atria is recorded as a P wave on the EKG. The intranodal pathways connect the SA node and the AV (atrio-ventricular) node. The intranodal pathways are preferential or semi-specialized pathways consisting of concentrations of normal myocardial cells and Purkinje cells. (The tissues between these cells consist mainly of collagen and fat which have high electrical resistance.) The AV node lies on the floor of the right atrium. Conduction through the intranodal pathways is rapid; conduction is then slowed in the AV node itself. The AV node serves only to transmit the impulse. Impulse conduction speeds up as it leaves the AV node passing to the bundle of His. From the bundle of His, the impulse passes rapidly down both the right and left bundle branches to the terminal Purkinje fibers. Ventricular depolarization or activation then occurs, producing the QRS complex on EKG. Following depolarization, the mechanical activity of muscle contraction occurs, producing a pulse. Cellular recovery (repolarization) follows depolarization and is evidenced on the EKG as a T wave. It is during the repolarization phase that the ventricles fill with blood. The next electrical impulse arrives when filling is completed and ventricular depolarization again occurs. *Each cardiac cycle consists of depolarization and recovery (repolarization).*

*IMPORTANT NOTE: The SA node is the normal pacemaker of the heart because it has the *fastest* rate of impulse formation and discharge. The SA impulse reaches slower potential pacemakers and discharges their immature impulses before they have the opportunity to discharge spontaneously. Sounds complicated, right? The important thing to remember is that the *fastest* pacemaker always controls the heart rate . . . just like the *fastest* runner controls the race! It's also helpful to know that the SA node is influenced by both the sympathetic and parasympathetic nervous system . . . thus, the sinus rate of discharge fluctuates with nervous stimulation.

Practice Exercise 1

Now it's your turn.

The electrical impulse normally originates in the sinoatrial node and travels across the heart to initiate myocardial muscle depolarization. Trace and label the parts of the conduction system on this diagram.

The activation phase of the cardiac cycle is known as ___depolarization___.

The recovery phase of the cardiac cycle is known as ___repolarization___.

Normally, the SA (sinoatrial) node fires ___60___ to ___100___ times per minute.

✔ For **Feedback 1**, refer to page 37.

Input Section 1.2: The P Wave and P-R Interval

All electrical activity can be recorded. As an electrical impulse travels across the myocardium initiating depolarization, a monitoring device will display various wave forms.

Sinoatrial
(SA) node

Atrial excitation begins in the sinoatrial (SA) node, spreading through specialized conducting pathways to activate the right and left atria. The monitor will display a wave form that usually looks like this.

P

For reasons unknown to me, this is called a P wave! Owing to the direction of electrical activation, P waves are *normally upright* in leads I, II, aVF, and V_3-V_6. P waves are normally inverted in leads aVR and may be inverted in leads V_1 and V_2. P waves may be upright, flat, diphasic, or inverted in leads III and aVL.

The P wave represents depolarization of both the right and left atria. Remember, muscle contraction follows electrical depolarization.

So, whenever a P wave is observed, the "monitor observer" will know that depolarization of the atria has occurred.

Since the impulse originates in the sinoatrial node and since the SA node is the heart's natural pacemaker, the P wave should be the *first* wave form one sees in each cardiac cycle.

Atrial Depolarization = ⌒

We now have a P wave, telling the monitor observer that atrial depolarization has occurred. Not unlike other muscles, after activation there must be a rest or recovery (repolarization) period. And, just as you might suspect, during this rest period no work is done. No work presents on the monitor as a straight line known as the P-R segment.

Atrial depolarization (the P wave) is followed by a straight line (the P-R segment) which represents both atrial recovery time and transmission of the impulse through the AV junction, to the ventricles. Taken together, the P wave and the P-R segment, make up the P-R interval. The P-R interval (the combined P wave and straight line) thus represents atrial activation and recovery and, the further conduction of the impulse through the AV junction, through the bundle of His, down the bundle branches to the Purkinje fibers. The P-R interval begins at the initial P wave deflection and terminates at the beginning of the QRS.

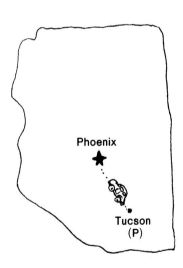

A number of factors influence the P-R interval. Though they will be discussed in a later section, for now, a simple analogy will be used. Suppose that I live and work in Tucson, but must also drive to Phoenix because I have a second job there. My work in Tucson corresponds to atrial work, so I'll call my Tucson work "P." Then, I jump in my VW and drive to Phoenix. The time it takes me to both do my work in Tucson and then drive to Phoenix could be called my Tucson-Phoenix interval. This corresponds to the "P-R interval" which is the time it takes for the sinus impulse to activate (do work in) the atria, for the atria to recover, and for the impulse to travel through the A-V junction to the ventricles.

Using this analogy further, it's easy to understand that my Tucson-Phoenix interval could vary depending on how fast I work, how fast I drive—or, if there is highway construction. Similarly, the P-R interval could vary depending on the rate of impulse conduction or pathway obstruction.

Practice Exercise 2

Let's review!

A. Atrial excitation (in the healthy heart) begins in the ___SA node___.

B. As this impulse spreads across the atria, it causes atrial muscle contraction following ~~the~~ depolarization___.

C. The monitor picture associated with atrial depolarization is the ___P___ wave.

D. Okay, now draw a P wave.

E. In the healthy heart, the ___P wave___ will note the beginning of each cardiac cycle.

F. The P-R interval looks like this: (draw one)

P-R I

G. The P-R interval represents the time it takes the impulse to depolarize the atria and travel from the atria, through the ~~intranodal pathways~~ AV Node to the ventricles.

✔ For **Feedback 2,** refer to page 37.

Input Section 1.3: The QRS Complex

So, now what??
So far, our EKG complex looks like this.

P

P-R interval

The sinoatrial-generated impulse has traveled to the ventricles.

The next major event in the cardiac cycle is ventricular depolarization (the traveling impulse reaches and activates the ventricles). Ventricular depolarization is identified on the monitor as a QRS complex, a Q wave, an R wave and an S wave. The QRS complex is predominantly upright in leads, I, II, III, aVL, aVF, V_4, V_5, and V_6. (Refer back to pages 5, 6, and 7.)

These waves (QRS) represent depolarization of the ventricular muscle. The first downward (negative) deflection is the Q wave.

The R wave is the first upward (positive) wave or deflection . . .

. . . and, if a negative deflection (below the baseline) follows an R wave, it is labeled an S wave.

Now, the monitor picture looks like this.

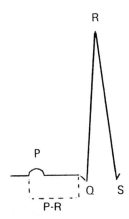

The P waves tells us the atria have depolarized. The P-R interval represents the time it takes for atrial depolarization and for the SA impulse to travel from the SA node through the atria, through the AV junction, through the bundle of His, down the bundle branches to the Purkinje fibers. And voila! When the traveling impulse reaches the Purkinje fibers, ventricular depolarization occurs—shown on the monitor as the QRS. Ventricular muscle contraction normally follows electrical depolarization.

Depending upon which EKG lead one is examining, one may not observe an actual Q wave. In other words, the QRS may look like this. There is no observable Q wave (initial negative deflection). Technically speaking, this is an "Rs" wave . . .

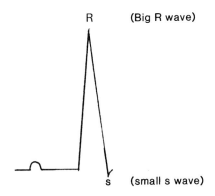

. . . but it is referenced as a QRS wave.

Likewise, in predominantly negatively deflected leads—V_1, V_2, and V_3—the QRS will appear different owing to the placement of the electrode, the proximity to the heart muscle and the direction of the depolarization wave. (Refer back to p. 8.)

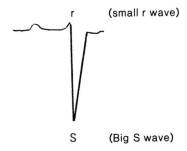

Though the above wave form is also referred to as a QRS complex, technically there is only a small r and a large S wave! An R wave is the first upward deflection, and an S wave is a negative-downward deflection that follows, regardless of wave size.

Practice Exercise 3

A. Draw and label the waves representing ventricular activation or depolarization.

B. Ventricular depolarization begins when the SA initiated ~~impulse reaches~~ _The Purkinje fibers in (The ventricles) ← Specifically_

✔ For **Feedback 3,** refer to page 38.

Input Section 1.4: The ST Segment, the T Wave and U wave . . . (followed by a word about the QT interval and QRS interval and QRS-ST segment)

Only a few more *minor* details. Following ventricular activation (depolarization), there must be a period of rest or recovery (repolarization).

Simple physiology—cells work—they get tired—they rest! So, the remaining portions of a normal EKG cycle appear as illustrated below.

The ST segment (straight line between the S wave and T wave) represents an early phase of ventricular muscle recovery. During this time, the ventricular cells are in a state of "inaction" (refractory state), unresponsive to any further electrical stimulation. The ST segment begins at the J point (junction of the end of the QRS with the beginning of the ST segment) and ends at the beginning of the T wave.

The T wave is the recovery phase (repolarization) following ventricular activation (depolarization). The top (apex) of the T wave is the earliest time the ventricles can respond to another electrical stimulus.

Various pathologies and conditions producing changes in the ST segment and T wave will be studied in later Sections. Whew!!

Occasionally, a U wave may be visible following the T wave. If visible, the U wave is smaller than the T wave, though oriented in the same direction. The U wave is thought to represent repolarization of the Purkinje fibers.

The QT interval represents the total time for ventricular depolarization and repolarization. It further represents the absolute refractory period. The QT interval is measured from the intiation point of the QRS to the termination point of the T wave. The QT interval should measure no greater than ½ of the R-R interval (the distance between two R waves). The QT interval interval is also discussed on page 126, 264, and 305.

Let's do the whole thing—an entire EKG cycle! When I see this complex on the monitor, I can now intellectually describe the whole physiologic process.

Ready? Okay . . . . "My good man/woman, EKG monitor interpretation is based on simple application of a basic physiologic principle. Ion shift at the myocardial cell membrane level allows one to record electrical potential via specially designed electrodes. Atrial excitation begins at the SA node and spreads down the conduction

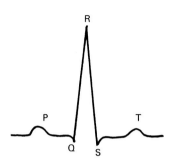

system. The initially recorded wave, the P wave, represents depolarization of the atria. The straight line following the P wave represents time for atrial repolarization and impulse conduction to the ventricles. The QRS complex represents ventricular depolarization. Following ventricular depolarization is the repolarization phase evidenced by the ST segment and T wave!"

> Remember, the EKG is simply a representation of the electrical events occurring within the myocardium!

Sounds fairly intellectual, right?!

Practice Exercise 4

A. Label each wave.

P.S. If you are unsure, look at the top of the page!

B. Atrial excitation begins in the ___SA Node___.

C. The P wave represents ___Atrial depolarization___.

D. The P-R interval represents ___time in between atrial depolarization + ventricular depolarization (time it takes atria to depolarize & impulse to travel to the ventricles)___.

E. The QRS represents ___ventricular depolarization___.

The Q wave is the first ___downward___ deflection.

The R wave is the first _____ positive _____ deflection.

The S wave is the _____ ~~se~~ downward _____ deflection following the R wave.

F. The ST segment represents _____ repolarization of ventricles → early phase of this _____.

G. The T wave represents _____ ventricular repolarization _____.

H. The PQRST complex represents one _____ cardiac cycle _____.

✔ For **Feedback 4,** refer to page 38.

Input Section 1.5: Paper Time

Now that the PQRST cycle has been more or less exhausted, we need to think about EKG paper— henceforth, this will be referred to as "paper time." In order for this whole process to make good sense, some convention of measure must be applied. EKG recording paper is run at a standard speed of 25 mm. per second to standardize the measurement of the various electrical events. EKG paper is subdivided both horizontally and vertically with 1 mm. and 5 mm. (dark lines) spaced lines. The vertical lines represent time intervals, much like a clock!

So, moving horizontally across the EKG paper denotes *time*. One must understand the concept of paper time in order to calculate heart rate from the EKG paper.

In the following illustration, notice the three second marker intervals at the top of the EKG paper. Every three seconds this mark will appear. The distance between three of these markers is 6 seconds.

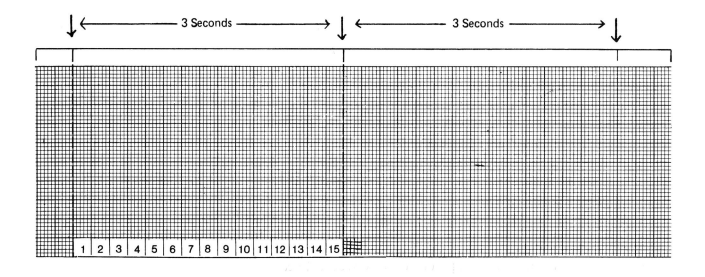

Each larger square represents *0.20 seconds.* That makes sense if one counts the number of large squares between each three second marker. (See bottom illustration page 24.)

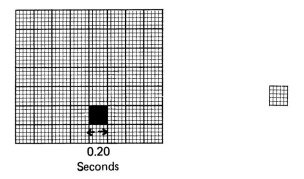

0.20
Seconds

There are 15 large squares between each three second marker (15 × 0.2 seconds each = 3.0 seconds).

Now look at one of the smallest squares. Each small square represents *0.04 seconds.*

Again, that makes sense if one counts the number of small squares moving across one big square. There are five small squares (5 × 0.04 seconds = 0.2 seconds or one large square).

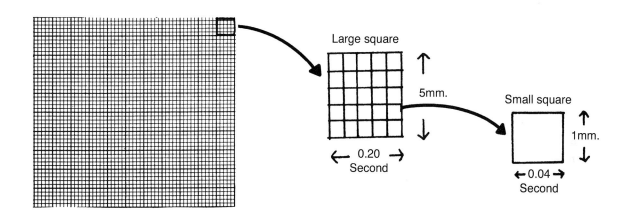

Large square

5mm.

0.20
Second

Small square

1mm.

0.04
Second

Practice Exercise 5

Paper time is actually quite easy . . . if you practice!

Before looking back, complete the following statements.

A. Moving horizontally across EKG paper denotes ___time___.

B. Every ___3___ seconds I will see a time marker on the EKG paper.

C. The amount of time between three of these time markers is ___6___ seconds.

D. Each large square represents ___.20___ seconds.

E. I understand that there are 15 large squares (0.20 seconds) between two ___3___ second markers.

   Therefore, ___3___ seconds lapse between those markers (15 × 0.20 seconds = ___3.00___).

F. The smallest square on the EKG paper represents ___0.04___ seconds.

.20
15
10.0
2.00

3.00

G. There are __5__ small squares (in one row) within a large square.

H. There are __~~15~~ 30__ large squares in a six second time interval. ~~12043~~ 0.04

I. Three small squares represent __~~60~~ .12__ seconds. .12

J. Four small squares represents _____ seconds. .16

K. Five small squares represent __.20__ seconds, which is the same as __one large box__.

L. How much time is represented by five big squares? ~~5 seconds~~ 1 seconde.

M. How much time is represented by 13 big squares? ~~2.6 seconds~~ 2.6 seconds

   . . . If you can answer question N without looking back, you have a sound understanding of paper time.

N. How much time has elapsed when there are five big squares and three small squares?

__1.12 seconds__   1 second + .12 ÷ .04 / 3

✔ For **Feedback 5,** refer to page 39.

Input Section 1.6: Measuring P, P-R, and QRS Intervals

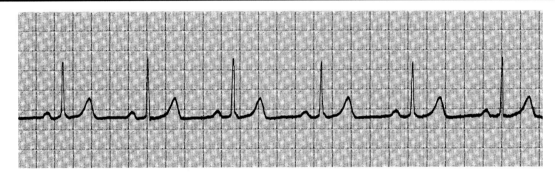

   Although we will not go into great detail, it is important to think about *atrial activation.* You will remember that the P wave represents atrial depolarization (depolarization of both the left and right atria).

   The *normal* P wave does not exceed 0.11 seconds in duration (less than three small squares) or more than 2.5 mm. in height. Any increase in duration or amplitude suggests *atrial hypertrophy.* Though it is not always possible to distinguish right from left atrial hypertrophy on an EKG, one can make several generalizations. Basically, atrial hypertrophy represents an enlargement of one or both of the atrial chambers due to excessive strain or workload.

   With left atrial hypertrophy (often seen in mitral stenosis), one may observe a wide, notched P wave called *P mitrale,* best seen in leads I and II. Following is an example of left atrial hypertrophy.

P-R segment = .12-.20 seconds

Right atrial hypertrophy is most commonly associated with chronic pulmonary disease. P waves associated with right atrial hypertrophy are usually tall (greater than 2.5 mm. in height) and *peaked* in leads II, III, and AVF.

Though the duration and amplitude of P waves is interesting, I do not expect you to commit this to memory . . . however, you should be aware that abnormalities may occur in the P wave itself! *Whew!*

Remember the P-R interval? The P-R interval represents the time required for atrial activation, atrial recovery and impulse transmission through the AV node, across the bundle of His, down the bundle branches, to the Purkinje fibers.

In a healthy adult heart, the impulse will travel from the sinus node to the Purkinje system in 0.12 to 0.20 seconds.

To be within normal limits then, the P-R interval must measure 3-5 small squares in width or between 0.12 and 0.20 seconds in duration.

Look at the following EKG strip. The P-R interval is almost 4 small squares wide. The P-R interval is measured from the beginning of the P wave to the beginning of the Q wave . . . or if there is no Q wave, to the beginning of the upward R wave. (For assistance with measurement, see the diagrams at the top of page 28.)

The P-R interval in the above strip is *almost* 0.16 seconds in duration (.04 × 4 = 0.16 seconds).

That means the P-R interval is within normal limits. In other words, the impulse is traveling through the conduction system at a healthy speed.

As a contrast, examine this next strip. Here the P-R interval measures 0.24 seconds (6 × .04 = 0.24) indicating a *delay* in impulse conduction or a *conduction defect*.

And, as you might guess, an abnormally short P-R interval represents *accelerated* impulse conduction. For now, we are only concerned with the accurate measurement of the P-R interval. Pathology will be discussed later in the text.

CORRECTLY MEASURING THE P-R INTERVAL AND QRS DURATION

The P-R interval is measured from the beginning of the P wave to the beginning of the QRS . . . in this instance, to the beginning of the Q wave.

In this example, the P-R interval measurement is taken from the beginning of the P wave to the beginning of the R wave (the beginning of the R wave upstroke).

Remember, *to be within normal limits the P-R interval must measure 3–5 small squares in width, or 0.12 to 0.20 seconds in duration.*

We will be concerned with one other major paper time measurement. The QRS, you will recall, represents ventricular depolarization. Unless a conduction defect is present (abnormal, slow conduction), the QRS will measure *less* than 3 small squares wide, or less than 0.12 seconds in duration. The QRS is measured from the beginning of the Q wave to the end of the S wave. If a Q wave is not present, measure the distance between the R and S waves. Please refer to the above diagrams.

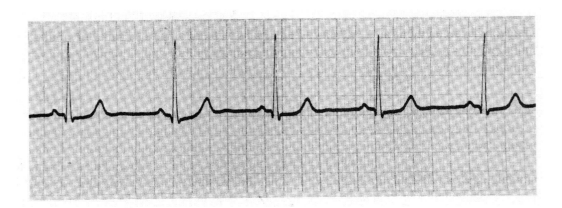

In the above rhythm strip, the QRS measures *approximately 0.10 seconds or 2½ small squares*. Therefore, ventricular depolarization occurs within the expected period of time (*less than 0.12 seconds or less than 3 small squares*).

Practice Exercise 6

A. To be within normal limits, the P-R interval must measure ___3___ to ___5___ small squares in width or ___.12___ to ___.20___ seconds in duration.

B. P-R interval less than ___3___ small squares in width or greater than ___5___ small squares in width represents an abnormality in the impulse conduction.

C. Evaluate the boxed cardiac cycle at the top of next page. The P-R measures ___5___ small squares or ___.20___ seconds.

D. The QRS waveform represents _ventricular depolarization_

E. To be within normal limits, the QRS must measure _____3_____ small squares

less than _.12_ seconds in duration.   _slightly less than 3_

F. The QRS in the above boxed cardiac cycle measures _____ small squares which

is _____.08_____ seconds. _slightly less than .12 seconds_

✔ For **Feedback 6,** refer to page 40.

Input Section 1.7: Calculating Heart Rate

Now, let's try some *fun* things with heart rate!

There are several methods for calculating heart rate from a cardiac monitor. Probably the most accurate method is to count the number of beats or cardiac cycles in a one minute (60 second) time interval. If you think in terms of three second time markers, that's a *long* EKG strip. Though this method is cumbersome, it should be used *when the rhythm is **irregular*** and an accurate heart rate is needed. (This is much like taking an apical pulse—if it is irregular, one must count it for one full minute.)

> Note: When in doubt about any heart rate, take the patient's pulse . . . and remember, an apical pulse is usually the most accurate.

When we are dealing with a *regular* rhythm, the process of calculating heart rate can be simplified. Every three seconds a marker appears on the EKG paper. *Count the number of EKG complexes or cardiac cycles in a six second time interval. Multiply that number by 10* to find the number of complexes in one minute. That number is the approximate heart rate.

Figure the heart rate in the following EKG strip. Note the circled three second markers.

70 bpm

In the previous strip there are 7 complexes within a six second time interval.

Therefore, 7 × 10 equals 70.

This patient's heart rate is *approximately* 70 beats/minute.

The fastest method to calculate a *regular* heart rate involves memorizing the following numbers: *300, 150, 100*; *75, 60, 50*. Say them to yourself—300, 150, 100; 75, 60, 50. Repeat them again. Now close your eyes and repeat them.

No kidding! Close your eyes and repeat the numbers!

The next item you must know is how to recognize an R wave. The R wave is the first upward deflection in a QRS complex.

This is an R wave. *Remember* what it looks like.

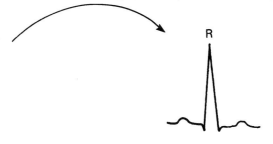

Find an R wave that falls on a *heavy vertical* line on the EKG paper (see arrow).

Notice that the R wave of beat 6 falls on a heavy vertical line. *Do not* count this line, but beginning with the next heavy vertical line, count 300. You may count either to the right or to the left of the complex. In this example, we will count to the left! The first heavy vertical line after the R wave is 300. Continuing on to the left, the next heavy vertical line is 150. The third heavy vertical line is 100. The fourth heavy vertical line is 75. Before the fourth heavy vertical line is another R wave. That means that this patient's heart rate is between 75 and 100, but closer to 75. Once you have become familiar with this method, it will serve to allow you a rapid estimate of the patient's heart rate. Using this method, one does not need to be concerned with the three second time markers!

Figure the heart rate in the next sample EKG strip.

Find the R wave that falls on a heavy vertical line . . . it has to be beat 7 moving from left to right. In this example, you are forced to begin counting vertical lines to the left of the R wave. *Remember,* do *not* count the vertical line on which the R wave falls. Begin counting on the next vertical line to the left, 300, 150 and so forth.
What did you get? Me too!
This patient's heart rate falls between 100 and 150.

Now close your eyes and repeat the six numbers you have memorized.
Actually, you can use any wave (other than an R wave) that you wish when figuring heart rate in this manner. It's just that R waves are usually the easiest waves to spot. ☺

> *Remember:* This method should *only* be used when the rhythm is **REGULAR** and it is an estimate of heart rate.

If you are wondering why this method works, it is because there are 1500 small EKG squares per minute. If you count the number of small EKG squares between two R waves (12 in the above example), and divide 1500 by that number, you will get the precise heart rate.

$$12\overline{)1500} \quad 125$$

Practice Exercise 7

Now try some practice! Figure the heart rate on each of the following EKG strips. Do not look back until you have completed the exercise.

A. Reference the strip at the top of the next page then decide if the rhythm is regular. Imagine all the tall upright waves (R waves) are sticks lying in a row.

Decide if they are evenly spaced. Answer the following questions:

Each marker at the top of the EKG paper represents ___3___ seconds.

There are ___5___ complexes in the six second time interval displayed. Therefore, ___5___ × 10

equals ___50___. The approximate heart rate is ___50___ beats/minute.

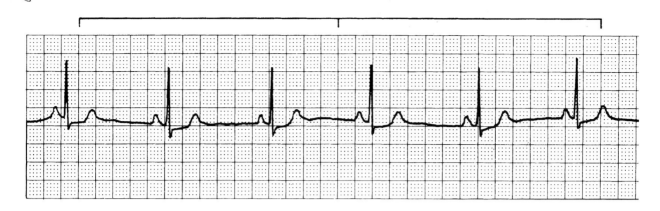

B. Calculate the heart rate on EKG strip below.

Heart rate = ~~approx 70 bpm~~ (Irregular)

_____

C. Remember the six numbers you memorized? . . . 300, 150, 100; 75, 60, 50. Calculate the heart rate of the strip below using that method. Step one consists of finding an R wave that falls on a heavy vertical line.

Beat __4__ falls closest to a heavy vertical line. The next heavy vertical line to the left is counted as __300__. The next heavy vertical line is counted as __150__, *etc.* The heart rate falls between __75__ and __100__ beats per minute.

D. Using the same method, calculate the heart rate in the following strip.

The heart rate is *between 100 - 75 bpm, but closer to 100 bpm*

(Irregular heart rate)

✔ For **Feedback 7,** refer to page 40.

A Brief Review

I forgot to tell you . . . if you get tired, you can interrupt your study at any point. That's why the material is organized in this fashion. You can stop and go as you please. You're almost an expert now anyway!

Following is a brief review summarizing what we have covered thus far!

1. The sinus node is the pacemaker in the normal heart. Thus, the term sinus rhythm implies that the electrical impulse originates in the sinus node.

2. The P wave is the first wave formation in the normal EKG complex. The P wave represents depolarization of the atria. The P waves seen on an EKG strip should all appear identical, and should be equidistant to the following QRS complexes.

3. The P-R interval of each EKG complex represents the time necessary for the sinoatrial impulse to travel from the sinus node through the AV junction to the ventricles. In normal conduction, that time should be *0.12–0.20 seconds.* Now, how many small EKG squares is that? Remember, each small square represents 0.04 seconds . . . so, 0.12 seconds equals three small squares, and 0.20 seconds equals five small squares. Thus, a normal P-R interval will measure between *3–5 small squares* in width or 0.12–0.20 seconds in duration.

4. The QRS represents depolarization of the ventricles. Every normal rhythm should have a QRS preceded by a P wave and followed by a T wave . . . all occurring in a regular fashion. The normal QRS should measure *less* than *0.12 seconds,* or less than 3 small EKG squares. (If the QRS is 3 or more small squares in width or duration, it indicates a defect or delay in the conduction system.)

5. The T wave represents the recovery state after ventricular depolarization. The T waves should all be upright and appear identical. The ST segment will be flat, neither elevated nor depressed.

6. A normal heart rate is 60–100 beats per minute. Typically, the sinus node will initiate an impulse 60–100 times per minute, and each time, the impulse will be conducted down through the AV junction, through the bundle of His, down the bundle branches to the Purkinje fibers to initiate ventricular depolarization.

Input Section 1.8: Sinus Rhythm

Now, let's think about a sinus rhythm or a normal rhythm. This next strip illustrates a sinus rhythm.

A sinus rhythm will have all of the following identifying features.

Rate:	60 to 100 beats per minute
Rhythm:	Regular
P Waves:	A P wave will precede each QRS complex. All P waves will be uniform in appearance.
QRS:	All QRS complexes will appear uniform in configuration.
Conduction:	Each P wave will be followed by a normal QRS complex.

Sinus rhythm is given its name because it originates in the sinoatrial node. The SA node is the normal pacemaker of the heart because it has the highest inherent rate of discharge or automaticity (60 to 100 times per minute). Though other tissues have pacemaking capability, their inherent rates of impulse-formation are significantly less than the sinus rate. ***Thus, the fastest pacemaker always assumes control of the rhythm!***

Here is another example of sinus rhythm.

In the above strip, the heart rate is between 75 and 100, but closer to 100 beats per minute. Various pathologies (which will be discussed later in the text) occur even when the rhythm is normal! Notice that the T waves of this strip are inverted as compared to the sinus rhythm example at the top of the page.

Practice Exercise 8

Reference the above rhythm strip when answering these questions.

A. The heart rate in this strip is ___75-100___ beats per minute.

B. The rhythm is (regular)/irregular (circle one).

C. Each QRS complex is *preceded* by a ___P___ wave.

Do all the P waves look uniform or alike? __✓__ yes _____ no (check ✔ one)

D. Is each P wave followed by a normal QRS complex? __✓__ yes _____ no (check ✔ one)

E. Do all QRS complexes appear uniform? __✓__ yes _____ no (check ✔ one)

F. VOILA! This is a ___sinus___ rhythm!

✔ For **Feedback 8,** refer to page 42.

Input Section 1.9: Interpreting Dysrhythmias

Following is some introductory information for Section 2!

In order to accurately interpret dysrhythmias, there are *five* basic steps one must follow. As you become more proficient in EKG interpretation, you may combine, reorder . . . or even think of new steps. However, for now, it will assist you to follow these five steps when analyzing any rhythm!

1. *First, determine whether the rhythm is regular or irregular.* If the rhythm is irregular, try to determine what makes it irregular. Are there early (premature) beats? Are there pauses? Are abnormal beats

present? The simplest method for determining rhythm regularity is to measure the distance between two consecutive R waves (R-R interval) and compare that distance with other R-R intervals in the strip (examine the R-R intervals in the previous strip). In a regular rhythm, the R-R intervals will all measure the same.

2. **Second**, *determine the heart rate*. Remember . . . if the rhythm is irregular, it is necessary to count the rate for one full minute. (In the previous strip, the rate is 90.)

3. **Third**, *one must evaluate atrial activity. What atrial activity is evident?* Are there P waves that occur uniformly across the monitor tracing? Are the P waves alike in appearance? If no distinct P waves are present, is there any evidence of atrial activity, or is the baseline preceding the QRS flat? If atrial impulses are present, are they regular or irregular? Is the atrial activity occurring so rapidly that there are more atrial deflections than QRS complexes? If actual atrial wave forms are difficult to identify, does the baseline appear chaotic?

4. **Fourth**, *determine ventricular activity. What ventricular activity is evident?* Are the QRSs of normal duration (less than 0.12 seconds)? Do the QRSs occur uniformly across the monitor tracing? Does a QRS follow every P wave or atrial wave deflection?

5. **Finally**, it is important to *determine the relationship between atrial and ventricular activity.* Is each P wave producing a QRS, or are there P waves that are not followed by QRS complexes? Is each QRS preceded by a P wave, or is there evidence of independent ventricular activity? Is the P-R interval of all conducted beats constant, does it vary, or is there no established relationship?

The above five steps will be repeatedly followed as various rhythm abnormalities are explored.
The above five steps will be repeatedly followed as various rhythm abnormalities are explored.
The above five steps will be repeatedly followed as various rhythm abnormalities are explored.
The above five steps will be repeatedly followed as various rhythm abnormalities are explored.
The above five steps will be repeatedly followed as various rhythm abnormalities are explored.

Remember: One need not apply a sophisticated name to any rhythm. A simple descriptive analysis (answering the questions in the above five steps) conveys the most accurate information!

MOVING TO SECTION 2 ...

ACME VAN LINES

✔ Feedback 1

Very good!

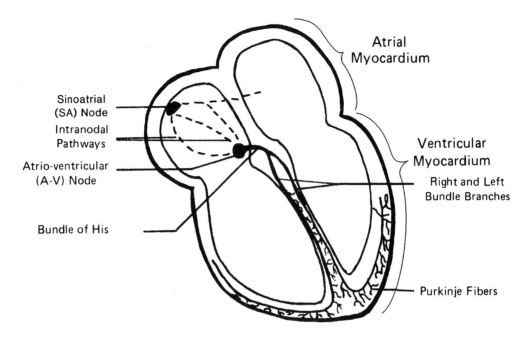

The impulse originates in the sinoatrial (SA) node and travels down the intranodal pathways, activating the atria. The impulse then travels through the AV node, slowing slightly. Impulse conduction speeds up as it leaves the AV node, passing to the bundle of His. From the bundle of His, the impulse travels rapidly down the right and left bundle branches to the Purkinje fibers.

Each cardiac cycle consists of two phases—activation or depolarization, and recovery or repolarization. Normally, the SA node fires 60 to 100 times per minute.

✔ Feedback 2

If your answers look like this, you're doing a super job!

A. Atrial excitation (in the healthy heart) begins in the sinoatrial or SA node.

B. As the impulse spreads across the atria, it causes atrial muscle contraction following depolarization.

C. The monitor picture associated with atrial depolarization is the P wave.

D. (a "P" wave.)

E. In the healthy heart, the P wave will note the beginning of each new cardiac cycle.

F. (a P-R interval)

G. The P-R interval represents the time it takes for the impulse to depolarize the atria and travel from the atria, through the <u>AV node</u> to the ventricles.

P.S. If your answers varied from these, review the material one more time!

✔ Feedback 3

A. If you have drawn a QRS complex, good for you!

 = Ventricular Depolarization

B. Ventricular depolarization begins when the SA initiated impulse reaches the ventricles (after traveling through the atria, through the AV junction, through the bundle of His, down the bundle branches to the Purkinje fibers). Ventricular muscle contraction follows electrical depolarization.

✔ Feedback 4

Excellent work! Your answers should be similar to mine.

A.

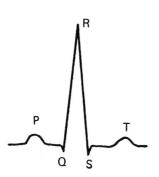

B. Atrial excitation begins in the <u>SA (sinoatrial) node</u>.

C. The P wave represents <u>atrial depolarization</u>.

D. The P-R interval represents <u>the time for atrial recovery and the time necessary for the impulse to pass from the SA node through the AV node, through the bundle of His, down the bundle branches to the Purkinje fibers.</u>

E. The QRS represents <u>ventricular depolarization</u>.
The Q wave is the first <u>downward</u> deflection.
The R wave is the first <u>upward</u> deflection.
The S wave is the negative or <u>downward</u> deflection following the R wave.

F. The ST segment represents <u>the early phase of ventricular muscle recovery (repolarization)</u>.

G. The T wave represents the <u>recovery phase following ventricular activation (repolarization)</u>.

H. The PQRST complex represents one <u>cardiac cycle</u>.

The following summary is included to tie together any loose ends.

Remember, wave forms may be either positive or negative depending upon which lead one is viewing.

P-Wave—Artial excitation starts at the SA node and spreads through both atria. The P wave represents depolarization of the atria. If P waves are present, and of normal size and shape, it can be assumed that the stimulus began in the SA node.

P-R Interval—The period of atrial repolarization is represented by the P-R interval. It also represents the time for the impulse to pass from the SA node, through the AV junction, through the bundle of His, down the bundle branches to the Purkinje fibers. The normal P-R interval is usually between 0.12–0.20 seconds.

QRS Complex—These waves represent depolarization of the ventricular muscle. The initial *downward* deflection is the Q wave. The R wave is the first positive or *upward* deflection. The S wave is the *downward* wave following the R wave. The normal QRS duration is less than 0.12 seconds.

ST Segement—This segment represents the early phase of repolarization (recovery of the ventricular muscle).

T wave—The recovery phase following ventricular activation.

Note: Electrical depolarization occurs before cardiac muscle contraction . . . and, electrical repolarization follows cardiac muscle contractions.

✔ Feedback 5

How did you do? Probably excellent, as usual! I hope your answers match mine.

A. <u>time</u>

B. <u>3 seconds</u>

C. <u>6 seconds</u>. That may be confusing, but I 3 I 3 I there are only two 3 second intervals between three markers!

D. <u>0.20 seconds</u>

E. 15 large squares between two <u>3</u> second markers. Therefore, <u>3</u> seconds lapse between these markers (15 squares × 0.20 seconds [per square] = 3.0).

0.04 = little square
0.20 = big square
duh .

F. 0.04 seconds

G. <u>5</u> small squares

H. <u>30</u> large squares in a 6 second time interval

I. <u>0.12</u> [0.04 seconds (one small square) $\times$ 3 small squares = 0.12 seconds]

J. <u>0.16</u> [0.04 seconds (one small square) $\times$ 4 small squares = 0.16 seconds]

K. <u>0.20</u> seconds which is the same as one large square

L. <u>1.0</u> second [0.20 seconds (per big square) $\times$ 5 big squares = 1.0 second]

M. <u>2.6</u> seconds [0.20 seconds (per big square) $\times$ 13 big squares = 2.6 seconds]

N. <u>1.12</u> seconds. There are two ways to figure this.
1. You could figure the 5 big squares first
   0.20 seconds per big square $\times$ 5 big squares   = 1.0 second
   Then figure the small squares:
   0.04 seconds per small square $\times$ 3 small squares = <u>0.12</u> seconds

                                    Total = 1.12 seconds

or

2. You could simply say there are a total of 28 small squares.
   So, 0.04 seconds per small square $\times$ 28 small squares = 1.12 seconds

✔ Feedback 6

If your answers match mine, you're doing a great job! If they don't, a little more practice is in order!

A. To be within normal limits, the P-R interval must measure <u>3</u> to <u>5</u> small squares in width or <u>0.12</u> to <u>0.20</u> seconds in duration.

B. A P-R interval less than <u>3</u> small squares in width or greater than <u>5</u> small squares in width represents an abnormality in the impulse conduction.

C. The P-R interval of the EKG cycle measures <u>5</u> small squares or <u>0.20</u> seconds (the upper limit of normal).

D. The QRS wave form represents <u>ventricular depolarization</u>.

E. To be within normal limits, the QRS must measure <u>LESS than 3</u> small squares or less than <u>0.12</u> seconds in duration.

F. The QRS of the boxed cardiac cycle measures <u>slightly less than three</u> small squares which is <u>slightly less than 0.12</u> seconds.

✔ Feedback 7

Keep up the good work!

A. Each marker at the top of the EKG paper represents <u>three</u> seconds. There are <u>5</u> complexes in the six second time interval displayed. Therefore, 5 $\times$ 10 equal <u>50</u>. The approximate heart rate is <u>50</u> beats/minute, though it is very close to 60! This is just an estimate.

8

B. If you calculated a heart rate of approximately 70, you are

Incorrect!!!

A heart rate estimation method cannot be utilized when a rhythm is <u>irregular</u>. Had one observed a full 60 second trace, he/she would have noticed that this was just a brief slow period in the rhythm. The patient's actual heart rate was 90 beats per minute! *Remember, when a rhythm is irregular, one must count the number of EKG complexes in a <u>full</u> minute! Or, better yet, physically count the patient's pulse.*

C. Beat 4 falls closest to a heavy vertical line. The next heavy vertical line to the left is counted as <u>300</u>. The next vertical line is counted as <u>150</u>, etc. The heart rate falls between <u>75</u> and <u>100</u> beats per minute.

D. Did I catch you? The 300, 150, 100; 75, 60, 50 method will <u>not</u> be an accurate estimate of heart rate because this rhythm is irregular. One would need to count the number of EKG complexes or cycles in one <u>full</u> minute to determine the heart rate.

P.S. Here is a little "cheat sheet" to hang near your monitors. Count the number of small squares (small boxes) between two R waves of a regular rhythm, then read across the chart to determine heart rate.

A Trusty Guide for Determining Heart Rate

No. of Boxes	Heart Rate	No. of Boxes	Heart Rate
5	300	25	60
6	250	26	57
7	214	27	55
8	187	28	53
9	166	29	52
10	150	30	50
11	136	31	48
12	125	32	47
13	115	33	45
14	107	34	44
15	100	35	42
16	94	36	41
17	88	37	40
→ 18	83	38	39
19	79	40	37
20	75	44	34
21	71	46	32
22	68	48	31
23	65	50	30
24	62		

Count the number of *small* EKG squares between two R waves on the following strip.

In this strip there are <u>18</u> small squares between R waves. Looking back to the Trusty Guide (page 41), one can quickly see that the heart rate is <u>83</u>.

REMEMBER, this method of determining heart rate applies *only* when the rhythm is *regular*!

In the event that you are wondering how this Trusty Guide came into being, the story is as follows. There are 1500 little tiny EKG squares in one minute. So, if one counts the number of small squares between two R waves (i.e., 18 in the previous example) and divides that number into 1500, one arrives at the heart rate. Remember this method works *only* when the rhythm is regular.

$$18\overline{)1500}^{\,82}$$

✔ Feedback 8

Excellent work!

A. The heart rate in this strip is *approximately 90* beats per minute.

B. The rhythm is **regular.**

C. Each QRS complex is preceded by a <u>P</u> wave. All the P waves look uniform.

D. Each P wave is followed by a normal QRS complex.

E. All the QRS complexes appear uniform.

F. This is a **sinus rhythm!**

Notes

Notes

Sinus and Atrial Dysrhythmias

Objectives

When you have completed Section 2, you will be able to describe or identify

1. a method for interpreting dysrhythmias
2. sinus arrhythmia
3. sinus bradycardia
4. sinus tachycardia
5. wandering atrial pacemaker (W.A.P.)
6. premature atrial contractions (P.A.C.s)
7. atrial tachycardia and re-entry mechanisms
8. atrial flutter
9. atrial fibrillation
10. atrial flutter-fibrillation
11. sick sinus syndrome (brady-tachy syndrome)
12. Wolff-Parkinson-White Syndrome (bypass re-entry mechanisms)

45

Input Section 2.1: Steps for Interpreting Dysrhythmias

You're back! From this point forward, the content will build upon principles learned in the first section. All abnormal rhythm patterns explored will be compared to sinus rhythm.

Sinus rhythm

You will remember, sinus rhythm is a *regular* rhythm with a rate of 60–100 beats per minute. Each QRS complex is preceded by a P wave. All P waves are uniform in appearance. All QRS complexes are uniform in appearance and each P wave is followed by a QRS.

As we begin to interpret the various abnormal rhythm patterns, *five* steps will be followed.

1. *Determining rhythm regularity.* If the rhythm is irregular, one must determine what makes it irregular. Are there early (premature) beats? Are there unexpected pauses? Are abnormal beats occurring? The simplest method for determining rhythm regularity is to measure the distance between two consecutive R waves (R-R interval) and compare that distance with other R-R intervals. In a regular rhythm, the R-R interval measurement will remain constant (as illustrated in the bottom diagram on page 48).

2. *Determining heart rate.* Remember . . . if the rhythm is irregular, it is necessary to count the rate for one full minute.

3. *Determining atrial activity.* Are P waves occurring uniformly across the monitor tracing? Are the P waves alike in appearance? If no distinct P waves are present, is there evidence of atrial activity, or is the baseline preceding the QRS flat? If atrial impulses are present, are they regular or irregular? Is the atrial activity occurring so rapidly that there are more atrial deflections than QRS complexes? If actual atrial wave forms are difficult to identify, does the baseline appear chaotic?

4. *Determining ventricular activity.* Are the QRS complexes of normal duration (less than 0.12 seconds)? Do the QRSs occur uniformly across the monitor tracing? Does a QRS follow every P wave?

5. *Determining the relationship between atrial and ventricular activity.* Is each P wave producing a QRS, or are there P waves that are not followed by QRS complexes? Is each QRS preceded by a P wave, or is there evidence of independent ventricular activity? Is the P-R interval of all conducted beats constant, does it vary, or is there no established relationship?

Practice Exercise 1

Study the above strip and then answer the following questions.

A. The heart rate is ___75___ beats per minute.

B. The rhythm is (regular) / irregular (circle one).

C. Each QRS complex is preceded by a ___P wave___.

D. All P waves are ___uniform___ in appearance.

E. Each P wave is followed by a ___QRS complex___.

F. All QRS complexes are ___uniform___ in appearance.

G. The P-R interval is ___constant___ and measures ___.18___ seconds.

H. Therefore, this is a ___NSR___ rhythm!

To interpret any rhythm, I use the same five principles.

1. First, I determine if the rhythm is ___Regular___.

2. Second, I must determine the heart ___rate___.

3. I next determine ___atrial___ activity.

4. Then I look to determine ___ventricular___ activity.

5. The final step involves determining if a relationship exists between ___atrial___ and ___ventricular___ activity.

✔ For **Feedback 1,** refer to page 80.

Input Section 2.2: Sinus Arrhythmia

The first dysrhythmia to be explored is *sinus arrhythmia.*

A sinus arrhythmia is a *slightly* irregular rhythm that is initiated by the SA node. Usually the slight variation in rhythm is related to **respiration.** The heart rate will increase slightly with inspiration, and decrease slightly with expiration. A sinus arrhythmia is a normal finding in children and young adults. A *slight* sinus arrhythmia may be found throughout adulthood. Sinus arrhythmia is usually the result of increased vagal tone.

Sinus arrhythmia may also be found with conditions such as rheumatic fever, atelectasis, infectious diseases, and so forth. Last, but not least, a sinus arrhythmia may be seen in patients receiving digitalis. Any factor which *increases* vagal tone will exaggerate a sinus arrhythmia.

Looking closely at this rhythm strip, you will note the following:

1. The heart rate falls somewhere between 60 and 100 beats per minute.

2. **The rhythm is irregular.**

3. The P waves are all uniform in appearance.

4. The QRS complexes are all of normal configuration and duration.

5. Each P wave produces a QRS. The P-R interval measures approximately 0.16 seconds and is consistent across the strip (so, atrial activity is related to ventricular activity!).

☆ **The only abnormal finding is that the rhythm is *slightly* irregular, showing irregular spacing of the normal P waves.**

The easiest method for determining rhythm irregularity is to measure the distance between two P waves (P-P interval) and then compare that distance to the distance between two other P waves (other P-P intervals).

OR

Measure the distance between two R waves (R-R interval) and then compare that distance to the distance between two other R waves (other R-R intervals).

Easy, huh?

The following strip demonstrates the time measurement between each R-R interval. One can easily see the slight irregularity, though everything else appears normal.

| 1.2 sec. | 1.0 sec. | 1.04 sec. | 1.04 sec. | .96 sec. | .98 sec. |

Remember, each small square on the EKG paper represents 0.04 seconds.

To review then, a sinus arrhythmia is simply a sinus rhythm that is slightly irregular! *No treatment is required* though it is important to determine the underlying causative factor.

Practice Exercise 2

Okay, now it's your turn! Review the next two rhythm strips, then answer the questions following each strip.

1.

A. The heart rate in this strip is **approximately** ___70___ beats per minute.

B. The P waves are all ___uniform___ in appearance.

C. A ___P___ wave precedes each QRS complex.

D. The QRS complexes are ___uniform___ in appearance.

E. A ___QRS complex___ follows every P wave.

F. The rhythm is regular/irregular (circle one).

G. This is a ___sinus___ rhythm.

2.

A. The heart rate in this strip is **approximately** __90__ beats per minute.

B. The P waves are all __uniform__ in appearance.

C. A __P__ wave precedes each QRS complex.

D. The QRS complexes are __uniform__ in appearance.

E. A __QRS complex__ follows every P wave.

F. The rhythm is regular/~~irregular~~ (circle one).

G. This is a __sinus arrhythmia__ rhythm.

3. Usually the irregularity found in sinus arrhythmia is related to __respirations__.

✔ For **Feedback 2,** refer to page 80.

Input Section 2.3: Sinus Bradycardia

Bradycardia is a term used to describe a heart rate less than 60 beats per minute. *Sinus bradycardia* is a normal rhythm with the exception that the heart rate falls below 60. The impulse originates in a normal fashion from the sinus (SA) node, but the impulses are fired at a slower rate due to vagal stimulation of the cardiac regulatory center.

Commonly, *sinus bradycardia* is the normal rhythm of athletes and other persons accustomed to regular physical exercise.

It may also occur during normal sleep. Sinus bradycardia can be induced by exerting pressure on the carotid sinus or the eyeball. Relating to pathology, a slow rate is commonly associated with increased intracranial pressure or in conjunction with

Obstructive disease (intestine, kidney, bladder)
Myxedema
Myocardial infarction
Drug actions (digitalis, morphine, anesthesia, or quinidine)

Here is a rhythm strip demonstrating a *sinus bradycardia.*

☆1. The rate is approximately 48 beats per minute (I referenced the chart on page 41).

2. The rhythm is regular.

3. The P waves are all uniform in appearance and precede each QRS complex.

4. The QRS complexes are uniform in appearance (and measure 0.10 seconds).

5. Each P wave produces a QRS. The P-R interval measures approximately 0.18 seconds and is consistent across the strip. Thus, atrial activity is assumed to be related to ventricular activity.

☆ **The only abnormality is that the heart rate is approximately 48, which falls below the lower limits of normal, 60 beats per minute. So, we have a sinus bradycardia.**

Using the five principles for dysrhythmia interpretation, one could say:

➤ The rate is approximately 48 per minute.

➤ The rhythm is slow and regular.

➤ The atria are activated regularly. P waves precede each QRS complex and they are uniform in appearance.

➤ There is a QRS complex following each P wave. The QRS complexes are occurring regularly at a rate of 48 per minute. All QRS complexes appear uniform and measure 0.08 seconds.

➤ There is a definite relationship between atrial and ventricular activity because each P-R interval is 0.18 seconds. In other words, the impulse originating in the sinus node moves down the conduction system to activate ventricular tissue in the same amount of time during each cardiac cycle.

Usually sinus bradycardia is observed and not treated. Treatment will be initiated only if the patient becomes symptomatic (mental confusion or disorientation, lethargy, loss of consciousness, and so forth). Should the patient become symptomatic, a physician should be notified immediately.

In most instances, intravenous (IV) atropine is the drug treatment of choice to increase the heart rate when symptoms are acute. (One must closely monitor urinary performance following the administration of atropine, as atropine is a smooth muscle relaxant.) If unresponsive to atropine, transcutaneous pacing is typically initiated.

If a patient is receiving digitalis and his heart rate falls below 50, it is likely digitalis will be discontinued. The *managing* physician should always be made aware of the digitalized patient with a sustained sinus bradycardia. Digitalis preparations *should be held* until the physician is notified; additional administration of digitalis may further slow heart rate or result in various forms of heart block.

Practice Exercise 3

A. The term bradycardia implies that the heart rate is less than _____60_____ beats per minute. Here are two strips for you to inspect.

B. The first strip demonstrates a sinus rhythm. Explain how the second strip is both similar to and different from the first. (Use the principles previously discussed!)

Approx 40 bpm is less than 60. Everything else characteristic of NSR.

The second strip demonstrates a ___Sinus bradycardia___(rhythm).

✔ For **Feedback 3,** refer to page 81.

Input Section 2.4: Sinus Tachycardia

Tachycardia is a term used to describe a heart rate *greater than* 100 beats per minute. *Sinus tachycardia* is a regular sinus rhythm with a rate greater than 100 beats per minute. *Usually a sinus tachycardia will not exceed the rate of 160 per minute.*

Sinus tachycardia is usually directly related to diminished vagal tone and may be exaggerated by increased sympathetic tone. Some of the more common causes of sinus tachycardia are exercise, excitement, anemia, fear, heart failure, pain, fever, shock, infection, and drugs—such as IV demerol, atropine or epinephrine, and foods—such as coffee or tea, and tobacco! Most authorities feel that for each Fahrenheit degree the temperature rises, the heart rate will increase approximately eight to ten beats per minute. I bet you didn't know that!

The following rhythm strip demonstrates a sinus tachycardia.

Using the five principles for dysrhythmia interpretation, one could say:

☆1. The rate is rapid, approximately 115 beats per minute.

2. The rhythm is regular.

3. The P waves are all uniform in appearance.

4. The QRS complexes are all uniform in appearance and duration.

5. Each P wave precedes the QRS by the same interval. In other words the P-R interval is constant, measuring approximately 0.14 seconds.

☆ The major abnormality is that the heart rate is 115, which falls above 100 beats per minute. Thus, we have a *sinus tachycardia*. (I have used the Trusty Guide on page 41 to determine the heart rate!)

If a heart rate of exactly 100 accompanies a sinus rhythm, it is usually called a *borderline sinus tachycardia.*

Should one find a patient's heart rate greater than 100 beats per minute, one must assume the role of *detective* to discover the underlying cause. The treatment for sinus tachycardia consists of *treating its cause* (i.e., lowering an elevated temperature or treating congestive heart failure, as examples).

If the patient has extreme anxiety, is cyanotic, has labored breathing or complaints of chest pain, a physician should be notified immediately. The increased heart rate associated with a sinus tachycardia results in increased myocardial oxygen consumption, though hemodynamic imbalance usually does not occur.

$$6 \overline{)300} \frac{50}{}$$

✒ Practice Exercise 4

A. Examine this rhythm strip closely, then describe *all* that you see!

Regular Rhythm
P waves uniform + precede QRS complexes
QRS complexes uniform
Rate = 50 bpm
Sinus Bradycardia
PRI = .16   QRS = .08

This rhythm is a __Sinus Bradycardia__ .

B. Again, critically analyze the following strip and describe your findings.

$$2\overline{)300}$$

Regular Rhythm
P waves uniform + precede QRS complexes
QRS complexes uniform
Rate = 150
PRI = .12
QRS = .08

This rhythm is a __Sinus tachycardia__ .

C. The treatment for sinus tachycardia consists of ___~~____~~ *treating the cause =*
lowering temp, treating anxiety, treating heart failure

GOOD WORK!

✔ For **Feedback 4,** refer to page 82.

Input Section 2.5: Wandering Atrial Pacemaker (W.A.P.)

Before moving forward, we should look briefly at *wandering atrial pacemakers.* Basically, a *wandering atrial pacemaker* rhythm is a variation of a sinus rhythm that has no clinical significance. Rather than seeing uniform P waves across the EKG strip, the *P waves tend to vary in appearance.* This P wave variation suggests that the pacemaker is wandering within the sinus mechanism and the surrounding atrial tissue.

Commonly, a *wandering atrial pacemaker* is observed when the sinus rate slows. You will remember that other tissues within the atria have pacemaking capabilities . . . , *but* it is always the pacemaker with the *fastest* rate of discharge that controls the rhythm. In a wandering atrial pacemaker rhythm, various pacemakers (located within the atria) are discharging at similar rates. Thus, no single pacemaker site is dominant.

As you look at the above strip, you will notice that the rhythm is slightly irregular. (If you are unsure, measure the P-P or R-R intervals.) Looking further, the P waves tend to vary in shape or contour. Because of this variation, we assume that no single pacemaker within the atria is dominant. *How do I know that the various pacemakers are located within the atria?* . . . because each cardiac complex begins with a P wave . . . and P waves represent atrial depolarization! ☺

The other fact one should be aware of is that the P-R interval may vary throughout a wandering atrial pacemaker rhythm. Since the P-R interval represents the time for impulse conduction from the pacemaker site through the system to the Purkinje fibers, it makes sense that if the pacemaker site changes, so will the time for impulse conduction!

Since ventricular activation is usually unaltered, the QRS complexes are of normal duration (less than 0.12 seconds). Owing to the fact that a wandering atrial pacemaker is a variation of normal, no treatment or intervention is required. Whew! Typically, a wandering atrial pacemaker is associated with pronounced pulmonary disease.

Practice Exercise 5

Without looking back, draw a rhythm strip demonstrating wandering atrial pacemaker. Sounds like fun . . . right?

✔ For **Feedback 5,** refer to page 82.

Input Section 2.6: Premature Atrial Contractions

We are now going to begin exploring *ectopic* activity. . . . electrical stimuli originating outside the normal conduction system.

A *premature atrial contraction,* henceforth to be known as a P.A.C., is an atrial impulse arising from an ectopic or abnormal atrial focus. As the name implies, the P.A.C. is *premature* in its relationship to the underlying sinus rhythm. In addition to occurring early or prematurely, the P.A.C. has an *abnormal appearing P wave.* In other words the P wave looks distinctly different from the P wave of the sinus rhythm since the route of atrial depolarization is different for the abnormal beat. That may sound confusing, so inspect the following rhythm strip.

The first thing one notices is that the rhythm is *irregular.* Beat 3 and beat 10 occur early or prematurely. This is a technical interpretation based solely on quick "eyeball inspection"! You will notice the premature beats (3 and 10) have P waves . . . but, they look distinctly different from the other P waves in the strip. P.A.C.s may have P waves that are inverted, slurred, taller or wider than the normal P wave. On this strip, the P wave of the P.A.C. appears flat.

Premature atrial contraction is one of the few logical names used in EKG interpretation! Because the P.A.C. falls early interrupting the underlying rhythm, it is called *premature.* And because there is a P wave we know the atria have depolarized.

A premature atrial impulse is *usually* conducted normally through the AV junction on to the ventricles. Do you know how I know that? *Voila!* because the P-R interval of the P.A.C. is usually between 3–5 small EKG squares (0.12–0.20 seconds) and because its QRS is usually narrow (*less than* 3 small squares). However, be advised that multiple rhythm abnormalities often occur together. It is not uncommon that the QRS associated with a P.A.C. will be widened, 0.12 seconds or greater. This is referred to as a P.A.C. that is *aberrantly* conducted, meaning that conduction is outside the normal conduction pathway.

In the following strip, every other beat is a P.A.C. (bigeminy P.A.C.s). Notice that the P waves of the premature beats tend to be less pronounced than the P waves of the sinus beats. For future reference, *bigeminy* is a term describing ectopic events occurring regularly in an every other beat pattern.

P.A.C.   P.A.C   P.A.C   P.A.C.   P.A.C

Premature atrial contractions may arise from a single focus (location) or several foci within the atria. All P.A.C.s arising from a single focus will have similarly appearing P waves. Conversely, if P.A.C.s arise from different sites, the appearance of their premature P waves will vary. When P.A.C.s arise from a single focus, there is a *tendency for a constant coupling interval.* So what is a *coupling interval?* Well, it's simply the interval or distance between the P.A.C. and the previous sinus beat. (This business about coupling intervals is for your trivia file .)

Coupling
Interval

P   P   P
   T   T   T

Sinus Beat   P.A.C.

Examine the following rhythm strip. Notice that the *coupling interval* is constant and the P waves of the P.A.C.s appear similar. We therefore assume that the P.A.C.s are arising from the same ectopic atrial site.

Coupling interval

P.A.C.   P.A.C.

The other obvious finding associated with P.A.C.s is the slight pause or delay occurring before the next sinus beat.

This pause tends to partly compensate for the prematurity. In other words, the P.A.C. firing prematurely disrupts the regular sinus cycle; the pause allows time for the sinus mechanism to reset the rhythm.

Premature atrial contractions may be observed in healthy individuals or may be associated with heart disease. P.A.C.s associated with rheumatic heart disease may be a forerunner to atrial fibrillation. P.A.C.s may also be noted in patients with pulmonary disease, right heart disease, and myocardial infarction. Drugs such as epinephrine and digitalis, stimulants such as coffee, tea, alcohol, tobacco, or emotional distress or fatigue may likewise precipitate P.A.C.s. To be on the safe side, always notify a physician when a patient begins having P.A.C.s and when they begin increasing in frequency! *The significance of P.A.C.s is the significance of the underlying clinical condition.* However, P.A.C.s. may precipitate rapid atrial dysrhythmias which will be covered later in this Section! Treatment, if indicated, typically involves the administration of propranol or digitalis.

Examine this next strip.

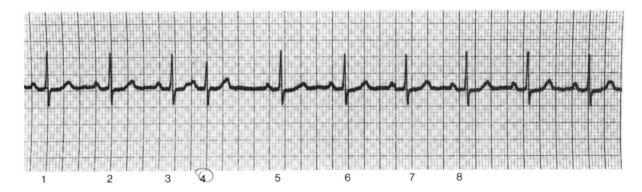

The P waves are *not* uniform in appearance. The P wave of beat 4 is premature in its relationship to the underlying rhythm and appears different from the other P waves. If you look closely, you will notice that the premature P wave falls on the T wave of the preceding beat. A P wave precedes every QRS complex. The QRS complexes are uniform in appearance, but do not occur regularly. There is a pause following the complex initiated by the premature P wave. The underlying rhythm is a sinus rhythm interrupted by a lone P.A.C.

Detecting P.A.C.s is usually not difficult. However, confusion may arise if, for some reason, a premature atrial impulse fails to be conducted. That sounds like a mouthful, so inspect this next strip closely.

First, examine atrial activity. Refer back to the previous strip and locate all of the P waves. You will note that a premature P wave (appearing distinctly different from the other P waves) follows after beat 3. What is this? Well, it's a P wave—and P waves represent atrial depolarization. It occurs prematurely. So it's a premature atrial contraction that *fails to conduct* to the ventricles. In other words, since a QRS does not follow the premature atrial impulse, one concludes that the impulse was blocked or interrupted enroute to the ventricles. So this is an example of a *blocked P.A.C.* Like conducted P.A.C.s, there is a pause following the blocked P.A.C.

P.S. If this is confusing to you, it may help to remember that you will never find two T waves occurring together!

Note: If a well-defined "bump" follows the T wave—most likely, it is a P wave!

Blocked P.A.C.s are most commonly associated with two phenomena, digitalis toxicity and tissue refractoriness. When blocked P.A.C.s are observed, make certain to check whether the patient is receiving a digitalis preparation, and observe for other digitalis toxicity signs and symptoms (discussed later in the text). When associated with digitalis administration, blocked P.A.C.s should be reported to the *managing* physician.

Look closely at this second strip. Notice the blocked P.A.C. This strip is a tough one! By looking closely, however, you will notice that the T wave of the fourth complex is distorted . . . it has an extra "bump." This extra "bump" is assumed to be a P wave! In other words, the premature P wave is sitting on the downslope of the T wave. Thus, we again have a blocked P.A.C.!

In this example, the premature atrial impulse does not conduct to the ventricles because the cardiac tissue has not fully recovered or repolarized. In other words, if the myocardial cells do not have sufficient time to repolarize, they may be refractory to (unable to receive) the next stimulation. (The patient belonging to this rhythm strip had a digitalis level of 4.7ng/ml.!!) **Ugh!** It is important to note that digitalis toxicity may be the culprit in either instance! A serum digitalis level is required to determine precise concentrations and to rule out digitalis toxicity. When digitalis toxicity is suspected, further doses of the drug are usually discontinued or held.

Enough on the subject of blocked P.A.C.s Let's try some practice.

Practice Exercise 6

A. Now, try your hand at interpretation! Describe all that you see.

Irregular Rhythm
Rate approximately 80 bpm
P waves uniform + precede each QRS complex
QRS complexes are uniform + follow each P wave
~~Sinus~~
PRI = .20
QRS = .10
~~Sinus Arrhythmia~~ PAC – sinus rhythm underlies
Beats 2, 6, + 10 are early

B. Circle the blocked P.A.C.s and indicate any suspicions you may have.

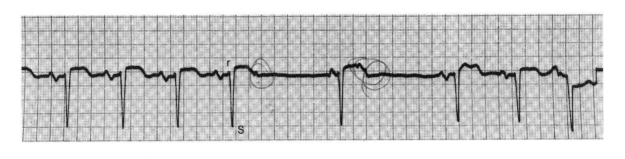

_____

_____

_____

_____

_____

It sometimes helps to sing a few bars of **"keep on smiling. . . ."**

✔ For **Feedback 6,** refer to page 83.

Input Section 2.7: Atrial Tachycardia and Re-entry Mechanisms

You now have a basic understanding of ectopic atrial activity, the P.A.C. When the atria are repeatedly and rapidly stimulated by an ectopic pacemaker, an atrial tachycardia results. Atrial tachycardia can be initiated by: a single ectopic atrial pacemaker (P.A.C.) firing rapidly and repeatedly; multiple ectopic atrial pacemakers firing rapidly and repeatedly; or, a circus-like stimulation (re-entry phenomenon) of the atria.

Although the SA node is the heart's natural pacemaker, it rarely fires faster than 160 beats per minute. A regular, rapid (faster than 160 beats per minute) rhythm with clear P waves is assumed to be initiated by an ectopic atrial pacemaker.

Atrial tachycardia rate 166.

Atrial tachycardia is basically a rapid and *regular sustained* rhythm with a rate between *160 and 220* per minute. In addition to occurring in a sustained fashion, atrial tachycardia may both begin and end abruptly. When this occurs, the short runs of atrial tachycardia are said to be occurring in *paroxysms.* Hence, short bursts or runs of atrial tachycardia are referred to as P.A.T. (*paroxysmal atrial tachycardia*).

Atrial tachycardia may be associated with coronary artery disease, valvular disease (e.g., rheumatic mitral disease) . . . or may be found in otherwise healthy individuals! In fact, any of the following factors may precipitate atrial tachycardia: emotional stress, drug actions of digitalis or quinidine, coffee, tea, tobacco, alcohol, and so forth.

Most patients with a sustained atrial tachycardia experience a fluttering sensation in the chest along with light-headedness due to the rapid ventricular rate. The rapid heart rate reduces cardiac output because the volume of blood ejected with each contraction *(stroke volume)* is decreased as a result of the shortened ventricular filling time. That sounds a bit complicated! Actually it's a great deal like your average household toilet. If you stand there flushing your toilet 180 times per minute, you can imagine what happens . . . not much! You must allow time (between flushes) for the reservoir to refill; otherwise, there's not much action or "toilet output" at the bottom. . . . Right? . . . Just like cardiac output—there must be an appropriate ventricular filling time.

This decrease in cardiac output can lead to left ventricular (LV) failure. The rapid rate also increases the oxygen demand and consumption of the cardiac muscle which, in turn, may cause ischemia of the myocardium and may precipitate an anginal attack (chest pain).

Examine the rhythm strip of atrial tachycardia found at the top of the next page.

The first two-thirds of the above rhythm strip demonstrate atrial tachycardia at a rate of approximately 200 per minute. The rapid rhythm breaks spontaneously into a sinus tachycardia (approximate rate of 115 per minute). You will recall that characteristically, atrial tachycardia has a heart rate that falls between 160 and 220 per minute. Whenever one finds a rapid rhythm with *clearly distinguishable upright P waves* occurring before the QRSs, the rhythm is assumed to be of atrial origin! You will notice that the QRS complexes in both the atrial tachycardia and the sinus tachycardia are of normal duration (narrow), since ventricular activation occurs normally. A word of caution: Because underlying pathology may complicate electrical activity, one may find an atrial tachycardia with a widened QRS known as atrial tachycardia with *aberrancy*.

Atrial tachycardia may terminate abruptly without treatment. If it persists, a physician should be notified immediately. If the patient is alert, he or she may be asked to perform the *Valsalva maneuver*. This maneuver requires that the patient hold his breath and bear down—it's basically like having a bowel movement. This maneuver increases vagal tone which may terminate the rapid rhythm. Another technique for increasing vagal tone (a vagotonic maneuver) is to place a *cold* or *ice* compress on the patient's face. By stimulating a vagal response, the AV junction may slow its rate of impulse conduction, thereby slowing the heart rate. This application of cold or ice water to the face stimulates the *mammalian diving reflex*, a primitive reflex that stimulates the trigeminal nerve (cranial nerve V) which activates the vagues nerve (cranial nerve X) which may result in slowed conduction! If these techniques are unsuccessful, synchronized cardioversion or, alternatively, beta blockers, calcium channel blockers, amiodarone, sotalol or digoxin may be administered. When the patient's condition is rapidly deteriorating, synchronized cardioversion is the treatment of choice, though amiodarone or diltiazem represent treatment options.

Always alert the *managing* physician to even brief periods of atrial tachycardia.

Multifocal Atrial Tachycardia (MAT)

Rather than a single ectopic site (P.A.C.) firing repeatedly, atrial tachycardia may also be precipitated by multiple ectopic sites or foci firing repeatedly. Multifocal atrial tachycardia is the terminology used when a rapid, irregular rhythm (greater than 100 beats per minute) presents with **at least 3 morphologically different (different in appearance) P waves**, signifying at least three different ectopic atrial sites or pacemakers. Depending upon the tachycardic rate, one may observe an isoelectric baseline between the differently appearing P waves. Typically, the QRS complexes are within normal limits, though they may appear widened with a very rapid rate.

Multifocal atrial tachycardia. Notice the rapid rate and variation in P wave morphology.

As with all dysrhythmias, a name is less important than an accurate description of the rhythm!

Multifocal atrial tachycardia is most often observed in the elderly with coronary artery disease in conjunction with chronic lung disease. It may also be associated with hypokalemia, pulmonary embolism, pneumonia and congestive heart failure. Treatment, if indicated, is based on the clinical condition. Beta-blockers, calcium channel blockers or amiodarone are drug options when CHF is absent and cardiac output is not significantly compromised. Treatment options for patients with CHF or compromised cardiac output (ejection fraction <40%) include amiodarone or diltiazem (a calcium channel blocker). Owing to the multiple atrial foci, cardioversion is rarely successful.

Adding to both diagnostic and treatment complexity, atrial tachycardia and upcoming atrial dysrhythmias (atrial flutter and atrial fibrillation) may be precipitated or caused by a *re-entry mechanism*. A re-entry mechanism results from an abnormal (accessory) connection between normal conducting fibers in the atria, creating a circular conducting pathway. *Under certain conditions*, a stimulus will travel rapidly and repeatedly around the circular pathway (circuit), like a race car around a race track, rather than down the normal conduction pathway. A stimulus traveling this rapid, circular pathway can precipitate atrial tachycardia. When atrial tachycardia is caused by this circular activation of atrial tissues, treatment involves disrupting the abnormal circuit, as discussed on page 67.

A re-entry dysrhythmia caused by an accessory circuit is a *DIFFICULT* concept (even for the experts!). The following example of *re-entry mechanics* attempts to demystify cardiac physiology and is included as optional, higher level reading. You may **skip** down to **TREATMENT OF RECURRENT ATRIAL OR SUPRAVEN-TRICULLAR TECHYCARDIA . . .** or take two deep breaths and read on !

Atrial Re-Entry Mechanisms
 (Advanced Study)

Re-entry type dysrhythmias arise from one of two types of conduction system anomalies, both formed during embryonic development:

(1) accessory circuitry (an abnormal connection between conducting fibers which creates a localized abnormal conduction path or circuit) located anywhere within the conduction system

(2) actual bypass tracts (around the normal conduction system) that connect the atria directly to the ventricles.

The second type of anomaly will be discussed near the end of this Section. Here, we will focus on accessory circuitry in the atria.

The presence of an accessory conducting circuit (an abnormal connection between two conducting fibers) predisposes *the owner* to various rapid atrial or supraventricular dysrhythmias. In effect, this extra circuitry, under specific conditions, can precipitate a rapid, *circus-like* stimulation of the atria which, in turn, produces a rapid ventricular rate. A *right-timed* P.A.C. coupled with unequal refractoriness in a portion of the circuit, are the usual conditions necessary to initiate a circus movement atrial tachycardia. **Circus movement tachycardias** are often abbreviated as CMTs.

DIAGRAM
1

In normal healthy conduction, a sinus impulse travels through the atria along specialized conducting fibers or tracts, producing atrial depolarization (ᴡᴡ), then travels across the AV node (slowing slightly) and the bundle of His, down the right and left bundle branches, out to the Purkinje fibers to initiate ventricular depolarization (ᴡᴡ). See Diagram 1.

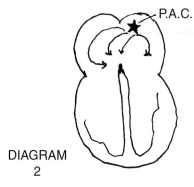

DIAGRAM
2

When a P.A.C. arises from an excitable focus (somewhere in either atria), the stimulus progresses (propagates) across the atria, traveling along the specialized fibers or tracts (atrial excitation pathway) from the point of ectopic origin to the AV node. From there, the remainder of the conduction sequence is normal. See Diagram 2.

DIAGRAM
3

Suppose, however, an anomalous connection exists between two specialized conducting fibers or tracts of the P.A.C. conduction route. Refer to the dotted line (. . . . . .) in Diagram 3. Even though this abnormal connection exists, conduction is uninterrupted (progressing around and out of the circuit) when the tissues are in a uniform state of recovery (repolarization or receptivity). Refer to Diagrams 3 and 4.

P.A.C.

DIAGRAM 4   CONNECTION PATHWAY

EARLY P.A.C.

A

BLOCK
B

DIAGRAM 5

Certain conditions, however, will cause the anomalous connection to behave as a *true* electrical circuit. In this instance, an early timed P.A.C. finds one "leg" or conducting fiber of the circuit in a *not-yet-recovered* or not fully repolarized state. That portion of the circuit is refractory or unable to receive a stimulus until fully recovered. In other words, a forward moving (antegrade) stimulus attempting to activate that "leg" or fiber (labeled **B**) would be blocked temporarily (unidirectional block). It is this temporary blockage that creates *electrical circuit behavior*. Refer to Diagram 5.

(O)

A

NOW UNBLOCKED
B

Diagram 6

In this situation (a blockage secondary to refractory tissue), the wave of excitation travels normally across the fully repolarized (unblocked) leg (labeled **A**) of the circuit causing depolarization of atrial cells as it moves forward toward the AV nodal pathway. However, because of the abnormal circuitry, the wave of excitation also flows backward (retrograde) toward the blocked area (labeled B). If, by this time, the tissue in the blocked area is fully recovered, the moving stimulus activates the once blocked area, causing depolarization. The wave of excitation slows slightly during depolarization, then continues on to the point of (**O**)rigin (See Diagram 6).

So, now back at the point of origin (**O**), the whole cycle can begin again. Ugh!! If the atrial tissues in "leg" A of the circuit are fully recovered from the previous stimulation, the progressing wave of excitation (pre-excitation) will assume control of the rhythm, continuing a counter-clockwise loop around the circuit, producing a rapid atrial tachycardia. The rapid rate is a result of the accelerated pace of atrial activation created by the anomalous circuit. Whew!

If, however, the atrial tissues in "leg" A are not fully recovered (partial state of repolarization) when the stimulus comes around the circuit, the circus-like activation will cease! In other words, the abnormal stimulation is interrupted and the normal underlying pacemaker resumes control of the rhythm.

You *may* want to ponder this *demystified cardiac physiology* again over coffee (or other stimulants)! **The important points to remember are covered below.**

- Anomalous circuitry (a re-entry mechanism) within the atrial conduction system may be responsible for rapid, atrial dysrhythmias, often described as *circus-like* atrial activation.

- Timing is everything!! In the presence of abnormal circuitry, refractory tissue can both start (see "leg" B, diagram 5) or terminate (see "leg" A, diagram 6) circus like atrial activation.

- A re-entry mechanism is also referred to as a *pre-excitation* syndrome.

- A re-entry mechanism (anomalous conducting circuit) can only be determined by invasive studies.

IF YOU FEEL SUSCEPTIBLE TO UNIDIRECTIONAL BLOCK,

PLEASE UNDERSTAND AND YOU ARE PROGRESSING IN A NORMAL, ANTEGRADE (FORWARD) FASHION!!

Finally, examine this strip.

The heart rate in the above strip is approximately 187 beats per minute which makes me think of atrial tachycardia. But, where are the P waves? P waves may or may not be there! If *definite* P waves are not observable, one cannot call the rhythm *atrial* tachycardia. So what will we call it? How about just describing what we see?

This is a rapid, regular rhythm with a heart rate of 187 beats per minute. The QRS complexes are borderline, measuring slightly less than 0.12 seconds. Oftentimes, rapid regular rhythms with normal duration QRSs are referred to as *supraventricular* (SVT) rhythms. The term *supraventricular* implies that the rhythm originates above the level of the ventricles.

Treatment of Recurrent Atrial or Supraventricular Tachycardia

Patients with recurrent tachydysrhythmias or those unresponsive to drug therapy are often studied in the electrophysiology lab. These studies are called electrophysiology studies and abbreviated EP studies. The EP lab is much like a cardiac catheterization lab. The patient is placed on an x-ray table with fluoroscopic capability (ability to shoot a moving, real time x-ray). However, the EP lab also has sophisticated electrocardiography equipment that allows for the precise anatomic location of dysrhythmias.

A venous cutdown, usually femoral, is performed allowing for the insertion of special catheters into the femoral vein. A catheter is threaded into the vein and venous flow helps to advance the catheter up through the abdominal vena cava up to the superior vena cava into the right atrium, and eventually into the right ventricle. This special catheter is capable of reading endocardial (from within the heart chambers) electrical activity. These "inside" EKGs identify the abnormal depolarizations or bypass pathways causing the tachydysrhythmia.

Once the site of pathology is confirmed, *radiofrequency ablation* (RFA) is employed. RFA delivers high frequency energy via a catheter inserted into the heart. RFA destroys the tissue causing the dysrhythmia. In particular, RFA is incredibly effective in terminating dysrhythmias caused by a re-entry phenomenon. Ablation destroys the tissue allowing reentry to occur. Following ablation of the tissue, the cardiologist again attempts to induce the rhythm. If the abnormal rhythm cannot be induced, the treatment is considered successful.

Ablation is considered curative for most SVTs. However, in some patients, continued drug therapy (anti-arrhythmics) is necessary.

In Summary of Atrial Tachycardia

If this is your first foray into EKG interpretation, the lengthy discussion of atrial tachycardia may have drained your battery! *Not to worry.* Since re-entry phenomena and multifocal ectopic activity reappear throughout the text, it seemed fitting to sensitize you early on! The following brief (and simple) summary captures the highlights of atrial tachycardia.

Atrial tachycardia originates in one of three ways:

1. A single ectopic atrial focus fires rapidly and repeatedly (rapid fire P.A.C.s), assuming control of the rhythm by virtue of its accelerated rate (faster than the sinus pacemaker). You will recall that the fastest pacemaker controls the rhythm. The monitor picture shows a rapid (characteristically, 160–220 beats per minute), regular rhythm with uniform P waves.

2. A rapid, regular atrial rhythm can be precipitated by an initiating P.A.C. when an abnormal conduction circuit is present. The abnormal circuit allows the wave of excitation (initiated by the P.A.C.) to rapidly and repeatedly activate the atria in a circus-like fashion (requires a *right-timed* P.A.C.and the presence of anomalous circuitry). The monitor picture shows a rapid (characteristically, 160–220 beats per minute), regular rhythm with uniform P waves.

The monitor cannot distinguish single focus versus re-entry atrial tachycardia since the electrical activity appears the same!

3. A rapid, slightly irregular atrial tachycardia can be precipitated by multiple ectopic sites firing rapidly (characteristically, 160–220 beats per minute). Rather than appearing uniform, at least three different P wave presentations will be visible.

QRS Morphology

In the normal healthy heart, the QRS is narrow, measuring less than 0.12 seconds. Typically, the QRS associated with atrial (or supraventricular) tachycardia occurs within normal limits (WNL). However, rapid atrial (or supraventricular) stimuli may encounter the conduction pathway only partially recovered (partially repolarized) between repeat stimulations. When conducting tissues are partially refractory, impulse conduction occurs more slowly, requiring more time. Thus, one may find a widened QRS associated with rapid atrial and supraventricular dysrhythmias. This widening of the QRS secondary to conduction pathway refractoriness is known as **aberrancy** (atrial tachycardia with aberrancy.)

These concepts will be revisited throughout the text! Now, on other rapid atrial dysrhythmias!

Practice Exercise 7

Just relax. Okay, now study the strip at the top of page 68. Describe everything that you see using the questions on the next page as a guide.

$$7\,\overline{)1500} \quad 219.4$$
$$-\,14$$
$$\underline{-19}$$
$$\quad 300$$

30

A. Describe the rhythm pattern and cardiac complexes
   Regular
   P before QRS; QRS following P

B. What is the heart rate? *app 214 bpm*

C. What can you say about atrial activity?
   present - one ectopic focus rapidly + repeatedly firing

D. What can you say about ventricular activity? *rapid*

E. This rhythm is *atrial tachycardia* .

F. Treatment is aimed at slowing down the heart rate. A method that might be used is the Valsalva maneuver. Describe this maneuver. *hold breath + bear down*

G. Atrial tachycardia may be precipitated by which of the following events or conditions? (Check all that apply.)
   ☑ A P.A.C. firing rapidly and repeatedly
   ☑ A P.A.C. entering a re-entry circuit
   ☑ Emotional stress
   ☑ Stimulants
   ☑ EKG practice exercises *ha ha*

H. Explain the difference between atrial tachycardia and multifocal atrial tachcardia.
   multifocal atrial tachycardia can originate from multiple ectopic foci

I. Describe RFA and its therapeutic use. _____

_____

_____

_____

_____

✔ For **Feedback 7,** refer to page 84.

Input Section 2.8: Atrial Flutter

Remember the normal conduction system?

Before we go any further, you must commit the following to memory.

The AV node *is physiologically unable* to conduct greater than approximately 220 impulses per minute. (This is a *general* rule.) If the heart rate exceeds 220 impulses per minute, some of the impulses will not be conducted through to the ventricles. This is called a normal *physiologic block.* Physiologic block is a protective mechanism that *guards* the ventricles from the effects of rapid stimulation!

Atrial flutter is a rapid *regular* atrial rhythm that arises from an excitable ectopic site (focus) in the atria or results from a *re-entry circuit* around the tricuspid valve of the right atrium.

It is important to remember that the fastest pacemaker will control the heart rate. The *atrial rate* in atrial flutter is usually between *220–350* impulses per minute. Following what we said above, all of these impulses will not be conducted to the ventricles because the AV node is incapable of conducting more than 220 impulses per minute.

The rapid *atrial* impulses of atrial flutter appear *saw-toothed* in shape and are labeled "F" waves. ("F" waves stand for flutter waves.) Flutter waves are continuous—they never stop. Consequently, they may even distort the QRSs! Flutter waves are more pronounced in leads II, III, and aVF . . . in other leads, the "saw-toothed" appearance is less visible.

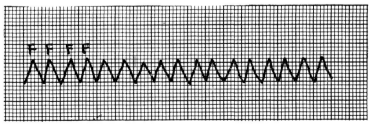

Saw-toothed atrial flutter waves

Since the AV node is unable to conduct greater than 220 impulses per minute, certain flutter impulses will not be conducted, or will be blocked from reaching the ventricles. *Usually,* only ½, ⅓, or ¼ of the atrial impulses will be conducted through the AV node to the ventricles.

To make this easy to understand, *let's say that the atrial flutter rate is 300* (300 F waves per minute).
If ½ of those atrial impulses are conducted (2:1 conduction), the ventricular rate will be 150.

In other words, for every two flutter waves, there is one QRS. The first flutter wave is blocked; the second flutter wave conducts to the ventricles producing ventricular depolarization (a QRS).

If ⅓ of those impulses are conducted (3:1 conduction), the ventricular rate will be 100.

For every three flutter waves, there will be one QRS. The first two flutter waves are blocked; the third one conducts to the ventricles producing ventricular depolarization.

Or, if 1/4 of those atrial impulses are conducted (4:1 conduction), the ventricular rate will be 75.

For every four flutter waves, there will be one QRS. The first three flutter waves are blocked; the fourth flutter wave conducts to the ventricles producing ventricular depolarization.

So, the atrial activity appears saw-toothed in leads II, III, and aVF. There are flutter waves *rather than* P waves! The QRS complexes are normally *narrow* (less than 0.12 seconds), and the ventricular rhythm is *usually regular.* If, however, the degree of *physiologic block* in the AV node varies, the ventricular rhythm may be somewhat irregular. In other words, the AV node may arbitrarily allow flutter impulses to be conducted to the ventricles.

The above monitor tracing indicates atrial flutter with variable physiologic block in the AV node (irregular atrial flutter). As you can see, with variable block the ventricular response is irregular. You know what this means . . . to determine an accurate heart rate one would need to count for one full minute! ☺

Regardless whether the QRS complexes occur regularly or irregularly, the rhythm is atrial flutter. *The diagnosis of atrial flutter is based on the rapid, regular, continuous atrial impulses occurring at a rate of 220–350 per minute.*

When describing atrial flutter, it is important to specify the rate at which the atrial flutter waves are occurring and indicate both the *rate* and *regularity* of the ventricular response.

Atrial flutter is commonly associated with rheumatic heart disease, particularly with mitral stenosis, coronary artery disease, corpulmonale, hypertensive heart disease, hyperthyroidism, and diabetes.

Following is a strip demonstrating atrial flutter with a regular ventricular response (4:1 atrial flutter—four flutter waves for every QRS).

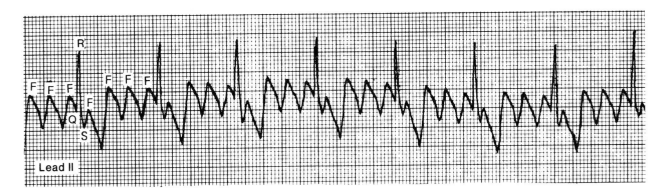

Let's describe what is happening!

Oh! I forgot to tell you something. This is going to sound *truly* illogical, but . . . if I turn an atrial flutter tracing upside down, it's easier for me to see the flutter waves. When no one is watching, try it!

Okay. Lets analyze the atrial activity.

Well, there are no P waves. Instead, there are rapid, saw-toothed continous flutter waves. To calculate the atrial flutter rate, use the "300, 150, 100; 75, 60, 50" method. Find a *flutter wave* that falls on a heavy vertical line. Do not count that vertical line. The next one is 300 . . . right?

So, the atrial flutter rate in the above strip is 300! Because physiologic block limits the AV node capacity of conducting greater than 220 impulses per minute, some of those 300 impulses will be blocked or will not conduct. If you look closely, there are four flutter waves for every QRS (4:1 conduction).

What about ventricular activity? The ventricular rate is regular at a rate of 75 per minute. The QRS complexes are within normal limits (less than 0.12 seconds). In atrial flutter, the *ventricular rate is usually between 60–150 per minute*. Atrial and ventricular activity are related because the interval between the conducted flutter wave and its QRS is always constant.

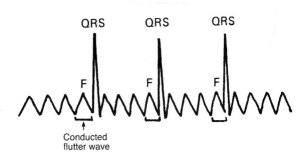

The distance between the atrial flutter wave preceding each QRS and the QRS measures the same indicating that atrial activity is related to ventricular activity. In other words, the atrial impulse (flutter wave) prior to the QRS, conducts down through the AV node to the ventricles producing ventricular depolarization (QRS).

Vagotonic maneuvers, such as carotid pressure or the Valsalva maneuver, may interrupt atrial flutter . . . or may assist in the diagnosis of atrial flutter.

Look at this next strip!

← Carotid Massage →

Note the prominent flutter waves during carotid massage. Carotid message is a rarely employed "physician-only" procedure owing to the risk of embolisin. More commonly, adenosine will be administered. Adenosine produces transient AV block allowing better visualization of flutter waves.

Atrial flutter may be treated in a variety of ways, but the *object* of initial treatment is to slow the rapid ventricular response. Similar to the discussion of atrial tachycardia, a rapid heart rate may predispose the patient to a diminished cardiac output, LV failure, ischemia, and angina. If the patient is acutely symptomatic, the best method of treatment is synchronized cardioversion using a low current setting. The DC (direct current) cardioversion interrupts the chaotic firing of the ectopic atrial focus, allowing the sinus pacemaker to resume control.

In a more stable clinical presentation, drugs such as verapamil, diltiazem or amiodarone may be administered to slow the ventricular response. These drugs produce further block in the AV node, reducing the number of conducted atrial impulses. In other words, the drug effect might change a 2:1 conduction to a 3:1 or 4:1 conduction pattern. (For example, an atrial flutter rate of 300 in a 2:1 conduction pattern would produce a ventricular rate of 150. If the increased block resulted in a 3:1 conduction pattern, three flutter waves per QRS, the ventricular rate would be 100. In a 4:1 conduction pattern, the ventricular rate would be 75.)

$$2\overline{)300} = 150; \quad 3\overline{)300} = 100; \quad 4\overline{)300} = 75$$

If the ventricular rate is well tolerated, initial drug therapy may be focused on terminating the ectopic rhythm. Drugs such as procainamide, disopyramide, propafenone, sotalol, amiodarone, flecainide, ibutilide or dofetilide may be given in attempt to convert the rhythm. As this text goes to press, a new antiarrhythmic drug, dronedarone (a non-toxic derivative of amiodarone) is being used on an experimental basis.

NOTE: Prior to drug therapy, it is important to determine whether the patient is currently taking digoxin. Though rare, digoxin toxicity can cause atrial flutter!

If atrial flutter is recurrent and found (through electrophysiologic studies) to be associated with a re-entry mechanism, the treatment of choice is ablation (discussed on page 67) which destroys the anomalous conducting pathway.

Only one other major point to make about atrial flutter. This is really a secret . . . a method to impress your friends!

BONUS ➤

> Any time you observe a regular rhythm with a heart rate between 150–190, *always* think about atrial flutter!
> (See the rhythm strip below)

Flutter waves may be hiding . . . see for yourself!

Finally, note the atrial flutter waves occurring at a rate of 250 per minute in the next strip. The two leads (lead II and V_1) are presented to make the point that atrial activity is best viewed from leads II, III and aVF. You will notice that the flutter waves are indistinguishable in lead V_1.

Practice Exercise 8

/ 1300

Atrial flutter is a fun rhythm to detect.

A. Use your skills to describe this strip in detail! _____

ventricular rate = 100 bpm
atrial rate = 300 bpm →varying ventricular response
                        rate 2:1 + 4:1 alternating
QRS= 0.08

_____

B. The atrial rate in atrial flutter varies between ___~~200~~ 220___ and ___350~~___~~ impulses per minute. Characteristically, the ventricular rate will vary between ___60___ and ___150___ beats per minute. The AV node is unable to conduct greater than ___220___ impulses per minute. Beyond this rate, a ___~~ventricular~~ physiologic___ block occurs.

✔ For **Feedback 8,** refer to page 85.

Input Section 2.9: Atrial Fibrillation

By now, you may be feeling a bit overwhelmed! That, however, is a natural reaction. Knowing that you are nearing the end of Section 2 may improve your outlook! Atrial fibrillation is an easily identified dysrhythmia.

Atrial tachycardia
atrial flutter
atrial fibrillation

Atrial fibrillation

The above strip demonstrates *atrial fibrillation* (sometimes abbreviated as "A fib"). There are no P waves; instead there are *bizarre* and *irregular* atrial deflections referred to as fibrillation or "f" waves. The "f" waves have no rhythmic pattern; thus *atrial activation is chaotic.* The "f" waves in atrial fibrillation occur at a *rapid and irregular rate* which varies from 400–600 impulses per minute. In atrial fibrillation, the baseline appears to *undulate.*

We must refer back to the discussion concerning physiologic block. Owing to physiologic block, the AV node is incapable of conducting more than 220 impulses to the ventricles per minute. Thus, the 400–600 atrial impulses per minute cannot all be conducted. Most usually, this physiologic block will permit 120–160 impulses through to the ventricles each minute. However, if associated with a re-entry mechanism (an anomalous conduction circuit), the ventricular rate may be faster. The ventricular response (QRSs) associated with atrial fibrillation will occur irregularly due to the fact that the AV node has varying refractory periods (rest periods) following conducted impulses. Thus, the R-R interval will *always* vary, as depicted in the above tracing. Because the "f" waves occur *continuously,* they may deform the QRS complexes, the ST segments, and the T waves!

In atrial fibrillation, there is no coordinated activation process in the atria. The tissue within the atria is electrically fragmented into various stages of excitation, refractoriness (resting state), or responsiveness. In other words, the tissues are "out of phase" with each other. Normally, all the fibers within a heart chamber will be in essentially the same electrophysiologic state—they will all be in a state of excitation, all in a state of refractoriness, or all in a partial state of responsiveness.

In many instances, the ventricular response rate will be rapid (120–160 beats per minute). Like previously discussed rapid rhythms a rapid ventricular response may decrease cardiac output and precipitate LV failure, ischemia, and chest pain. Remember the toilet analogy . . . page 61.

With uncontrolled atrial fibrillation, cardiac output is compromised because of both the rapid ventricular rate and the loss of synchronized atrial activation (atrial kick). It is common to find a *pulse deficit* associated with atrial fibrillation. A pulse deficit exists when the apical pulse is faster than the radial pulse, when the two pulses are counted simultaneously. When the cardiac output is compromised, not all cardiac contractions will be felt radially.

Let's try describing what we see, using the five steps for dysrhythmia interpretation.

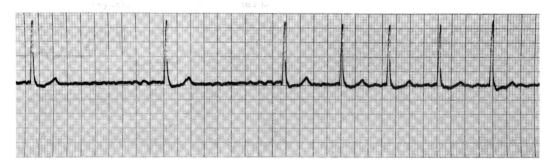

One can visually determine that the rhythm is irregular. As a matter of fact, atrial fibrillation is described as being *irregularly irregular*! In order to accurately determine heart rate, one would need to count the ventricular complexes (QRSs) over the course of one full minute. Preferably, the heart rate should be determined by simultaneously counting the patient's apical and radial pulses for one minute.

Next, evaluate atrial activity. There are no P waves, and thus, no P-R intervals. The baseline appears to *undulate*. There are rapid, small irregular atrial waves with no common pattern. An evaluation of ventricular activity reveals that the QRS complexes are normal in shape and duration (measuring less than 0.12 seconds), though they occur irregularly. The interval between the R waves (R-R interval) varies.

Evaluation of the relationship between atrial and ventricular activity reveals a *bizarre* conduction pattern. Most of the atrial impulses (fibrillation waves) that reach the AV node are blocked from further progression (owing to the fact that the AV node in unable to conduct greater than 220 impulses per minute). The atrial impulses that pass through the AV node are normally conducted, as demonstrated by QRS complexes of normal duration.

Atrial fibrillation is one of the most commonly observed dysrhythmias and its occurrence increases with advancing age. Symptoms associated with atrial fibrillation vary and may include palpitations, fatigue, dizziness, and congestive heart failure (CHF). Though an easily recognized dysrhythmia, the etiology of atrial fibrillation is more complex. It may occur in otherwise healthy individuals, may be associated with drug and alcohol toxicities, may result from electrolyte imbalances, or be associated with significant pathologies such as coronary artery disease, pulmonary disease, hypertensive heart disease or rheumatic heart disease. Whew!

Owing both to the underlying pathology and the duration of the pathology, the treatments for atrial fibrillation vary. **In all instances, the aim of treatment is the reduction of the rapid ventricular response and the restoring of hemodynamic equilibrium**. In emergent situations (hemodynamic collapse or evidence of ischemia), synchronized cardioversion will usually be the first line of treatment. In a stable clinical situation, efforts will be made to determine the duration of atrial fibrillation. If the dysrhythmia is of recent onset (usually less than 48 hours), synchronized cardioversion is the treatment of choice.

When the duration is unknown, diagnostic procedures are commonly conducted in an electrophysiology lab. Those procedures include a transesophageal echocardiogram (TEE) to rule out blood clot formation in the left atrium caused by the out-of phase atrial depolarization and the compromised atrial muscle contraction. When there is no evidence of thrombus formation, synchronized cardioversion, drug therapy, or procedures such as radiofrequency ablation (RTF, discussed on page 67) or cryotherapy (creates electrical barriers in the atria using laser cold probes) may be employed to convert or abolish the dysrhythmia. As an alternative to diagnostic studies, a patient may be placed on an anticoagulant (warfarin) for three to four weeks prior to cardioversion or chemical conversion. Drugs commonly employed for chemical conversion include flecainide, propafenone, procainamide, sotalol, amiodarone, ibutilide and others. The AFFIRM Substudy (J.American College of Cardiology, 2003: 42.) found that amiodarone is more effective at maintaining sinus rhythm and preventing the recurrance of atrial fibrillation when compared with sotalol or class I antiarrhythmic drugs.

Importantly, recent randomized controlled studies have demonstrated that restoring atrial fibrillation to a sinus rhythm does not improve the long term survival rate not reduce the incidence of stroke. Those study findings have shifted the treatment for long standing atrial fibrillation away from conversion to a **rate control strategy**. In other words, treatment is aimed at controlling the ventricular response rate to atrial fibrillation; the atrial fibrillation continues, but fewer atrial impulses are conducted through the AV junction to the ventricles resulting in a slower heart rate. Rate control drug therapy involves beta-blockers and calcium channel blockers. (The actions of beta-blockers and calcium channel blockers will be discussed in Section 13!)

☆ **The following are the important points remember.**

➤ Atrial fibrillation is an easily recognized, irregularly irregular rhythm.
➤ Atrial fibrillation has many causes.
➤ Long-standing atrial fibrillation predisposes the patient to risk of stroke.
➤ Generally, therapy is aimed at reducing the rapid ventricular response and restoring hemodynamic balance.
➤ Specific therapy depends on the underlying cause and the duration of the dysrhythmia.

Find one more example of atrial fibrillation on the top of the next page. Notice how the baseline *undulates*!

Notice the undulating baseline.

Practice Exercise 9

A. The atrial deflections in atrial fibrillation are known as _____F_____ waves. These atrial impulses occur ~~350~~ 400 to ___600___ times per minute. The AV node is unable to conduct greater than _220_ impulses per minute owing to a normal a _physiologic_ block.

B. If on a monitor tracing one sees *no clear P waves, an undulating baseline and a varying R-R interval,* one can suspect _atrial fibrillation_ .

C. Examine this rhythm strip closely. Then, describe what you see.

No clear P waves - undulations present
QRS complexes are irregular
QRS = 0.68
QRS complexes are irregular

✔ For **Feedback 9,** refer to page 85.

Input Section 2.10: Atrial Flutter-Fibrillation ("flutter-fib")

Occasionally, a rhythm strip will be encountered that looks suspiciously like atrial flutter (F waves observed across the strip). Yet, when one attempts to measure the rate and *regularity* of the F waves, they *do not* measure out! In other words, the F waves do not occur regularly. Oftentimes, this rhythm is referred to as *impure flutter,* or more commonly, *atrial flutter-fibrillation.* It is unclear whether such a phenomenon truly exists, or whether the classification has been created for convenience sake! In all probability, the underlying disorder is that of a coarse atrial fibrillation. Fortunately, treatment is similar for the two atrial dysrhythmias.

See what you think! Try measuring the regularity of the *flutter* waves on the next strip (top of page 77).

P.S. There is no practice exercise associated with input 10. Whew!

Input Section 2.11: Sick Sinus Syndrome (Brady-Tachy Syndrome)

Sick sinus syndrome is more a classification category rather than a specific diagnosis. Sick sinus syndrome is thought to be related to degeneration of the SA node cells, and is therefore usually found in patients with coronary artery disease and other degenerative processes. Because of this degeneration, the monitor picture of a patient with sick sinus syndrome displays such disorders as sinus bradycardia, sinus tachycardia, sinus pause, atrial or supraventricular tachycardia, escape beats, etc. In other words, the monitor tracing is a *"mixed bag"* of slow and rapid rhythms arising *above* the level of the ventricles (this means that the QRS duration is within normal limits indicating normal ventricular depolarization).

Let's look at a sample strip.

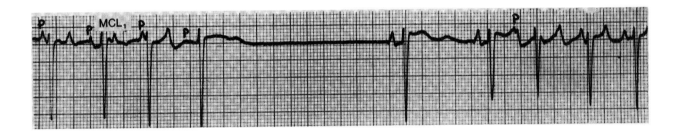

Notice the inconsistent and erratic nature of the sinus pacemaker. If you think this is a difficult rhythm strip, you are absolutely right!

Many times the patient exhibiting a sick sinus syndrome presents with a history of syncope or fainting and periods of fluttering sensations in the chest. In many cases, diagnosis is made from the analysis of continuous Holter monitor tracings (the patient wears a portable monitor while he or she goes about normal activities). Once sick sinus syndrome is identified, the object of treatment is to maintain a stable heart rate. Drugs such as atropine have little long term success in speeding up a slow sinus pacemaker discharge rate. Suppressive drugs utilized to slow rapid rhythms would further suppress the slow phases of the rhythm. Gets complicated, right?

Because of the varying nature of sick sinus syndrome, the treatment of choice involves the combination of a ventricular pacemaker (to augment heart rate during slow rhythms) and suppressant drugs (to control the rapid periods of the rhythm).

Since sick sinus syndrome is a collection of other dysrhythmias, there is no practice exercise! Such a deal!

Input Section 2.12: Bypass Re-Entry Mechanisms (Wolff-Parkinson-White Syndrome)
Advanced Study

Earlier in this Section, atrial re-entry mechanisms were considered as possible causes for atrial tachycardia, atrial fibrillation and atrial flutter. Here, we will consider an *example* large scale (global) re-entry mechanism caused by an accessory connection (**bypass**) between the atria and the ventricles. A bypass route connecting the atria and ventricles (bypassing the AV node) can be responsible for rapid supraventricular tachycardias (originating in either the atria of the AV junction). Wolff-Parkinson-White (WPW) Syndrome is one such re-entry dysrhythmia caused by an anomalous bypass between the atrial and ventricles.

Wolff-Parkinson-White (WPW) Syndrome is another one of those *somewhat complicated* re-entry or pre-excitation phenomena and is included here as **information, only!** An anomalous congenital connection (known as the Kent bundle) connects the atria and ventricles, bypassing the AV node. You will recall that impulses passing normally through the AV node are slowed before progressing down the conduction system. The presence of a by-pass pathway can expedite conduction. A WPW supraventricular tachycardia is often precipitated by a premature impulse, often arising in the atria. Conduction of that impulse follows both the normal and bypass conduction pathways, though traveling in different directions and at different times!

The majority of WPW tachycardias demonstrate a forward (antegrade) conduction over the AV node and bundle of His pathway and a backward (retrograde) conduction over the accessory path (Kent bundle) as demonstrated in the diagram below. The sequence begins with a premature beat. The impulse (wave of excitation) conducts from the point of origin through the AV junction, across the bundle of His and down the bundle branches to the Purkinje system. Somewhere in the ventricles, the wave of excitation also encounters the bypass connection and spreads rapidly backward along the bypass path to the atria where it again initiates atrial activation and the cycle begins again! This repeated cycle of rapid retrograde conduction (circus movement stimulation) increases the rate of atrial and ventricular conduction. Other than the rapid rate, EKG findings associated with retrograde conduction across the anomalous pathway are subtle. Inverted P waves may be observed in leads II, III and a VF and the lateral leads.

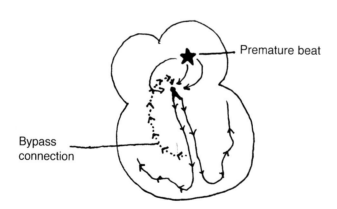

In other cases of WPW, an early-timed premature beat may find the normal conduction system refractory (not fully recovered). Because refractory tissues are immune to stimulation, the advancing premature stimulus is temporarily blocked. In this instance, the premature impulse travels rapidly forward (around the AV node) down the bypass pathway to initiate ventricular depolarization. The wave of excitation then enters the normal conduction system (Purkinje system) backwards or retrograde which causes depolarization of the remaining ventricular tissue. Examine the diagram at the top of page 79. Essentially, this sequence of stimulation produces a dual or double stimulation (one stimulus occurring earlier, traveling forward and faster; one stimulus traveling backward, later and slower) of the ventricles. The retrograde stimulus then continues propagating backward through the normal conduction pathway, back to re-excite the atria. The counter-clockwise rapid sequence then repeats, repeats, repeats, etc.

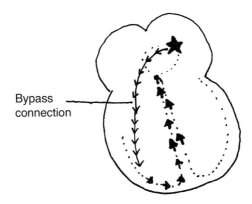

Bypass
connection

As you might suspect, this abnormal conduction and dual stimulation of ventricles produces characteristic EKG changes. In this conduction sequence, one finds a short P-R interval (less than 0.12 seconds), and a slurred beginning of the QRS (proximal limb of the QRS) known as a *delta wave*. The slurring of the initial portion of the QRS contributes to the widened QRS (a characteristic finding).

Delta wave

P

Perhaps an *imperfect* analogy may aid understanding of this type of abnormal conduction. Think of hotel or airport with a large continuous (timed) revolving door (large enough to accommodate several folks with luggage). Typically, even though the speed of the revolving door is timed or pre-set, one can make the revolving door move faster by pushing on the door. Next to revolving doors, a regular door exists (for bellmen to re-enter the lobby or terminal). For the purpose of this analogy, assume the bellman's door cannot be opened from inside the hotel or terminal.

OK. Father and rambunctious five year old exit the hotel, entering the revolving doors together. While the father walks at the pre-set pace of door revolution, the five year old slips past the rubber revolving door guard, exists first, runs back (retrograde) into the hotel through the bellman's door, re-enters the revolving door, pushing on the door to accelerate the pace of door revolution. (Thus the revolving the door has been both powered by the normal mechanism and by a bypass mechanism.) This is so much fun, the five year old continues to repeat the process, causing the door to revolve at a faster pace than intended. This rapid circus movement will likely continue until intervention occurs. Hope the analogy helped!

Other accessory pathways (other than the Kent bundle) can exit between the atria and ventricles, also creating rapid rhythm anomalies. As was noted earlier, one can only identify the presence of a re-entry mechanism (localized or bypass tract) through invasive diagnostic procedures. Often, it is the recurrence of a rapid supraventricular rhythm (or the inability to disrupt or control the rhythm with drug intervention) that prompts diagnostic and interventional studies and procedures.

There are three main therapeutic interventions for treating rapid WPW and related bypass re-entry dsyrhythmias. The most effective interventions are surgical ablation or radiofrequency ablation (RFA) which destroy or disrupt the anomalous bypass pathway, thereby disabling the abnormal atrial – ventricular conduction route. Drug therapy (a less effective alternative) intended to disrupt or slow rapid supraventricular dysrhythmias requires forethought. Drugs which act by slowing conduction across the AV node can exacerbate rapid conduction along the bypass tract. Thus, drug therapy often involves a combination of agents, those which block conduction in the accessory bypass path (class 1C or III drugs) combined with an AV nodal blocker.

The above discussion of accessory path anomalies is informational. You will be relieved to know, there is no accompanying practice exercise!

Concluding Note From the Management

In summary, a rapid, regular atrial or supraventricular dysrhythmia may be caused by a single ectopic focus firing repeatedly or by a circus-like stimulation in the presence of an accessory pathway. Invasive diagnostic procedures are necessary to determine the etiology!

✔ Feedback 1

If your answers are similar to mine, you have the basics down pat! If you are "shaky" on any of the points covered, review Section 1 one more time. (You'll be happy you did!)

A. The heart rate in this rhythm strip is approximately <u>70</u> beats per minute.

B. The rhythm is (regular.)

C. Each QRS complex is preceded by a <u>P wave.</u>

D. All P waves are <u>uniform</u> in appearance.

E. Each P wave is followed by a <u>QRS.</u>

F. All QRS complexes are <u>uniform</u> in appearance.

G. The P-R interval is *constant* and measures 0.12 seconds.

H. Therefore, this is a **sinus** rhythm.

The five principles used in dysrhythmia interpretation are:

1. First, determine if the rhythm is <u>regular.</u>

2. Second, determine the heart <u>rate.</u>

3. Next determine <u>atrial</u> activity.

4. Then determine <u>ventricular</u> activity.

5. The final step involves determining if a relationship exists between <u>atrial and ventricular</u> activity.

✔ Feedback 2

You're doing great!

1. A. The heart rate in this strip is **approximately** <u>70</u> beats per minute.

B. The P waves are all <u>uniform</u> in appearance.

C. A <u>P</u> wave precedes each QRS complex.

    D. The QRS complexes are <u>uniform</u> in appearance.

    E. A <u>QRS</u> follows every P wave.

    F. The rhythm is (regular)

    G. This is a **sinus rhythm.**

2. A. The heart rate in this strip is **approximately** <u>90</u> beats per minute.

    B. The P waves are all <u>uniform</u> in appearance.

    C. A P wave precedes each QRS complex.

    D. The QRS complexes are <u>uniform</u> in appearance.

    E. A <u>QRS</u> follows every P wave.

    F. The rhythm is (irregular)

    G. This is a **sinus arrhythmia.**

3. Usually, the irregularity found in sinus arrhythmia is related to <u>respiration.</u>

Just for review, here are the EKG criteria for a sinus arrhythmia.

EKG Criteria for Sinus Arrhythmia	
Rhythm:	Slightly irregular. The P-P interval or R-R interval varies in duration.
Rate:	60–100.
P waves:	Normal configuration.
QRS:	Normal configuration and duration.
Conduction:	Each P wave is followed by a QRS; the P-R interval is constant.

✔ Feedback 3

Nice work!

A. The term *bradycardia* implies that the heart rate is <u>less than 60 beats</u> per minute.

B. Rhythm strip 2 is similar to strip 1 in the following ways:

    1. In each strip, the P waves appear uniform.

    2. A P wave precedes each QRS.

    3. In each strip, the QRS complexes appear uniform.

    4. A QRS complex follows each P wave.

    5. The rhythm is regular in each strip.

Rhythm strip 2 differs from rhythm strip 1 in this way:

In rhythm strip 1 (sinus rhythm), the heart rate falls between 60 and 100 beats per minute.
In rhythm strip 2, the heart rate is <u>41</u> beats per minute, falling below the normal range of 60–100 beats per minute. (I have used the Trusty Guide on page 41 to determine the heart rate!!)
The second strip demonstrates a <u>sinus bradycardia.</u>

Just for review, following are the EKG criteria for a sinus bradycardia.

EKG Criteria for Sinus Bradycardia

Rhythm:	Regular.
Rate:	Less than 60.
P waves:	Normal configuration.
QRS:	Normal configuration and duration.
Conduction:	Each P wave is followed by a QRS; the P-R interval is constant.

✔ Feedback 4

What a pro!

A. The P waves are all uniform in appearance.
   A P wave precedes each QRS complex.
   A QRS complex follows every P wave.
   QRS complexes measure approximately 0.08 seconds in duration.
   The P-R interval is constant and measures 0.16 seconds.
   The rhythm is regular.
   The heart rate is <u>50</u> beats per minute.
   This is a <u>sinus bradycardia</u>!
   Did I fool you? Hope Not!!!

B. The P waves are all uniform in appearance.
   A P wave precedes each QRS complex.
   A QRS complex follows every P wave.
   The rhythm is regular.
   The heart rate is <u>150</u> beats per minute.
   QRS complexes (rS complexes) are approximately 0.08 seconds in duration.
   The P-R interval is constant and measures approximately 0.12 seconds.
   This is a **<u>sinus tachycardia</u>**.

C. The treatment for sinus tachycardia consists of <u>finding and treating its underlying cause</u> (i.e., fever, heart failure, anxiety, etc.).

Just for review, following are the EKG criteria associated with a sinus tachycardia.

EKG Criteria for Sinus Tachycardia

Rhythm:	Regular.
Rate:	100–160.
P waves:	Normal configuration.
QRS:	Normal configuration and duration.
Conduction:	Each P wave is followed by a QRS; the P-R interval is constant.

✔ Feedback 5

How did you do? Remember, in wandering atrial pacemaker (W.A.P.), all QRS complexes will be preceded by a P wave. . . . It's just that the P waves may look different! The rhythm will be slightly irregular owing to the varying atrial pacemaker. See my art on the next page!

This is what my *freestyle* W.A.P looks like

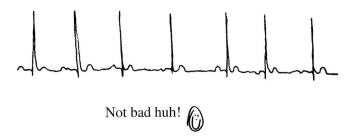

Not bad huh!

✔ Feedback 6

Nice work! If you are becoming frustrated, remember . . . **All great minds are frustrated!**

A. Beat 2, beat 6, and beat 10 are premature. The contour of the P waves in the premature beats is slightly different from the normal P waves. The underlying rhythm is a sinus rhythm. A QRS complex follows every P wave. All the QRS complexes are uniform in appearance, measuring approximately 2 1/2 small squares or 0.10 seconds. The P-R interval of the underlying rhythm measures approximately 0.20 seconds, the upper limits of normal. The P-R interval of the premature beats is slightly longer. A slight pause follows each P.A.C.

B. In this example, the premature atrial impulses occur during the repolarization phase of the preceding beats. Thus, the ventricular tissue is unable to respond to the stimulation. Therefore, the P.A.C.s are blocked or not conducted. The P-R interval of all conducted beats measures 0.24 seconds, indicating delayed conduction.

Non-conducted or blocked P.A.C.s interrupt a sinus rhythm.

Just for review purposes, here are the EKG criteria for P.A.C.s.

EKG Criteria for Premature Atrial Contractions	
Rhythm:	Irregular owing to the disruption caused by premature beats.
Rate:	Usually normal (60–100 beats per minute).
P waves:	The P waves appear prematurely and differ in contour from the normal P waves.
QRS:	Usually normal configuration and duration.
Conduction:	A normal QRS follows the abnormal P wave. There is a slight pause or delay before the next normal beat. This pause tends to partly compensate for the prematurity. (Of course, if the P.A.C. is blocked, it is not followed by a QRS!)

✔ Feedback 7

How did you do? Sometimes this material is difficult. If you feel a bit insecure, try reading the section one more time. 🙂

A. The rhythm is regular. There is a PQRST cycle in each cardiac complex.

B. The heart rate is approximately 200 beats per minute.

C. Each QRS is preceded by a P wave. All P waves look uniform.

D. Each P wave is followed by a QRS. All QRS complexes appear uniform. The QRS measures 0.12 seconds.

E. This rhythm is *probably* an <u>atrial tachycardia</u>, though if you answered <u>supraventricular tachycardia</u>, you are *absolutely* correct!

F. The Valsalva maneuver consists of having the patient hold his or her breath and bear down.

Just for review, here are the EKG criteria for atrial tachycardia.

EKG Criteria for Atrial Tachycardia	
Rhythm:	Regular.
Rate:	<u>160–220</u> beats per minute.
P waves:	May be buried in the QRS complexes or T waves and not visible; or may be similar to the contour of sinus P waves.
QRS:	Usually normal, but may be widened.
Conduction:	A ventricular complex follows each P wave by the same interval.

G. Atrial tachycardia may be precipitated by any of the following events or conditions.

    ☒ A P.A.C. firing rapidly and repeatedly

    ☒ A P.A.C. entering a re-entry circuit

    ☒ Emotional stress

    ☒ Stimulants

    ☒ EKG practice exercises 🙂

H. Atrial tachycardia is a regular, rapid rhythm (rate 160–220) with visible, uniform P waves. The dysrhythmia is a result of: a single ectopic site within the atria firing repeatedly; or, a P.A.C. entering an anomalous circuit, creating a re-entry phenomenon. The QRS is usually within normal limits. Multifocal atrial tachycardia is a rapid, irregular rhythm (rate >100 beats per minute) produced by multiple (at least 3) ectopic sites within the atria firing repeatedly. Distinctly different P waves are visible.

I. RFA, radio frequency ablation, is a treatment for supraventricular tachyarrhythmias. RFA involves delivering high frequency energy via catheter into tissue causing the dysrhythmia. RFA destroys the tissue causing the dysrhythmia. It is particularly effective in destroying anomalous conducting circuits responsible for re-entry tachycardias.

✔ Feedback 8

Excellent work!

A. There are no P waves. Rather, there are saw-toothed atrial waves ("F" waves) occurring regularly at a rate of 300 per minute. The QRS complexes occur irregularly owing to variable physiologic block. The QRS complexes appear uniform and measure approximately 0.08 seconds. One would need to count the heart rate for one full minute!

B. The atrial rate in atrial flutter varies between 220 and 350 impulses per minute. Characteristically the ventricular rate will vary between 60 and 150 beats per minute.

The AV node is unable to conduct greater than 220 impulses per minute. Beyond this rate, a physiologic block occurs.

Just for review, here are the EKG criteria for atrial flutter.

EKG Criteria for Atrial Flutter	
Rhythm:	Atrial activity occurs in a regular pattern. The ventricular rhythm may be regular or irregular, depending on the degree of physiologic block.
Rate:	The atrial rate ("F" waves) occurs between 220–350 per minute.
	The ventricular rate (QRSs) may vary from 60–150 depending on the number of impulses passing through the AV junction.
P waves:	There are characteristic atrial oscillations—"saw-toothed" waves ("F" waves) ranging between 220–350 per minute. *No isoelectric line is visible.*
QRS:	The QRS complexes appear uniform and usually measure less than 0.12 seconds.
Conduction:	Usually $\frac{1}{2}$, $\frac{1}{3}$, or $\frac{1}{4}$ of the flutter (atrial) impulses will be conducted to the ventricles.

✔ Feedback 9

What a Pro you are !

A. The atrial deflections in atrial fibrillation are known as "f" waves. These atrial impulses occur 400 to 600 times per minute. The AV node is unable to conduct greater than 220 impulses per minute, owing to a normal physiologic block.

B. If on a monitor tracing one sees no clear P waves, an undulating baseline and a varying R-R interval, one can suspect atrial fibrillation.

Interpretation

C. This rhythm is irregularly irregular. There are no clear P waves or P-R intervals. Atrial activity appears rapid and chaotic. The baseline appears to undulate. The QRS complexes are normal in shape and are less than 0.12 seconds in duration. The QRS complexes occur irregularly—the R-R interval varies. One would need a full minute strip to accurately determine heart rate. Most of the atrial impulses reaching the AV node are blocked. Those impulses passing through the AV node are conducted normally.

Just for review, here are the EKG criteria for atrial fibrillation.

	EKG Criteria for Atrial Fibrillation
Rhythm:	The ventricular rhythm is totally irregular.
Rate:	The heart rate varies according to the number of atrial impulses conducted through the AV node to the ventricles.
P waves:	No P waves or P-R intervals; instead, there are rapid, small, irregular waves ("f" waves).
QRS:	The QRS's are normal in shape and duration, but occur irregularly. The R-R interval varies.
Conduction:	The conduction is bizarre. Most of the atrial impulses which reach the AV node are blocked. Those impulses that pass through the AV node are normally conducted.

Notes

Notes

Junctional Escape and Ectopic Rhythms

Objectives

When you have completed Section 3, you will be able to describe or identify

1. junctional escape rhythms and junctional escape beats

2. premature junctional beats

3. junctional tachycardia

Input Section 3.1: Junctional Escape Rhythm

You're back again! Persistent creature, aren't you! Though there are several other abnormal atrial rhythms, those will be reserved for more advanced lessons! Whew!

The heart has many potential pacemaker centers—the SA node, the atria, the AV junctional tissues, and the ventricles. Only the *dominant* or the *fastest pacemaker* (highest automaticity) will normally control the heart. If the sinus node fails to discharge an impulse *or* if the sinus impulse fails to be conducted *or* if the sinus rate of discharge is inadequate, a lower and slower (more distal) pacemaker may assume the role of pacemaker. (Persistent or intermittent failure of the sinus mechanism may occur secondary to myocardial infarction, ischemia, hypoxia, vagal stimulation or degeneration of the SA node cells, as is often associated with sick-sinks syndrome.)

A lower or more distal pacemaker initiated rhythm is known as an *escape rhythm*—a safety mechanism of the heart. In some respects, a lower (escape) pacemaker resembles an emergency power generator that "kicks in" when the normal current fails. And, like a generator, the escape pacemaker is not necessary when normal electrical activity resumes.

When an escape rhythm is initiated in the AV junctional tissue, it is known as an *idiojunctional rhythm* or a *junctional escape rhythm*. This junctional pacemaker *usually* discharges an impulse 40–60 times per minute (though it may discharge slower or faster).

You are no doubt thinking that the term *escape* is a peculiar name for a rhythm. Basically, the term implies that a lower, more distal pacemaker has *escaped* from the control of the sinus node. In other words, although lower tissues have the ability to serve as pacemakers, their inherent rates of impulse discharge are slower than the sinus node. Therefore, the faster sinus impulse controls heart rate. In effect, the faster sinus impulse causes depolarization before lower, more distal pacemakers have the opportunity to generate pacemaking impulses! Only when the sinus pacemaker fails, slows or is interrupted will a lower pacemaker assume control of the rhythm.

An escape rhythm *always occurs* as a *secondary phenomenon*, never as a primary disorder. In other words, an escape rhythm serves as a safety mechanism when higher order pacemakers are disrupted or fail.

The previous rhythm strip (page 90) demonstrates an idiojunctional or junctional escape rhythm with a rate of 50 beats per minute. You will note that the rhythm is regular, there are no visible P waves and the QRS is of normal duration. One can expect to see a junctional escape rhythm *when the sinus pacemaker fails or is depressed*. If the patient has a sinus bradycardia (less than 60 beats per minute), his heart rate may be *slower* than the AV junctional pacemaker, which has the ability to initiate a rhythm at a rate of 40–60 beats per minute. In this case, the AV junctional pacemaker might become the dominant pacemaker because it has a faster rate. It is helpful to remember that the *AV node itself has no pacemaker fibers*. Only the lower portion of intranodal pathways and the bundle of His have pacemaker properties.

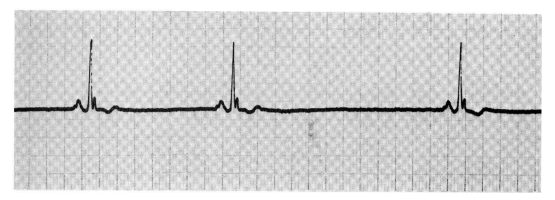

The above rhythm strip demonstrates a sinus bradycardia slowing to a rate of approximately 23 beats per minute! In a *healthy* heart, one would expect a lower, more distal pacemaker to come through, taking control of the rhythm.

Before going further, let's explore a junctional escape rhythm in detail.

The first thing one notices is that the rhythm is *regular*. The customary junctional heart rate is between *40 and 60 beats* per minute. What about atrial activity? You will recall that P waves denote atrial depolarization. In a true junctional rhythm, the P wave (if visible) is usually inverted $\overset{P}{\frown}$ in leads II, III, and aVF. (Atrial activity is usually most clearly evident in leads II, III and aVF). In a junctional escape rhythm, P waves may occur *before*, *during*, or *after* the QRS. Because of its location, the AV junctional pacemaker impulse will be conducted both in an antegrade (forward) and a retrograde (backward) fashion.

In other words, when the impulse originates in the AV junction, the impulse must travel upward and backward to activate the atria, and downward to activate the ventricles. The impulse traveling to the ventricles will be conducted in a normal forward fashion following the normal conduction pathway. In other words, the QRS will be *"of normal duration"* (less than 0.12 seconds).

Atrial activation, however, is a bit more complicated. To fully understand atrial activation, one must recognize that the junctional impulse must travel in a backward or retrograde fashion to initiate atria depolarization.

The junctional pacemaking impulse travels in the *opposite* direction of the SA impulse. Retrograde or backward activation of the atria results in abnormal P waves, usually inverted in leads II, III and aVF.

Now, we must do a bit of abstract thinking! The junctional impulse must travel both to the atria and to the ventricles. If the junctional impulse reaches the (1) atria before the impulse traveling downward reaches the (2) ventricles, a P wave will appear just before the QRS complex. The P wave occurring before the QRS tells the observer that atrial activation occurred before ventricular activation. The inverted nature of the P wave suggests that atrial stimulation occurred in a backward fashion.

Additionally, the P-R interval of the junctional beat will be of *short* duration, *less than* three small squares, or *less than 0.12 seconds*. Some authorities believe the P-R interval will be 0.10 seconds or less! No doubt you are wondering why the P-R interval is short! Since the AV junctional pacemaker is in close proximity to the atria, the impulse "travel time" is short. Therefore, the P-R interval is short!

It should be pointed out that a P.A.C. may also have an inverted P wave occurring before the QRS if it is initiated low in the atria. However, when an ectopic impulse (P.A.C.) arises low in the atria, a sufficient time interval is required for the impulse to travel through the conduction system—in other words, it would have a normal (0.12–0.20) or prolonged P-R interval!

To review then, the above diagram demonstrates that the atria depolarize first (the P wave), followed by ventricular depolarization (the QRS). Notice that the P wave is inverted and the P-R interval is short.

The following rhythm strip demonstrates a junctional escape rhythm with a rate of 55 per minute. Notice the inverted P waves and the shortened P-R intervals occurring before each QRS. P waves occurring before the QRS indicate that atrial depolarization precedes ventricular depolarization.

In contrast, let's suppose that the AV junctional pacemaker impulse reaches and activates the ventricles before it reaches and activates the atria.

The QRS represents ventricular depolarization. The P wave represents atrial depolarization. So when the ventricles depolarize before the atria, guess what we see?!

You're right. . . . the QRS coming before the P wave!

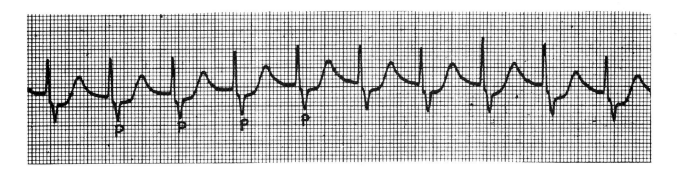

The above rhythm strip demonstrates a junctional escape rhythm, rate 88 per minute. Since the rate of this escape rhythm is faster than the inherent AV junctional rate (40–60), one might elect to call it an accelerated junctional escape rhythm or an accelerated idiojunctional rhythm. *It is important to specify the rate of any rhythm!*

Looking at the above strip, one can now intellectually say this is a junctional escape rhythm with ventricular depolarization occurring before atrial depolarization (because the QRS comes before the P wave). If this is confusing to you, it simply means that you're in the same boat with everyone else! Usually escape rhythms are regular. You will notice that the rate is approximately 88 per minute, somewhat faster than a typical junctional rhythm. It is important to remember that even though a junctional pacemaker has a common or inherent rate (40–60 per minute), the pacemaker is not limited to those rate parameters!

Before progressing further, examine the above rhythm strip again. The rhythm is regular. The rate is 88 per minute. **This is a pop quiz!** Why isn't the above rhythm a sinus rhythm? The answer, of course, is that there is no upright P wave. You knew that, right?!

Finally, what would you expect to find if the junctional pacemaker impulse reached and activated the atria and ventricles at almost the same time?

That's tough one! Take time to think before reading on.

If the impulse traveling backward or retrograde reaches the atria at the same time that the impulse traveling forward or antegrade reaches the ventricles, the P wave will not be obvious. It is said to be "buried" or "hiding" in the QRS.

P wave is hiding!

This "hiding" concept is a bit difficult to grasp, so let's move away from EKG's for a moment. Imagine that I'm in a shopping center, driving around in hopes of finding a parking space. I spy one, so I quickly drive toward it. However, I neglect to notice a big truck driving toward the empty space from the opposite direction!

Later, when a rescue helicopter pilot is viewing the accident scene, he only sees the truck!

The VW is buried or hiding! But, we know it's there! It simply is not visible because the truck is so large.

The monitoring electrodes have a distant view of activity much like the helicopter pilot! External monitoring electrodes "sense" internal electrical events, but "sense" only one electrical event when two events occur simultaneously. Thus, when atrial and ventricular depolarization occur at the same time, the monitoring electrodes will sense one electrical event and the monitor will record the larger QRS.

Does that help? Hope so!

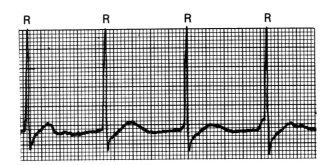

When I observe a monitor tracing like the one above, I know the rhythm *cannot* be of sinus origin because there are no upright ‿⌒‿ P waves occurring before the QRS complexes. Infact, there are no visible P waves!. Yet, the QRS is of normal duration (less than 0.12 seconds), so I know the ventricles were activated in a normal fashion. Therefore, this must be a junctional rhythm with P waves "hiding" in the QRS complexes. Thus, I conclude that atrial and ventricular depolarization have occurred during the same time frame. ☺

Some of the more frequently encountered causes of junctional escape rhythms are digitalis toxicity, hypoxia, acute infections, vagal influence, and myocardial infarction. A small artery nourishes the sinus node. In about 75% of the population, this small artery is supplied by the right coronary artery (RCA). It stands to reason that compromise of the RCA (disease or damage) may cause interruption of the sinus mechanism. This frequently results in a junctional escape rhythm (a lower, more distal pacemaker assumes control).

 If, for some reason, the SA node fails to discharge (sinus arrest) or if the impulse is blocked within the sinus mechanism (sino-atrial block), an AV junctional pacemaker may take over the rhythm, as evident in the following strip.

Notice that following complex 7, the sinus mechanism is disrupted, allowing an AV junctional pacemaker to escape or take control of the rhythm.

Here is another example.

This rhythm strip demonstrates failure of the sinus pacemaker. Notice that the first complex is a normal sinus beat followed by a 2.0 second pulse. A junctional escape pacemaker then emerges to assume control of the rhythm. Note that the rate of the junctional escape rhythm is approximately 37 beats per minute. (Though escape rhythms are generally regular, at *start up* one may observe some variation in rhythm regularity). There are no P waves visible either prior to or following the QRS. The QRS is of normal duration. Here, atrial and ventricular activation are occurring in concert (the P wave is hiding).

To review then, any disruption or failure of the sinus pacemaker may result in an escape rhythm (a safety mechanism). In order to determine the origin of the escape rhythm, one must look closely at *all* of the wave forms. If the QRS is of normal duration (less than 0.12 seconds), we will soon learn that the rhythm cannot be initiated in the ventricles. The absence of normal, upright P waves in leads II, III, and aVF indicates that the rhythm is probably not of sinus or atrial origin. In other words, the rhythm is most likely of AV junctional origin. If a P wave is observed, it will occur prior to, or after the QRS, and will be inverted in leads II, III, and aVF. If the inverted P wave occurs before the QRS, the P-R interval *must measure less than* 0.12 seconds to qualify as a junctional rhythm.

Looking at this next strip, you can see that the QRS occurs before the P wave, so ventricular depolarization occurs before atrial depolarization. Easy, huh?

If you remember the discussion on premature atrial contractions (page 56), you will recall there is a pause following the P.A.C. which allows the sinus pacemaker to reset itself. When a premature beat is followed by a long pause, a junctional escape beat may occur before the sinus pacemaker can regain control. Do you know why that occurs?

Well . . . the AV junction is behaving normally, conducting all impulses progressing down from the atria. Then unexpectedly, there is a pause—no impulse arrives at the AV junction. Since the AV junction can initiate pacemaker impulses 40–60 times per minute, it slips in a junctional beat (junctional escape beat) to ensure that the heart rate does not fall to an exceedingly unhealthy rate. Had the sinus pacemaker failed to resume control, the AV junctional pacemaker could have maintained the heart rate at 40–60 beats per minute!

The important point to remember is that escape beats or escape rhythms are *NEVER* primary phenomena. They always result *secondary* to another event or problem. Therefore, escape rhythms are never terminated. Abolishing an escape rhythm would be analgous to turning off the emergency generator when the power is out!! Rather, the aims of treatment are to support the escape pacemaker and to correct the primary disorder.

It is important to understand that a patient may experience a hemodynamic imbalance owing to both a slow heart rate and the loss of synchronized atrial activity (atrial kick). Therefore, it may be necessary to augment the heart rate using either atropine or a transcutaneous pacemaker. Atropine may promote an increase in the rate of AV junctional discharge, thereby increasing heart rate! Dopamine may also be added to the drug regimen to augment low blood pressure.

Are you ready to try some practice? Hope so!

Practice Exercise 1

Examine this strip closely. I'll help!

A. Is the rhythm regular? __slightly irregular → slow + regular__

The heart rate is approximately __24__ beats per minute.

Determine atrial activity. Are there P waves? __hidden in QRS__

_____

_____

Determine ventricular activity. __.12 seconds   —Normal ventricular Activity__

_____

_____

The QRS measures _____ seconds.

Because the QRSs are of normal duration, I know that the impulses are conducted normally __through the ventricles__.

This rhythm strip must be a __~~junctional ventricular escape~~__ rhythm. __junctional escape__

Since there are no obvious P waves, I must conclude that atrial and ventricular depolarization are occurring __simultaneously__. Thus, the P waves are hidden in the QRS complexes.

Now, try this one on your own. Describe all that you see! (I added a label to assist.)

B.   *Regular*
     50-60 bpm   *Junctional escape rhythm*
     inverted P wave
     PRI = short
     QRS = regular

✔   For **Feedback 1**, refer to page 103.

Input Section 3.2: Premature Junctional Beats

Junctional beats can occur either early (premature) or late (escape). Escape junctional beats occur secondary to failure or disruption of a higher pacemaker. Premature beats, on the other hand, usually represent irritability of the involved tissue and interrupt the normal or underlying rhythm.

A *premature junctional beat* is an impulse that arises in an excitable or irritable site or focus in the AV junctional tissue. You will remember that the AV node itself has no pacemaking capability! Like junctional escape beats, a premature junctional beat must travel both retrograde and antegrade to activate the atria and ventricles, respectively. In other words, an inverted P wave may occur before, during, or after the QRS complex.

The location of the P wave indicates the sequence of atrial activation.

An occasional premature junctional beat may be found in the healthy individual. However, recurrent premature junctional beats are usually associated with rheumatic heart disease or coronary artery disease. The significance of premature junctional beats is the significance of the underlying clinical problem.

Examine this rhythm strip carefully.

The first thing that catches the eye is an early or premature beat occurring earlier than the next expected sinus beat (see arrow). Before diagnosing the premature beat, notice that the underlying rhythm is a borderline sinus bradycardia with a rate of approximately 58 beats per minute. It is always helpful to determine the basic or underlying rhythm and rate before analyzing abnormal beats.

So what about this abnormal beat? Is there a P wave? Yes, there is a P wave, but it's upside-down or inverted. Ah-ha! Maybe this is a premature junctional beat! The P-R interval of the premature beat, measures a "hair" less than 3 small squares or 0.12 seconds. You will recall that to be qualified as a beat of junctional origin, *the P-R interval must be short*. The QRS of the premature beat appears similar to the QRS complexes in the normal underlying rhythm. This is to be expected since ventricular activation usually occurs in a normal fashion!

— Premature junctional beat

Because the premature junctional impulse travels normally down the conduction pathway, ventricular depolarization is unaltered. Therefore, the QRS complexes are of normal duration.

Now, analyze the following rhythm strip.

The underlying rhythm in the above strip is sinus rhythm, with a heart rate of approximately 75 beats per minute. If you have measured accurately, you will note that the QRS measures two small squares or 0.08 seconds. Beat 4 occurs prematurely. If you look closely at the premature beat, there is no obvious P wave, but the QRS is identical to the QRS complexes in the underlying rhythm. This must be a premature junctional beat! Because there is no obvious P wave in this premature junctional complex, we can assume that the atria and ventricles are depolarizing during the same period of time. In other words, the P wave is hiding in the QRS.

Next, examine this rhythm strip.

Here we see a premature junctional beat (the fourth complex) interrupting a borderline sinus tachycardia. You will notice that again, there is no evidence of a P wave occurring either before or after the premature beat. Thus, atrial and ventricular activation are occurring at the same time!

Usually premature junctional beats are merely observed and noted. If however, the patient becomes symptomatic, drug therapy may be initiated. Digitalis or propranolol are often the drugs of choice.

Practice Exercise 2

Now try some practice.
Describe everything that you see!

A. *#5 + #8 - interrupting underlying NSR*
No P waves present on premature beats
QRS = 0.06
P waves inverted after QRSes

B. _____

_____

_____

_____

_____

✔ For **Feedback 2**, refer to page 104.

Input Section 3.3: Junctional Tachycardia

When three or more rapid, ectopic junctional beats occur in succession, it is termed *AV junctional tachycardia*. It may be paroxysmal in nature, or it may persist. Usually the heart rate ranges between 120–200 beats per minute. If P waves are visible, they will occur before or after the QRS complexes. The QRS is *usually* of normal duration (less than 0.12 seconds) since the impulse is conducted normally through the ventricular conduction system. Junctional tachycardia may result from a single ectopic focus firing repeatedly. More commonly, however, junctional tachycardia occurs secondary to a re-entry circuit that allows a circus-like repeat stimulation.

Above are two rhythm strips demonstrating AV junctional tachycardia. Notice, the rhythms are *regular* and rapid.

Strip 1 demonstrates a heart rate of approximately 125 per minute. An inverted P wave precedes each QRS complex. The P-R interval is short, measuring less than 0.12 seconds. In this example, atrial depolarization occurs prior to ventricular depolarization.

Strip 2 shows a regular rhythm with a rate of 150 per minute. There are no P waves visible before or after the QRS complexes, and the QRS duration is within normal limits. In this instance, the atria and the ventricles are depolarizing at the same time (the P wave is hiding in a QRS).

We won't dwell on the subject of AV junctional tachycardia for one *good* reason! . . .

. . .When the heart rate is rapid, it is usually *impossible* to determine whether a P wave is related to the preceding QRS complex or whether it is occurring before the QRS. In fact, it is often difficult to discriminate the various wave forms when the heart rate is rapid!

Now, examine this strip.

In the above rhythm strip, the various wave forms are difficult to discriminate! I am uncertain if P waves are present. Because the duration of the QRS is within normal limits, I know this is either an atrial or a junctional tachycardia. Therefore, I am simply going to call this rhythm a supraventricular tachycardia with a heart rate of approximately 136 per minute. (I used the heart rate guide on page 41!)

Because often times, it is impossible to discriminate atrial tachycardia from an AV junctional tachycardia, the strip "tagged" as a *supraventricular tachycardia*. That simply means the heart rate is rapid, the QRS complexes are within normal limits (less than 0.12 seconds) and it is uncertain whether P waves are present. The term *supraventricular* indicates that the initiating pacemaker is above the ventricles, somewhere in the atria or AV junction (as evidenced by the narrow QRS, less than 0.12 seconds). Supraventricular tachycardia is one of the *few* terms worth remembering!

In any event, the clinical significance of AV junctional tachycardia is similar to that of atrial tachycardia. The rapid heart rate reduces cardiac output because the volume of blood ejected with each contraction is decreased as a result of the shortened ventricular filling time . . . just like the flushing-toilet analogy page 61. However, it is important to note that the patient with junctional tachycardia will be compromised from two points of view: (1) the rapid ventricular rate, and (2) the loss of appropriately synchronized atrial activity (atrial kick).

A decrease in cardiac output can lead to left ventricular failure, and may precipitate chest pain due to the increased oxygen demand and consumption of the cardiac muscle. The treatment for any rapid supraventricular rhythm (atrial tachycardia, junctional tachycardia) is similar. The object of treatment is to reduce the rapid ventricular rate and restore sinus rhythm. Typically, a beta blocker, a calcium blocker or amiodarone will be administered. Amiodarone is the drug of choice in the presence of poor cardiac output or congestive heart failure. If unsuccessful, or if the patient is compromised, synchronized cardioversion may be employed.

Practice Exercise 3

A Describe this rhythm strip in detail!

_____

_____

_____

_____

_____

_____

_____

_____

B. If one observes a rapid rhythm with narrow QRS complexes and no distinguishable P waves, one can

term the dysrhythmia a *supraventricular rhythm tachycardia*

✔ For **Feedback 3**, refer to page 105.

✔ Feedback 1

 ← Color this green!

Pass GO and collect $200.00. You're doing a great job!
Strip 1

A. The rhythm is *slow* and regular.

The heart rate is approximately <u>21</u> beats per minute . . . $70\overline{)1500}$ with quotient 21

I don't see any P waves anywhere!

The ventricular complexes are occurring regularly and they all appear uniform.

The QRS measures <u>0.08</u> seconds.

Because the QRSs are within normal limits, I know that the impulses are conducted normally through <u>the ventricles</u>.

This rhythm is a <u>junctional escape</u> rhythm.

Since there are no obvious P waves, I must conclude that atrial and ventricular depolarization are occurring <u>in the same period of time</u>. Thus, the P wave is hidden in the QRS complex!

P.S. Treatment would consist of speeding up the heart rate!

Strip 2. . . . Hope your answers are <u>similar</u> to mine!

B. The rhythm is <u>regular</u>.

The heart rate is between <u>50–60</u> beats per minute.

An upside-down or <u>inverted</u> P wave precedes each QRS complex. All the inverted P waves appear uniform. The P-R interval is <u>short</u>, less than three small squares, or <u>less than 0.12 seconds</u>.

The QRS complexes are occurring <u>regularly</u>, and all are <u>uniform</u> in appearance.

The QRS measures slightly less than 3 small squares.

Because the QRSs are less than 3 small squares, I know that the impulses are conducted normally through the ventricles.

This is a <u>junctional escape rhythm</u>. The inverted P waves occurring <u>shortly</u> before each QRS complex indicate that the junctional pacemaker activates the atria before reaching and activating the ventricles.

Just for review, here are the EKG properties of a junctional escape rhythm.

Properties of an Idiojunctional or Junctional Escape Rhythm

- The rhythm is usually regular
- The pacemaker impulse formation is usually slower (40–60 beats per minute) than that of the sinus pacemaker.
- It occurs secondary to failure or disruption of the sinus pacemaker.
- If visible, P waves are inverted or upside down in leads II, III, and aVF.
- P waves may occur before, during, or after the QRS.
- The QRS complexes occur regularly, are uniform in appearance, and normally measure less than 0.12 seconds.

Extra! Extra! Bonus on next page!

Bonus

I saw this elderly patient today and she wasn't feeling well at all! I thought you might enjoy looking at her monitor tracing with me.

Beats 2, 3, and 4 tell me that her underlying heart rhythm is a sinus bradycardia with a heart rate of less than 50 beats per minute. Apparently, her sinus node was feeling a bit "under the weather," so it periodically failed to fire an impulse. Consequently, the good ol' AV junction came through to save the day!

Beat 1 demonstrates a junctional escape beat that has no P wave. So, in this instance, the atria and ventricles were depolarizing in the same period of time. (The P wave is hiding in the QRS.) Beats 2, 3, and 4 demonstrate the underlying sinus bradycardia. Beat 5 shows a junctional escape beat with a retrograde P wave (the P wave follows the QRS). Thus, in this instance, the ventricles have depolarized before atrial depolarization occurs. The last beat (6) is similar to beat 1.

This patient has a pacemaker that wanders from the AV junction to the sinus node and back to the AV junction! More than likely, this patient has a sick sinus syndrome relating to degeneration of the sinus node.

✔ Feedback 2

Nice work!

A. The underlying rhythm is a sinus rhythm, with a rate of approximately 80 per minute. Beats 5 and 8 are premature, interrupting the underlying regular rhythm. Inverted P waves occur after the premature beats. The QRSs of the premature beats are within normal limits. This must be premature junctional beats interrupting a sinus rhythm! Because the P waves of the premature beats occur following the QRS, I know that atrial depolarization occurred after ventricular depolarization.

B. The underlying rhythm is a sinus rhythm with a heart rate of approximately 75 beats per minute. The QRS complexes measure 0.08 seconds. Beat 4 is premature, interrupting the underlying regular rhythm. The premature beat does not have an obvious P wave. The QRS of the premature beat appears like the QRS complexes in the sinus rhythm. This is a premature junctional beat with atrial and ventricular depolarization occurring during the same period of time (the P wave is hiding in the QRS!).

Note: See the top of page 105 for a quick review of premature junctional beats.

Just for review, a premature junctional beat has the following properties:

Properties of a Premature Junctional Beat

- The premature beat interrupts the underlying rhythm; thus, the rhythm is irregular.

- An inverted P wave may occur before, during, or after the QRS complex of the premature beat.

- The QRS of the premature beat is usually similar to the QRS complexes of the underlying rhythm.

✔ Feedback 3

How are you doing? Fine, I hope!

A. This is a regular rhythm with a heart rate of approximately 115 beats per minute. The QRS complexes appear uniform and measure approximately 0.08 seconds. Inverted P waves follow each QRS complex, indicating that ventricular depolarization occurs prior to atrial depolarization. This is an AV junctional tachycardia!

B. If one observes a rapid rhythm with narrow QRS complexes (less than 0.12 seconds) and no distinguishable P waves, one can term the dysrhythmia a supraventricular tachycardia.

To review then, an AV junctional tachycardia is a regular rhythm with a rapid rate. The P waves may occur prior to, during, or after the QRS complexes. The QRS complexes appear uniform and usually measure less than 0.12 seconds.

Notes

Ventricular Ectopic and Escape Rhythms

Objectives

When you have completed Section 4, you will be able to describe or identify

1. premature ventricular contractions (P.V.C.s)

2. fusion beats

3. ventricular tachycardia

4. ventricular re-entry mechanisms

5. torsades de pointes

6. ventricular flutter

7. ventricular fibrillation

8. pulseless electrical activity (PEA)

9. ventricular escape rhythm

Input Section 4.1: Premature Ventricular Contractions

Now, back to the art of dysrhythmia interpretation!

This section addresses ventricular ectopic and ventricular escape rhythms. Sounds ominous, doesn't it? Actually, ventricular abnormalities are relatively easy, compared to what has been dealt with previously!

Probably everyone is familiar with ventricular extrasystoles or premature ventricular contractions (P.V.C.s). Ectopic ventricular excitation originates below the bifurcation of the bundle of His, outside the normal conduction system.

P.V.C.s represent abnormal electrical stimulation arising from an excitable focus or site, somewhere in either ventricle. There is no failure of the normal or underlying rhythm, merely additional premature beats arising from an irritable focus.

As the name *premature ventricular contraction* implies, P.V.C.s interrupt the normal rhythmic cycle. In addition, they may be coupled or related to the preceding sinus beats. You'll remember (from page 57) that a *coupling interval* is the distance between the premature beat and the preceding sinus beat. Remember?

Following is a rather dramatic illustration of P.V.C.s interrupting a normal rhythm. Notice that the coupling interval is constant. One can expect the coupling interval to be constant when the P.V.C.s are uniform in appearance, indicating that the ventricular stimulus arises from a single focus or location.

Note the constant coupling interval illustrated below

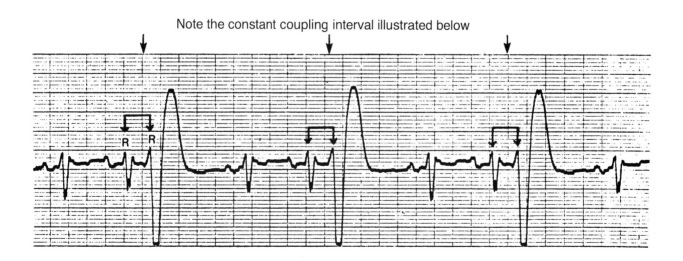

Most usually, P.V.C.s are extremely obvious owing to their *bizarre* appearance. One need know very little about interpreting EKGs to recognize the abnormality!

To confirm that these abnormal beats are indeed P.V.C.s, *they must prematurely interrupt the underlying rhythm, have a widened QRS (0.12 seconds or greater) and have no observable P wave prior to the wide QRS.*

Atrial depolarization is recorded on the monitor as a P wave   ; ventricular depolarization is recorded as the QRS complex.

Since a premature ventricular impulse originates in the ventricles outside the normal conduction pathway, ventricular depolarization will occur from the point of origin, much like a rock thrown into a pool of water. This abnormal activation of the ventricles causes the QRS to be wide and bizarre. Further, since the P.V.C. originates in the ventricles, there will be no P wave prior to the QRS. So where are the P waves??? . . . or when do the atria depolarize? *One of two things may happen:*

1. A sinus impulse may fire while the ventricular ectopic impulse is moving across the ventricles. If this happens, the P wave may be "buried" in the QRS complex. In this case, the atria and the ventricles are stimulated by two separate impulses—the atria by the SA impulse, and the ventricles by the ectopic impulse (the P.V.C.). On the EKG strip, no P wave is obvious in the abnormal cardiac cycle.

    When myocardial activation occurs in this manner, there is very little disruption of rhythmicity. In other words, in a regular rhythm, the P.V.C. falls almost where one would expect the next sinus impulse to occur.

In the above strip, note that no P wave occurs before or after the QRS. Rather, the P wave is buried in the QRS. When the P wave is "buried," there is no pause following the P.V.C and there is minimal disruption of the rhythm cadence.

2. The ectopic ventricular impulse may occur early in the cycle and be conducted backward (retrograde) through the AV junctional tissue across the atria before the sinus impulse fires. In this case, ventricular depolarization occurs prior to atrial depolarization. So, one would see a wide, bizarre QRS complex followed by a P wave, as demonstrated below.

You will also notice, when retrograde conduction occurs, a long pause follows the premature beat. This pause is called a *compensatory pause*, and measures the distance of two normal R-R intervals. This pause allows the sinus pacemaker to reset the rhythm.

If this is difficult to understand, just remember that a P wave will never occur before the premature ventricular beat. A P wave may occur during or after the wide, bizarre QRS complex. You're probably wondering why I did not say that to begin with . . . right? **Right!**

The important point to remember is that all P.V.C.s indicate ventricular irritability. The visible presence or absence of a P wave merely indicates the sequence of atrial activation.

Now that you have an understanding of the P waves (atrial activation), we need to address the subject of the "widened" QRS. *All premature ventricular contractions will have a QRS measuring 0.12 seconds or greater.* A ventricular ectopic impulse (P.V.C.) initiates ventricular depolarization from the point of origin in either the right or left ventricle. The wave of excitation behaves much like a stone thrown into a pool of water, progressing outward. The wave of excitation thus travels outside the normal conducting pathway, requiring more time to achieve ventricular depolarization.

You will remember that moving horizontally across the EKG paper denotes time.

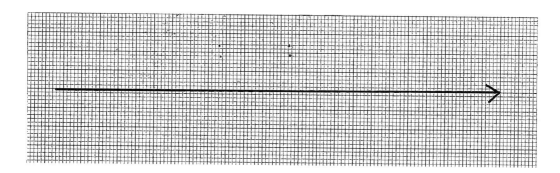

Thus, because the abnormal stimulus (P.V.C.) takes longer to achieve ventricular depolarization, the QRS will be widened—0.12 seconds or greater. (The speed of impulse movement through the myocardium varies from 0.5 to 1.0 meters per second, while the specialized conduction pathways conduct much faster, from 1.0 to 4.0 meters per second!) It should be noted that the wave of excitation produced by a P.V.C. originating in the right ventricle spreads generally from right to left. When viewed from a right precordial lead (V_1), the wave of depolarization moves away from the positive $\oplus$ electrode. The resulting QRS will be wide and negative in appearance. Conversely, when a P.V.C. arising from the left ventricle (spreading generally from left to right) is viewed from lead V_1, the QRS will be wide and positively directed, moving toward the positive $\oplus$ electrode.

To review then, a premature ventricular contraction (P.V.C.) presents as a wide, bizarre QRS that interrupts the underlying rhythm. A P wave will never occur before this abnormal QRS, but may occur during or following the QRS.

P.V.C.s can occur in normal hearts, especially during periods of fatigue or emotional distress. Likewise, persons who drink caffeine products or smoke may have P.V.C.s. (If you have ever experienced your heart "skip a beat," you may have experienced a P.V.C.!) When listening to a heart beat or feeling the pulse, you may hear or feel a pause following an early beat.

Persons taking such drugs as pronestyl, digitalis, or drugs with known proarrhythmic effects, and persons with low serum potassium levels may experience P.V.C.s. Hypoxia may also result in ectopic ventricular activity. Manipulating the heart tissue itself (open heart surgery) or catheters situated within the heart chambers (pacemaker catheters, cardiac catheterizations, Swan-Ganz catheters) may predispose to ectopic ventricular activity.

In healthy persons, P.V.C.s are relatively harmless. However, in patients with existing heart disease and especially myocardial infarction, *P.V.C.s may **warn of ventricular tachycardia or ventricular fibrillation***. Ischemic tissue is thought to release a *substance* which is capable of increasing the automaticity of the Purkinje fibers. Thus, patients with ischemic disorders are prone to P.V.C.s.

Amiodarone administered intravenously is the current treatment of choice for ectopic ventricular activity. A bolus of amiodarone, usually 150 mg. I.V. is given over ten minutes to establish a blood level, followed by a continuous infusion. (Though amiodarone is preferred treatment, both lidocaine and procainamide remain acceptable alternatives.)

Usually, antiarrhythmic therapy is instituted when any of the following five scenarios are present:

1. P.V.C.s occurring with increasing frequency . . . (frequent P.V.C.s suggest increasing ventricular irritability and serve to decrease cardiac output.)

2. P.V.C.s occurring in rhythmic patterns, e.g., bigeminy P.V.C.s, where every other beat is a P.V.C.; trigeminy P.V.C.s, where every third beat is a P.V.C.; quadrigeminy P.V.C.s, where every fourth beat is a P.V.C., and so forth.

Ventricular bigeminy . . . or bigeminy P.V.C.s. Notice that
all the P.V.C.s appear uniform or monomorphic or unifocal (identical).

Ventricular trigeminy . . . or trigeminy P.V.C.s.
(Another example of trigeminal P.V.C.s can be found at the bottom of page 108.)

3. P.V.C.s falling close to the T wave of the preceding beat.

A P.V.C. falling on or near the T wave of the preceding beat is known as *the "R on T" phenomenon*. In the following strip you will notice that the T wave is inverted (upside down). That is significant too, as you will learn in a later section. The T wave is *vulnerable* to any electrical stimulation, particularly in the ischemic heart. A P.V.C. falling on a vulnerable T wave may precipitate ventricular tachycardia or ventricular fibrillation. (The apex of the T wave represents the earliest time the ventricles can respond to another stimulus.) Frequently, the ischemic heart is in various stages of repolarization. A P.V.C. occurring during this period can initiate depolarization of individual ventricular segments resulting in ventricular fibrillation.

A P.V.C. falling on a vulnerable T wave produces a run of ventricular tachycardia!

(We'll discuss this later in more detail.)

4. P.V.C.s originating from *more* than one irritable site or focus.
   In other words, P.V.C.s are different in appearance. Commonly, this is referred to as **multiformed, multifocal or multidirectional P.V.C.s**.

Sometimes this business of single and *multiformed* (or *multidirectional*) P.V.C.s is a bit confusing. So, to clarify the subject, I've borrowed an explanation from the Obstetrics Department! (If you can think of the ventricles as being a mama, you're all set!)

When twins develop from separately fertilized eggs, they appear uniquely different owing to their fraternal or **multiformed** relationship.

Multiformed (also known as polymorphic or multifocal) *P.V.C.s* originate from various irritable sites (or foci) within the ventricles, and appear uniquely different!

When, however, twins develop from a *single* fertilized egg, they appear identical.

Single origin P.V.C.s originate from the same irritable site (or focus) in either ventricle and are essentially identical in appearance.

. . . Yes, I know, these analogies are a bit far-fetched . . . but, **I bet you remember them**!

(Multiformed twins)

5. Two P.V.C.s occurring together, referred to as *paired P.V.C.s*, or a *couplet* of P.V.C.s. is also an indication for antiarrhythmic therapy.

In the above example an ectopic focus in the ventricles has discharged two impulses in rapid succession. This clues us that the ventricular ectopic site is *extremely* irritable. (If it continues to initiate rapid impulses, the ectopic pacemaker will assume control of the heart rhythm!!)

To review then, the following situations or patterns are usual indications for antiarrhythmic therapy.

1. P.V.C.s increasing in frequency

2. P.V.C.s occurring in rhythmic patterns, e.g. bigeminy, trigeminy, etc.

3. P.V.C.s falling close to the vulnerable T wave

4. multiformed P.V.C.s

5. paired P.V.C.s

The reader should be aware that drug therapy and the indications for drug therapy continue to evolve, based on accumulated clinical data and new drug clinical trials. **For the most current recommended drug therapy, one should consult the American Heart Association's Advanced Life Support text**. As an example, past practice supported drug prophylaxis for dysrhythmias associated with acute myocardial infarction (AMI). Current practice does not favor the administration of prophylactic antiarrhythmic drugs in the presence of AMI.

When P.V.C.s occur, they should be thought of as a **warning signal** until determined otherwise. They warn the observer that life threatening ventricular dysrhythmias may be imminent.

A physician should *always* be made aware when his or her patient begins experiencing P.V.C.s—the number per minute, their appearance (unifocal or multifocal), and their location in the cardiac cycle (i.e., falling near the vulnerable T wave). Most importantly, the care giver must directly evaluate the patient's clinical picture!

Before leaving the subject of premature ventricular contractions, the term "interpolated" ventricular extrasystoles or interpolated P.V.C.s should be mentioned. When a P.V.C. occurs between two normally conducted sinus beats, and the rhythm of those sinus beats is not disrupted, the P.V.C. is said to be *interpolated*. In other words, the P.V.C. is *sandwiched* between two normal beats!

Interpolation results when the retrograde (backward) conduction of the P.V.C. is blocked from reaching and activating the atria by refractory tissue above the ventricles.

Commonly, the sinus beat following the interpolated P.V.C. will have a *prolonged* P-R interval owing to refractoriness of the AV node. The AV node has not fully recovered from the premature ventricular stimulation . . . thus, conduction takes longer! Interpolated P.V.C.s are only observed in slow rhythms.

Interpolated P.V.C.s have the same significance as other P.V.C.s. I thought you might find them interesting!

Important Note

Excess digitalis will frequently result in ectopic ventricular activity. In this instance, lidocaine and other antiarrhythmic drugs have little or no effect. Digitalis should be withheld when digitalis toxicity is suspected. Typical therapy involves correcting electrolyte imbalances and supporting the patient. Magnesium, in particular, may counter ventricular dysrhythmias associated with digitalis toxicity. In severe cases, dilantin or Digiband may be administered.

☒ Single formed (monomorphic)
☐ Multiformed (polymorphic)

☐ Single formed (monomorphic)
☒ Multiformed (polymorphic)

Practice Exercise 1

How about some practice!

A. Describe this rhythm strip in detail.

_____

_____

_____

B. Describe the abnormality in this rhythm strip.

_____

_____

_____

_____

_____

C. In the following rhythm strip, _____*every other beat*_____ is a premature ventricular
contraction. This is known as _____*trigeminy*_____ .

✔ For **Feedback 1**, refer to page 135.

Input Section 4.2: Fusion (Dressler) Beats

To complicate life a bit further, we need to explore *fusion or Dressler beats*. So what's a fusion beat??
In normal conduction, the ventricles are activated by a sinus impulse traveling down the conduction system.

When a premature ventricular contraction (P.V.C.) occurs, it initiates myocardial depolarization in a backward or retrograde fashion distorting the QRS complex.

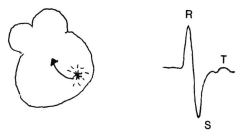

If a sinus impulse is initiated at the same time an ectopic focus in the ventricles initiates an impulse, ventricular depolarization (the QRS) will be produced by a double stimulation. That sounds confusing, so let's try an example. Let's say that the SA node initiates an impulse which activates the atria (producing a P wave), and that impulse travels 1/4 of the way across the ventricles, beginning ventricular depolarization.

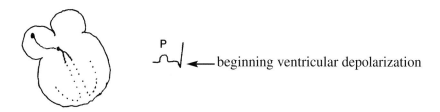

beginning ventricular depolarization

At the same time, a ventricular ectopic focus initiates an impulse (P.V.C.) causing retrograde or backward depolarization of the lower portion of the ventricles.

These two impulses, one traveling antegrade (forward) and one traveling retrograde (backward), collide somewhere in the ventricles.

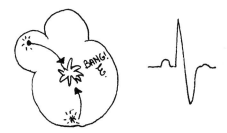

Thus, ventricular depolarization (the QRS) has been initiated by a double stimulation!

So what will the QRS look like? The QRS will resemble both the normal QRS and a wide, bizarre P.V.C. This "fused" QRS will be wider than the normal QRS, but less wide than a P.V.C.

Woops! I forgot something! What about a P wave? Will the fusion beat have a P wave? Of course! . . . because the SA impulse traveled through the atria (initiating atrial depolarization), through the AV junction into the ventricles before colliding with the premature ventricular impulse. So, the fusion beat will have a P wave, and that P wave will be equidistant from other P waves . . . in other words, the P-P interval will remain constant. Because of the double ventricular stimulation, the P-R interval, if visible, is abnormally short . . . the sinus impulse travels only part way down the conduction system! Examine this next rhythm strip.

The above underlying rhythm is sinus rhythm, though it is difficult to tell! The rhythm is interrupted by frequent P.V.C.s and an occasional P.A.C. Beats 2 and 7 are P.V.C.s—they are wide and bizarre and have no preceding P waves. But what about beats 4 and 9? They resemble the P.V.C.s, except that they are not as wide. And, there are P waves preceding the QRSs! The P waves occur right on time! Beats 4 and 9 represent fusion beats *(collision beats)!* Notice that the P-R interval of the fusion beats is shorter than the P-R interval of the underlying rhythm.

I almost forgot to tell you, fusion beats are also known as Dressler beats.

In review then, in order to identify a fusion beat, two phenomena must exist.

1. There must be a supraventricular pacemaker that conducts normally, producing normal QRS complexes.

2. There must be an ectopic ventricular focus, producing wide, bizarre QRS complexes.

Then . . . if a beat with an abnormally short P-R interval and a QRS complex somewhere in between the shape and duration of the normal and the ventricular ectopic QRS is observed, it must be a fusion beat!

Amiodarone or lidocaine therapy will not only abolish the P.V.C.s, but will also abolish the fusion beats. Remember, a fusion beat is, in part, a P.V.C.!

Practice Exercise 2

Step right up and try your luck!

A. Study this rhythm strip. Then label all the beats.

FUSION
Pwave

PVC   *PVC*

B. A fusion beat is ___between a PVC + sinus beat_____

_____

_____

_____

_____

_____

_____

✔ For **Feedback 2,** refer to page 136.

Input Section 4.3: Ventricular Tachycardia

Now, for some excitement . . . *Ventricular Tachycardia*!

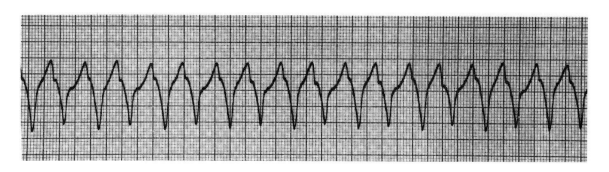

Ventricular tachycardia is most always associated with organic heart disease. It is probably one of the most difficult diagnoses to make, largely because one must make an instantaneous decision. The *important* fact is that ventricular tachycardia is a ***life-threatening*** dysrhythmia! Treatment *must* be initiated immediately when ventricular tachycardia is suspected.

The following criteria *help* to establish the diagnosis of ventricular tachycardia. (Refer to the rhythm strip at the bottom of the previous page).

1. The rate is usually rapid, between 140–200 beats per minute.

2. The P waves are usually buried in the QRS complexes making them obscure.

3. The QRS complexes are wide and bizarre.

4. The ventricular rhythm is *basically* regular.

Important Notice

Because virtually every criteria for ventricular tachycardia can be argued, **one must initiate treatment and *then* argue specific points**.

In ventricular tachycardia, the ventricles may be stimulated by an ectopic ventricular pacemaker firing repeatedly. Or, more likely, ventricular tachycardia is initiated by a single P.V.C. The repetitive ventricular stimulation is the result of a reentry mechanism within the ventricular myocardium.

To truly differentiate between ventricular and supraventricular activity, one must recognize atrial activity and its relationship to the QRS complexes. In ventricular tachycardia, the P waves (*if visible*) bear *no* relationship to the QRSs.

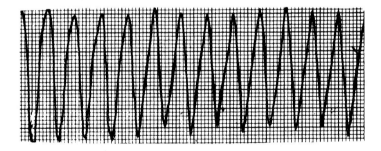

That's a difficult concept to grasp, so let's simplify it a bit! Let's say that the good ol' sinus pacemaker is firing along at a rate of 70. But, because an ectopic ventricular pacemaker is discharging an impulse at 180 times per minute, it takes control of the heart beat. (*The fastest pacemaker controls heart rate.*)

When the sinus impulses occur, they find the ventricular tissue refractory (or unable to respond) to further stimulation.

So, the P waves, *if visible*, bear no relationship to the QRSs. Usually, P waves are not visible—they're hiding within the QRS complexes! ☺

Long ago and far away, Schamroth (1971) suggested that the *best* evidence to support a ventricular tachycardia is the presence of a fusion beat during a tachycardia with bizarre QRS complexes. To refresh your memory, the third complex is a fusion beat.

This above strip demonstrates two sinus beats followed by a fusion beat and a P.V.C. The P wave of the fusion beat occurs on time . . . it does not occur early or late. The QRS of the fusion beat is wider than the normal QRS, but less wide than the P.V.C. Remember, a fusion beat is the result of a normal beat and a P.V.C. colliding!

You'll remember that a fusion beat produces the QRS by double stimulation—one impulse originating in the atria, and one from an ectopic site or focus in the ventricles. A "run" of ventricular tachycardia may begin or end with a fusion beat, or a fusion beat may be seen in the tachycardia itself.

Fusion beat

Ventricular tachycardia beginning with
a fusion beat.

Fusion beat

Ventricular tachycardia evidence of a
fusion beat.

Why does a fusion beat occur in the middle of ventricular tachycardia? Remember the P waves that are occurring at a slower rate, bearing no relationship to the QRSs? Well, a P wave happens to find the ventricular tissue polarized, so it initiates depolarization. But bang! Another ectopic impulse is fired. Thus, the two impulses collide, producing a fusion beat.

Fusion beat

A fusion beat is produced by a dual stimulation of the ventricles (sinus beat + P.V.C.). A P wave will be obvious, and the QRS of the fusion beat will not be as wide as the QRS of the ventricular beats. The P-R interval of the fusion beat will be abnormally short.

The presence of a capture beat is also evidence to support the identification ventricular tachycardia. So, what is a **capture beat?**

A capture beat is a fusion beat's Big Brother!

In essence, a capture beat is a normally conducted beat (a sinus beat) that manages to slip through during a ventricular tachycardia. One of those P waves firing along at a slower rate, bearing no relationship to the QRSs, finds the tissue polarized. So *it initiates and completes* normal conduction before the next abnormal ectopic ventricular beat occurs!

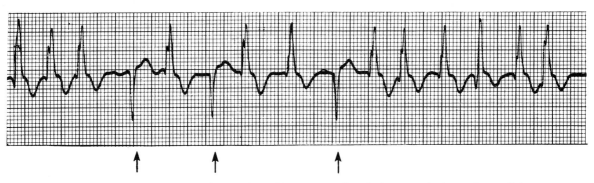

Capture Beats (three normally conducted beats occurring during ventricular tachycardia).

Because a capture beat conducts normally (in an antegrade fashion), the associated QRS has an entirely different contour than that of the PVC. The capture beat depolarizes the ventricles in an orderly, antegrade fashion. *A fusion beat is an incomplete capture beat!*

One must remember that ventricular tachycardia is a **life-threatening** dysrhythmia. It may rapidly progress to ventricular fibrillation; thus, treatment must be instituted *immediately*. If the patient is unstable (impaired cardiac function), amiodarone or lidocaine is administered intravenously followed by synchronized cardioversion. Synchronized cardioversion will be discussed in Section 7. Please reference Section 14 for antiarrhythmic drug details.

The patient with ventricular tachycardia may be alert, anxious, short of breath, and have a low blood pressure—or, he may be essentially unresponsive with no attainable blood pressure. When the patient is nonresponsive, direct defibrillation is applied. There is *no* time to waste! This is a "code arrest" situation.

Ventricular tachycardia may be sustained or paroxysmal in nature. It may suddenly appear and disappear without treatment.

Three or more P.V.C.s occurring together are considered ventricular tachycardia as evidenced in the following rhythm strip.

A P.V.C. falling on a vulnerable T wave (R on T phenomenon) may initiate a run of ventricular tachycardia as demonstrated in this next rhythm strip.

Though in the above examples, the ventricular tachycardia converted spontaneously, antiarrhythmic treatment is usually initiated. A discussion of drug therapy for sustained ventricular tachycardia can be found in Section 14.

 Practice Exercise 3

214
7 ⌐500
14
10
7
30

A. Describe this rhythm strip in detail (rate, rhythm, atrial activity and ventricular activity). Then, identity the probable treatment.

1 2   3   4 5 6 7   8 9 10 11 12 13   14 15

tx = amiodarone

Irregular Rhythm of PVCs/Ventricular tachycardia interrupting sinus rhythm
Bizarre + wide QRS Complexes
Runs of PVCS - 4+5
P waves only visible on sinus beats (3+ 8, +14)
Rate of tachy = approx 200-214 bpm

66
9⌐500
60
30
69

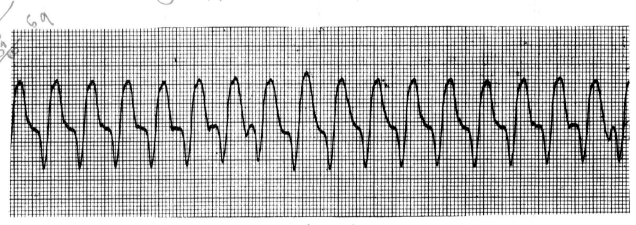

B. This above strip demonstrates ___Ventricular tachycardia___ with a heart rate of ___160___ beats per minute.

✔ For **Feedback 3**, refer to page 137.

INPUT SECTION 4.4: Ventricular Re-Entry Mechanisms
(Advanced Study)

At the beginning of this discussion (page 120), it was noted that ventricular tachycardia often occurs secondary to a re-entry mechanism (here we go again, here we go again, etc!) ☺ A ventricular re-entry mechanism is a localized aberration and may be located anywhere within the ventricular myocardium. Briefly, a ventricular re-entry mechanism behaves in the following example way.

Remember, a P.V.C. arises outside the normal conduction pathway and therefore must travel in a backward or retrograde fashion to initiate ventricular depolarization, as depicted in Diagram 1.

Diagram 1

When an anomalous connection exists between two ventricular conducting fibers, a circuit (of sorts) or communicating loop is formed (see dotted line in Diagram 2). Under certain conditions, [(1) an initiating P.V.C. and (2) unequal refractoriness in portions of the circuitry], the anomalous communicating loop will *behave as an electrical circuit*.

Diagram 2

P.V.C.

If a well-timed P.V.C. occurs and begins conduction through the anomalous circuitry, it may find certain of the tissues partially refractory (not fully recovered). Tissues in a state of refractoriness are unable to receive a further stimulation until fully recovered.

In this example, the tissues in "leg A" of the circuit are in a state of partial refractoriness. Thus, the wave of excitation produced by the P.V.C. progresses normally across "leg B" of the circuit, but is *blocked* from entering "leg A" From "leg B", the wave of excitation begins a retrograde activation of ventricular tissues **and** loops around the abnormal circuit (moving antegrade) to "leg A". See Diagram 3.

Block

P.V.C

Diagram 3

If the tissues in "leg A" of the circuit are now fully recovered, the wave of excitation causes depolarization of the once blocked tissues. The speed of excitation slows during depolarization, then moves further forward to the point of (O)rigin, as depicted in Diagram 4.

If, "leg" B is now fully recovered, the wave of excitation loops around again, repeating (and repeating) the same sequence. This repeated circus-like ventricular stimulation produces a rapid ventricular tachycardia.

Diagram 4

Diagram 5

If, however, the wave of excitation finds "leg" B refractory, the stimulus is blocked and the rapid ventricular rhythm subsides as depicted in Diagram 5.

Radiofrequency ablation (RFA) is often the preferred therapeutic intervention. RFA destroys the anomalous tissue responsible for re-entry.

Input Section 4.5: Torsades de Pointes (TdP)
🎓 (Advanced Study)

Torsades de pointes (TdP) is a rare polymorphic (multiformed) ventricular tachycardia associated with prolonged ventricular repolarization (a prolonged QT interval) resulting from variation in myocardial fiber recovery times. The term *torsades de pointes* (twisting of points) aptly describe the appearance. The wide QRSs vary in appearance, moving from upright (positive) to negatively directed complexes and back again, described as twisting around the baseline.

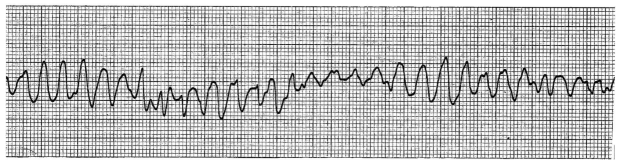

TdP commonly occurs in short bursts (5–15 seconds) and is therefore difficult to capture on 12 lead EKG. Characteristically, the rate ranges between 200 and 250 beats per minute. If the dysrhythmia persists, it may progress to ventricular fibrillation.

TdP can occur as an inherited disorder, a mutation in genes that control sodium and potassium channels. This type of disorder is termed an *inherited long QT syndrome*, discussed in Section 15. The dysrhythmia may also arise as a complication (**proarrhythmic** effect) of drugs that prolong the QT interval by blocking the potassium channel. This variation of TdP is termed an *acquired long QT syndrome*. (Drugs exhibiting a proarrhythmic effect are discussed below).

You will recall from Section 1, the QT interval is a measurement that represents the total time of ventricular depolarization and complete repolarization. Measurement begins at the Q wave and ends at the conclusion of the T wave. (If no Q wave is present, the measurement begins at the R wave). The QT interval is *best* measured in leads V_2, and V_3.

QT INTERVAL

In a normal healthy rhythm, the QT interval measures less than one-half of the R-R interval (refer to page 22 for a quick review). However, the QT interval varies with age, gender, heart rate and a number of other subtle factors. In a healthy state, the normal male QT interval averages 0.39 seconds; it is considered prolonged at 0.45 seconds. The normal female QT interval averages 0.41 seconds; it is considered prolonged at 0.46 seconds. Because the QT interval varies with heart rate, a formula (Bazet's formula) was derived to correct for heart rate variation.

$$\text{Bazet's formula} \qquad \mathbf{QTc} = \frac{\text{QT interval in seconds}}{\sqrt{\text{R} - \text{R interval in seconds}}}$$

QTc is the abbreviation utilized for a heart-rate corrected QT interval. Fortunately, QTc calculators are programmed into 12 lead EKG machines!

Another measure, QT dispersion (**QTd**) is used to determine variation in myocardial refractoriness. In this metric, the QT interval is measured on the same beat in all 12 EKG leads. The shortest QT interval measurement is subtracted from the longest QT interval measurement. The resulting difference is an indicator of the degree of variation (dispersion) in refractoriness. The greater the degree of dispersion, the presumed higher the risk for ventricular tachycardia or ventricular fibrillation associated with a proarrhythmic drug effect.

In general, patients presenting with a QT interval measurement of 600 milliseconds (0.06 seconds) or greater are presumed to have a higher risk. Unfortunately, however, a prolonged QT interval is only a moderate predictor of risk! To date, there are no absolute risk predictors.

Torsades de points is slightly more common in women than men. The dysrhythmia can be precipitated by ischemia, hypokalemia or hypomagnesemia (both conditions cause repolarization delay) or proarrhythmic drug effects (an arrhythmia worsens or a new arrhythmia appears). Some degree of TdP risk is associated with the proarrhythmia effects of the following antiarrhythmic drugs.

Class 1A drugs (procainamide, quinidine, disopyramide)
Class 1C drugs (encainide, flecainide)
Class III drugs (sotalol, amiodarone, ibutilide, dofetilide)

Additionally, albuterol (a bronchial dilator) and erythromycin have been associated with TdP.

The risk classification of drugs is continuously updated as clinical data are available. The most up-to-date information on drug induced arrhythmias can be found on the University of Arizona CERT International Registry for Drug Induced Arrhythmias. Information specific to QT interval prolongation can be accessed at www.qtdrugs.org/med-pros.

Treatment for TdP depends on the severity of symptoms. In paroxysmal TdP (sudden bursts), intravenous magnesium sulfate ($MgSO_4$) and potassium chloride (KCl) are typically the first treatment agents employed. Magnesium sulfate acts as an antiarrhythmic agent and can also be utilized to treat ventricular fibrillation unresponsive to other treatments. Sustained TdP requires immediate synchronized cardioversion.

Input Section 4.6: Ventricular Flutter

Ventricular flutter (as depicted on the previous page) is most usually a transition rhythm from ventricular tachycardia to ventricular fibrillation. The rate of ventricular flutter is greater than 200 beats per minute. Owing to this rapid rate, cardiac output is minimal. Ventricular flutter represents a medical emergency and is an indication for immediate defibrillation. The patient usually loses consciousness with the appearance of ventricular flutter.

Since ventricular flutter is a *transition* rhythm, we are going to *transition* to Input 7! There is no practice exercise associated with this dysrhythmia!

Input Section 4.7: Ventricular Fibrillation

That brings us to the lethal subject of ***ventricular fibrillation.***
Ventricular fibrillation is chaotic, uncoordinated, ineffective, ventricular depolarization.

Coarse ventricular fibrillation

In ventricular fibrillation, there is *total irregularity* of electrical activity. There is usually constant variation in the amplitude. **No PQRST** can be seen, and the baseline appears to wander. Ventricular fibrillation may be *coarse* (large waves) as seen above. Or, ventricular fibrillatory waves may be *fine* (more or less like atrial fibrillatory waves without QRSs).

Since there is *no* coordinated ventricular electrical activity, there is *no significant ventricular muscle contraction*. If one were to directly view the fibrillating heart, it would appear as a "bag of worms." Because the pumping action of the heart is lost, death occurs within minutes.

Usually, ventricular fibrillation does not just appear. Characteristically, myocardial irritability will first be evident—such as P.V.C.s. However, it has been demonstrated that ventricular fibrillation may occur spontaneously when associated with acute myocardial infarction. In most instances, ventricular fibrillation is a *terminal event*, and is associated with ischemic heart disease. It may, however, be induced by digitalis toxicity—particularly if digitalis intoxication is associated with hypokalemia. Ventricular fibrillation may also occur with *severe hypothermia*—when the body temperature approaches 28° centigrade. Further, electrical shock may induce ventricular fibrillation.

The only treatment for ventricular fibrillation is electrical defibrillation or nonsynchronized precordial shock. CPR should be instituted immediately. (Defibrillation will be discussed in Section 7.)

Commonly, one can anticipate successful defibrillation when the ventricular fibrillation occurs in a patient without heart failure or extensive myocardial damage and when the precordial shock is delivered within the first few minutes of the dysrhythmia. In the presence of fine ventricular fibrillatory waves unresponsive to initial defibrillation attempts, epinephrine may be administered. Epinephrine may convert fine fibrillatory waves to coarse waves, often more responsive to electrical shock.

* Precordial Shock

The above strip demonstrates ventricular fibrillation. Non-synchronized precordial shock
(defibrillation) interrups the chaotic rhythm and a sinus rhythm resumes.

Defibrillation may be unsuccessful in the patient with long-standing respiratory or cardiac disease. The efficacy of defibrillation is also comprised in morbidly obese persons.

* Precordial Shock

This strip demonstrates unsuccesful defibrillation.

One should bear in mind that the body *rapidly* converts to anaerobic metabolism with the cessation of circulation. There is a rapid buildup of lactic acid—resulting in metabolic acidosis. For this reason, buffering agents such as sodium bicarbonate may be administered following the establishment of adequate ventilation. Electrical intervention is more successful when the acidotic state has been corrected. *ACLS Guidelines* (American Heart Association) should be consulted for the latest, up-to-date treatments for code arrest.

Practice Exercise 7

Practice time again!

Describe these two rhythm strips in detail! Indicate the probable treatments or interventions.

A. ventricular fibrillation
undulating baseline - no PQRSTs present

181
8/1500
8
10
60

B. ventricular flutter tachycardia   (flutter = above 200bpm)
wide + bizarre QRS complexes approx 187 bpm

✔ For **Feedback 7**, refer to page 137.

Input Section 4.8: Pulseless Electrical Activity (PEA)

Yesteryear, Pulseless Electrical Activity (PEA) was known as electrical-mechanical dissociation (EMD). Either term is a descriptive designation of a phenomenon whereby electrical activity or electrical waveforms are visible on the monitor, but the patient or victim is pulseless. In other words, cardiac muscle contraction and perfusion do not follow electrical stimulation. PEA is a true cardiac emergency requiring immediate resuscitative measures, including CPR. In the presence of ventricular tachycardia (VT) or ventricular fibrillation (VF) wave forms, defibrillation is commonly the initial therapeutic intervention. When unsuccessful, intravenous epinephrine may be administered followed by further defibrillation attempts.

For rhythm patterns other than VT or VF, stimulating drugs such as epinephrine or atropine may be given in attempt to generate or speed up a slow pulse.

When the above measures fail to initiate a pulse, transcutaneous pacing is initiated.

In the adult patient, **hypoxia and respiratory failure** are the most common causes of pulseless electrical activity. Other causes include the following clinical conditions.

severe acidosis
severe hypovolemia
marked electrolyte imbalances
hypothermia
pulmonary embolism
tension pneumothorax

Beyond resuscitative measures, initial actions include diagnostic efforts to identify the precipitating cause of PEA. Once identified, therapeutic interventions are geared toward correcting or mitigating the underlying condition.

In summary of PEA, the patient is pulseless, despite the presence of electrical wave forms on the monitor. PEA represents a cardiac emergency requiring both life saving interventions as well as therapies to correct or improve the underlying clinical problem.

Practice Exercise 8

A. Indicate whether the following statements are True (T) or False (F)!

____T____ Pulseless Electrical Activity conveys the same message as Electrical-Mechanical Dissociation.

____T____ In PEA, rhythms or wave forms appear on the monitor.

____T____ CPR is the first line of intervention to treat a pulseless patient.

____T____ Treatment is focused on restoring adequate perfusion and correction of the underlying clinical disorder.

B. In the adult patient, ___hypoxia___ and ___respiratory failure___ are the most common causes of PEA.

C. Write a one sentence description of PEA._____

___wave forms are present on the monitor but the___

___patient is pulseless___

_____

_____

✔ For **Feedback 8**, refer to page 138.

Input Section 4.9: Ventricular Escape Beats and Rhythms

This is the *last* exercise of this section, so we'll keep it brief!

Since we have more or less exhausted the subject of ectopic ventricular rhythms, we now need to explore **ventricular escape rhythms.**

As previously discussed, the heart has many potential pacemakers, each with its own inherent rate of impulse formation. The more distal a pacemaker is located from the sinus node, the slower its inherent ability to pace or initiate impulses.

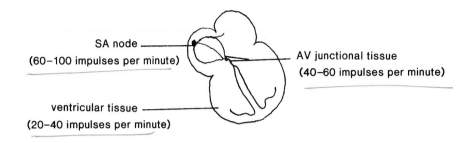

SA node
(60–100 impulses per minute)

AV junctional tissue
(40–60 impulses per minute)

ventricular tissue
(20–40 impulses per minute)

distal = lower

If the sinus node fails to discharge an impulse—or if the SA node discharges so slowly that the heart rate becomes inadequate—or if the sinus impulse fails to be transmitted, a lower (more distal) pacemaker may discharge spontaneously. That's a mouthful!

The SA node may be depressed by acute hypoxia, myocardial damage and/or reflex activity through the vagus nerve. In essence, an escape rhythm is a rhythm maintained by a pacemaker other than the sinus node, when the sinus node fails to activate the heart muscle or does so in an ineffective manner. Thus, an escape rhythm is never a primary phenomenon. An escape rhythm results *secondary* to another event or problem. Escape rhythms are *life saving mechanisms*. This should sound familiar (junctional escape rhythms were discussed on page 90)!

Escape rhythms are *generally* regular and may vary in rate from 10–100 beats per minute. If the escape rhythm is initiated in the AV junction it is called an idiojunctional rhythm (narrow QRS complex). If the escape rhythm originates in the ventricles (wide QRS, 0.12 seconds or greater) it is called an ***idioventricular rhythm*** or **a ventricular escape rhythm**.

Examine this example of an idioventricular rhythm.

The previous rhythm strip demonstrates a probable idioventricular rhythm with a heart rate of approximately 75 beats per minute. The rate is somewhat faster than the inherent ventricular rate (20–40 beats per minute), so it would be appropriate to term this rhythm an *accelerated* idioventricular rhythm. You will notice that the rhythm is regular. Escape rhythms are *almost* always regular! There are no P waves preceding the QRS complexes. Rather, *retrograde* P waves are obvious following each QRS indicating atrial depolarization followed ventricular depolarization. (Retrograde P waves are not always obvious in an escape rhythm.) Because no P waves occur before the QRS complexes, this cannot be a sinus rhythm. This cannot be a junctional (escape) rhythm because the QRS duration measures 0.12 seconds. Therefore, the rhythm is assumed to be of ventricular origin.

Examine this next example of a ventricular escape rhythm.

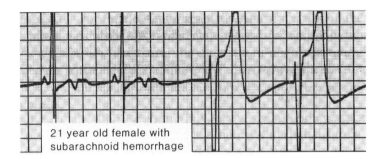

21 year old female with subarachnoid hemorrhage

The underlying rhythm here is a borderline sinus bradycardia. When the sinus pacemaker failed to initiate an impulse, a ventricular escape pacemaker assumed control of the rhythm. One might have expected an AV junctional pacemaker, rather than a ventricular pacemaker, to emerge thus commanding the escape rhythm. At times, however, a given pathology affects both the sinus and AV junction mechanisms, rendering them both incapable of effective impulse generation. Remember, escape rhythms never occur as primary disorders. When observed, escape beats or escape rhythms occur *late* in the cardiac cycle (as opposed to premature), coming *after* the next anticipated beat!

As with all ventricular impulses, *ventricular escape beats are widened, the QRS measuring 0.12 seconds or greater*. It simply takes a longer period of time for the ventricular escape impulses to depolarize the ventricles because they travel backward, outside the normal conduction system. Remember, moving horizontally across the EKG paper denotes time.

The patient with an *escape ventricular rhythm* may experience hemodynamic embarrassment owing to both the slow ventricular rate and the *loss of atrial kick*. In fact, persons with diseased myocardial tissue, particularly the patient with an acute myocardial infarction, may suffer greatly as a result of the ventricular escape rhythm, even if the heart rate is within a normal range. If the atrial contraction does not precede the ventricular contraction by the normal interval, one loses the *atrial kick*. The atrial kick is simply the residue of blood forced into the ventricles during atrial systole (contraction), just prior to ventricular systole (contraction). In other words, the atrial kick is an extra "umph" to the distended ventricles before they contract. This essentially *supercharges* the ventricles allowing for a more forceful contraction. When heart muscle damage is present, the absence of atrial kick may reduce cardiac output by as much as 25%. So, when a patient with heart damage presents with an idioventricular rhythm, he may exhibit shock symptoms owing to both the loss of atrial kick and the slow ventricular rate.

Treatment is *always* supportive in nature and is aimed at speeding up the heart rate and restoring hemodynamic equillibrium. If the SA node fires too slowly allowing a lower pacemaker to take control, treatment is focused on speeding up the rate of SA impulse discharge. Atropine is most usually the drug of choice.

If the sinus mechanism (or AV junctional tissues) cannot be successfully engaged as a higher order pacemaker, a transcutaneous pacemaker will likely be inserted until a transvenous pacemaker can be inserted under fluoroscopy. This is often necessary when an idioventricular rhythm is associated with extensive myocardial damage. (Myocardial damage associated with acute myocardial infarction will be discussed in Section 11.)

Thus, when an escape rhythm occurs secondary to failure or blockage of a higher pacemaker, treatment is aimed at speeding up the rate of ventricular impulse formation.

It is *important* to distinguish between ventricular escape beats or rhythms *and* P.V.C.s or ventricular tachycardia. Escape beats or escape rhythms are *life saving* while P.V.C.s or ventricular tachycardia may be *life threatening*.

Escape beats or escape rhythms are inscribed *late* in the cardiac cycle, occurring after the time of the next normal anticipated event.

Above, a ventricular escape rhythm emerges when the sinus pacemaker fails to initiate a timely impulse. Measure the P-P interval (see arrows) of the two sinus beats occurring at the end of the strip. Then, apply that same P-P measure to the beginning of the strip. The X indicates the location of the next expected sinus impulse. When the sinus impulse fails to fire on time, a lower more distal (ventricular) pacemaker assumes control.

P.V.C.s (or ventricular tachycardia) on the other hand, interrupt the underlying rhythm and are, therefore, inscribed *early* (prematurely) in the cardiac cycle, before the next anticipated beat.

A P.V.C. interrupts the normal underlying rhythm.

The *appropriate* treatment depends upon recognizing whether the abnormal beats are "premature" or "delayed" beats!

Of course, some rhythms are *simply* complicated! See for yourself.

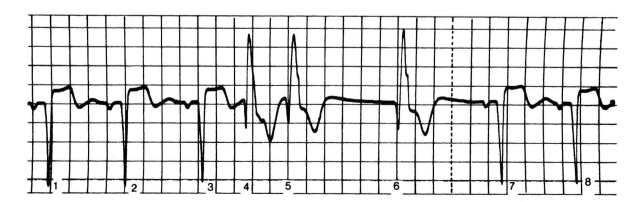

The previous rhythm strip belongs to a patient with an acute anteroseptal wall myocardial infarction. Notice that there is evidence of *both* "early" (*premature*) and "late" (*escape*) ventricular activity. Beats 4 and 5 are P.V.C.s; beat 6 is a ventricular escape beat. A situation like this is truly a *treatment dilemma*! Typically, amiodarone will be administered with a transcutaneous pacemaker available for backup.

Practice Exercise 9

A. Examine this rhythm strip carefully—then describe all that you see! What treatment might be employed?

Regular

wide QRS

no P

Rate approx 66 bpm

accelerated ventricular escape Rhythm

atropine given as tx

✔ For **Feedback 9**, refer to page 138.

✔ **Feedback 1**

You're becoming a Pro!

A. This is a sinus rhythm with a heart rate of approximately 90 per minute. Beat 6 is premature, interrupting the normal rhythm. The P-R interval of normally conducted beats measures slightly greater than 0.12 seconds. The QRS of normally conducted beats measures approximately 0.08 seconds. There is no obvious P wave in the premature complex. The QRS of the premature beat measures greater than 0.12 seconds. This is a P.V.C. and it occurs on the T wave of the preceding beat. This could initiate ventricular fibrillation!

B. The underlying rhythm is a sinus rhythm with an approximate rate of 80 beats per minute. Beat 2 and 5 occur prematurely, interrupting the underlying rhythm. Both of the premature beats have QRSs that measure 0.12 seconds or greater. The premature beats are P.V.C.s—but they do *not* look alike. So, we could say that there are multiformed P.V.C.s interrupting a sinus rhythm. The QRS of normally conducted beats measures approximately 0.10 seconds. The P-R interval of these beats measures approximately 0.14 seconds.

C. In this rhythm strip, *every other beat* is a premature ventricular contraction. This is known as *bigeminal P.V.C.s or ventricular bigeminy*!

To review then, premature ventricular contractions have the following EKG characteristics.

Characteristics of Premature Ventricular Contractions

- They occur prematurely, interrupting the underlying rhythm.
- There may be a P wave following the QRS.   *Not before*
- The QRS complexes are wide and bizarre in appearance, measuring 0.12 seconds or greater.
- There may be a compensatory pause following the premature beat.

✔ Feedback 2

We've got a winner folks!

A.   P.V.C.   Fusion Beat   P.V.C.

Sinus Beats   Sinus Beats

B. A fusion beat is an abnormal beat produced by a double stimulation. A sinus impulse is conducted normally through the atria (initiating atrial depolarization), through the AV junction, and into the ventricles initiating ventricular depolarization. At the same time, an ectopic ventricular focus fires (P.V.C.) initiating depolarization of the lower part of the ventricles. The sinus impulse and the ectopic ventricular impulses *collide* somewhere in the ventricles. Consequently, the QRS of the fusion

beat looks somewhere in between the normal sinus QRS and the P.V.C.!

Whew!

Remember, to truly identify a fusion beat, there *must* be both a sinus beat and a P.V.C. for comparison purposes. Fusion can only take place if the atrial impulse has started to penetrate the ventricles from above—so, *a P wave will always precede the abnormal appearing QRS!*

✔ Feedback 3

Dynamite!

A. The underlying rhythm is probably sinus rhythm. The underlying rhythm is interrupted by frequent bursts of ventricular tachycardia! P.V.C.s fall on the vulnerable T waves (R on T phenomenon) initiating short "runs" of ventricular tachycardia. The QRSs of the ventricular tachycardia are wide and bizarre. Amiodarone would be the probable treatment of choice.

B. This strip demonstrates ventricular tachycardia with a heart rate of 150 beats per minute.

Criteria That Assist In Identifying Ventricular Tachycardia

- The ventricular rhythm is *basically* regular.
- The rate is usually rapid, between 140--200 beats per minute.
- The P waves are usually buried in the QRS complexes, making them obscure.
- The QRS complexes are wide and bizarre.
- The ventricles are directly stimulated by an ectopic ventricular focus firing repeatedly or through a reentry process. Ventricular action is independent of atrial activity.
- Fusion or capture beats may be evident.

✔ Feedback 7

Nice work!!

A. There is no coordinated electrical activity in this strip. The activity is totally irregular. No PQRST can be seen. The baseline appears to wander or undulate. This is ventricular fibrillation. Treatment would consist of electrical defibrillation or nonsynchronized precordial shock. Until electrical defibrillation is administered and a sustaining rhythm is established, full cardiopulmonary resuscitation must be continued!

B. The rhythm is regular at a rate of approximately 187 beats per minute. No P waves can be identified. The atrial activity is probably hidden in the QRS complexes. The QRS complexes are wide (0.12 seconds or greater) and bizarre in appearance. This is most likely ventricular tachycardia. Treatment likely would consist of amiodarone administration or synchronized precordial shock. If the patient is unconscious, defibrillation may be used.

> **Criteria for Identifying Ventricular Fibrillation**
> - No PQRST can be observed.
> - Totally uncoordinated electrical activity.
> - The baseline appears to wander.
> - The baseline oscillations may be coarse or fine.*

*The rhythm strip on page 128 demonstrates a "coarse" ventricular fibrillation. The first practice exercise strip on page 130 demonstrates a "fine" ventricular fibrillation.

✔ Feedback 8

A. The following statements are all True (T)! 😊

    T   Pulseless Electrical Activity conveys the same message as Electrical-Mechanical Dissociation.

    T   In PEA, rhythms or wave forms appear on the monitor.

    T   CPR is the first line of intervention to treat a pulseless patient.

    T   Treatment is focused on restoring adequate perfusion and correction of the underlying clinical disorder.

B. In the adult patient, <u>hypoxia</u> and <u>respiratory failure</u> are the most common causes of PEA.

C. <u>PEA is a descriptive classification where wave forms are present on the monitor, but the patient is pulseless.</u>

✔ Feedback 9

How are you doing? Sometimes it's difficult to grasp ESCAPE rhythms . . . so, you may want to reread Input 9 one more time. 😊

A. The rhythm is regular with a heart rate of approximately 70 per minute. There are no P waves preceding the QRS complexes. The QRS complexes are wide, measuring greater than 0.12 seconds. This must be a ventricular escape rhythm! (One only sees an escape rhythm when higher pacemakers fail!) Typically, a ventricular escape rhythm will be slow, 20--40 beats per minute. One might call this rhythm an accelerated ventricular escape rhythm since the rate is 70 beats per minute.

    The treatment for this rhythm would depend on the cause. Any suppressant drugs (i.e., digitalis) would be discontinued. Treatment would be aimed at restoring a normal rhythm. One might attempt to speed up the SA node with atropine—or speed up a slow ventricular response rate with Isuprel or a transvenous ventricular pacemaker.

    Remember, there are no pacemakers distal to the ventricles! If the ventricular escape pacemaker fails, the patient's monitor picture may look like this. . . .

This straightline is referred to as *ventricular standstill* or *asystole*.

Notes

Notes

Conduction Disturbances and Heart Block

Objectives

When you have completed Section 5, you will be able to describe or identify

1. sinus arrest (sinus pause) and sinus block

2. atrial tachycardia with block

3. relevant history

4. first degree AV block

5. second degree AV block

   a. Mobitz type I—Wenckebach

   b. Mobitz type II

6. complete heart block

7. bundle branch block

You've come a long way!   I hope EKG interpretation has not become the focal point of your existence.

However . . . as was noted earlier, once you have a good grasp of the fundamentals, it is *repeated* practice that adds finesse!

We are now leaving the world of dysrhythmias to consider *conduction disturbances* and *heart block*. Before doing that, however, it is helpful to review the conduction system one more time.

You will notice that the bundle branch system looks somewhat different than in earlier drawings. That is because *in reality*, the left bundle branch has both an anterior and posterior division. Thus, the bundle branch system is composed of three fascicles (or little bundles) . . . the right bundle branch, the anterior fascicle of the left bundle branch, and the left posterior fascicle of the left bundle branch.

The important point to be made here is that *disease* or *toxic drug manifestations* may delay normal sinus impulse transmission or result in failure of impulse transmission from the atria to the ventricles (thus, the term *block*). This delay or interruption may occur anywhere within the conduction system!

Conduction disturbances and heart blocks are sometimes a bit confusing, so read carefully and proceed ahead!

Proceed Ahead . . .

Input Section 5.1: Sinus Arrest (Sinus Pause) and Sinus Block

---

Occasionally excessive vagal discharge, ischemic damage of the AV node, degenerative disease of the sinus mechanism or digitalis or other toxicity may interrupt the firing or conduction of the normal sinus impulse.

When this phenomenon occurs, a normal sinus rhythm may be interrupted by a pause or pauses.

Lead MCL₁

Though there are many abnormalities in the above strip, notice the pause following two normally conducted sinus beats. The pause is thought to result from failure (arrest) of the sinus mechanism.

As you inspect the previous tracing, recognize that such pauses would serve to give the patient an irregular pulse . . . therefore, one would need to count the heart rate for one full minute. If you look closely, you will notice that the next *anticipated* event during the pause is a P wave followed by a QRS. Because that anticipated P wave did not occur in a timely fashion, we assume that the sinus pacemaker did not initiate an impulse, or, if it did, it did not cause atrial depolarization. (Remember . . . the presence of a P wave tells us the atria have depolarized . . . therefore, the *absence* of a P wave tells us the atria did *not* depolarize.)

For purposes of definition, *sinus arrest* (or sinus pause) occurs when the sinus pacemaker fails to discharge an impulse at the expected time. The resulting pause is of *undetermined length*, as is demonstrated in the previous rhythm strip. Sinus arrest may be associated with degenerative disease of the sinus mechanism or drug toxicity. If the pauses are of significant duration, pacemaker therapy may be required.

Sinus block, on the other hand, exists when the sinus pacemaker initiates an impulse at the expected time, but that impulse is blocked within the sinus mechanism itself. In other words, the sinus impulse does not penetrate into the atria to initiate atrial depolarization. In this case, the resulting pause is usually predictable.

The X denotes the location of the next expected P wave.

Commonly, the pause associated with sinus block will be the same duration as the distance between two normally conducted sinus beats. SA block may be associated with vagotonia (athletes), digitalis administration, and rarely with hypokalemia. Usually, no specific treatment is required.

Interestingly enough, a true differential diagnosis between sinus arrest and sinus block cannot be established on the basis of an EKG alone . . . because all one observes is a pause (the absence of a P wave)!

Probably the best way to describe a strip like the one above is to call it a *sinus pause*, reporting the duration of that pause. (Remember, each small square represents 0.04 seconds!) In the above strip, 2.2 seconds elapse between the R wave prior to, and the R wave following, the pause.

Practice Exercise 1

Look at this strip closely . . . then describe all that you see!

_____

_____

_____

_____

_____

✔ For **Feedback 1**, refer to page 171.

Input Section 5.2: Atrial Tachycardia with Block

Remember atrial tachycardia? . . . We discussed this dysrhythmia on page 61. You will recall that atrial tachycardia is a rapid ectopic atrial dysrhythmia with an atrial rate of 160–220 per minute. Well, atrial tachycardia with rapid rates may be complicated by second degree AV block, the *physiologic* variety. This is the same *physiologic block* that we discussed earlier (page 69) . . . a protective mechanism that guards the ventricles from the effects of rapid stimulation.

Here is an artist's rendering of atrial tachycardia with block. Notice that there are two P waves for every QRS.

Atrial tachycardia with 2:1 AV block.
Ventricular rate = 100 (regular)
Atrial rate = 200 (regular)

Frequently, *atrial tachycardia with block* occurs as a manifestation of digitalis toxicity, and is therefore a contraindication for the continued administration of digitalis preparations.

Much like atrial flutter, the atrial rate in atrial tachycardia with block is described as a ratio to ventricular conduction, e.g., 2:1, 3:1, etc. In other words, there are two P waves for every QRS, three P waves for every QRS, and so forth.

In the event that you are wondering how atrial tachycardia with block differs from atrial flutter . . . remember, it's *ALL* in the atrial rate! By definition, if the atrial rate is regular at a rate of 160–220, the rhythm is atrial tachycardia. If, however, the atrial rate is regular at a rate of 220–350, the rhythm is atrial flutter!

Additionally, P waves become "saw toothed" in appearance at more rapid rates. Simple enough, right?

 Practice Exercise 2

Draw an example of 2:1 atrial tachycardia or atrial tachycardia with 2:1 block.

✔   For **Feedback 2**, refer to page 171.

Input Section 5.3: Early Studies and Relevant History

In the early days of electrocardiography, most conduction disorders were thought to occur primarily in the AV node. You will remember though that impulse transmission from the atria to the Purkinje system is electrically silent on the EKG. In other words, the P-R interval is electrically silent, representing impulse "travel time" from the atria to the Purkinje system.

P-R Interval

Looking only at the P-R interval, it is impossible to detect where in the conduction system a delay or block is occurring. In 1969, a technique to study impulse conduction was introduced—the His bundle electrogram (HBE).

Anatomically, the bundle of His lies under the membranous portion of the intraventricular septum. By positioning a catheter electrode in this area, actual depolarization of the bundle of His was recorded—allowing determinations to be made about the location of a block or delay. was In other words, the delay was determined to occur either above or below the bundle of His.

However, that was then, and this is now. Today sophisticated intracardiac electrophysiologic (EP) studies utilize multiple wires and techniques to identify questionable conduction anomalies.

In any event, the early His Bundle Electrogram studies demonstrated that conduction defects or blocks occurring above the bundle of His were usually *benign*, seldom progressing to complete heart block. Conduction defects or blocks originating below the bundle of His were more commonly associated with a *grave* prognosis!

Thus, the early HBE procedure refined the classification of heart blocks, and that knowledge continues to assist the modern practitioner. For the most part, heart (conduction) blocks can be classified in the following manner.

Heart blocks located above the bundle of His

- First degree AV block

- Mobitz Type I (Wenckebach) second degree AV block

- Complete AV block with a QRS of normal duration (less than 0.12 seconds)

Heart blocks located below the bundle of His

- Mobitz Type II second degree AV block

- Complete AV block with a widened QRS (0.12 seconds or greater)

Usually, AV conduction delays or blocks occurring *above* the bundle of His are *benign* (non-life-threatening) in nature and are frequently associated with ischemia or toxic drug effects. Conduction delays or blocks occurring *below* the bundle of His are *commonly* associated with extensive myocardial damage and therefore have poorer prognoses.

The above chart will be a useful reference as we continue on. In the event that you are confused, be assured you are progressing in a normal fashion!

Practice Exercise 3

How about some practice?

A. Label the parts of the conduction system.

B. Atrial depolarization is represented on the EKG as a _____ wave.

The P-R interval represents _____

_____

_____

_____

C. The QRS represents _____

Note: Remember, the P-R interval is electrically silent!

✔ For **Feedback 3**, refer to page 172.

Input Section 5.4: First Degree AV Block

First degree heart block is the terminology used to signify that the *P-R interval is greater than* the upper limits of normal.

 Your long-term memory should now be registering that the duration of a normal P-R interval is between 0.12–0.20 seconds, or 3–5 small EKG squares. The P-R interval represents the time it takes for the pacemaker impulse to travel across the atria, through the AV junction, down the bundle branches to the Purkinje system. Remember?

When the P-R interval is prolonged (measuring greater than 0.20 seconds) it is impossible by EKG to determine where in the AV conduction system the delay is occuring since the P-R interval is electrically silent. However, the prolongation indicates that something is holding up the show!!!

Here, it is helpful to understand earlier studies which demonstrated that first degree heart block (an abnormally long P-R interval) is *usually* due to a block somewhere *above* the bundle of His. First degree heart block is most usually a benign dysrhythmia.

Examine this rhythm strip.

You will notice that the P-R interval measures greater than 0.20 seconds (greater than five small squares). Specifically, the P-R interval measures 0.24 seconds. The P waves are of normal shape. The QRS is of normal configuration and duration (less than 0.12 seconds). *All* sinus impulses reach and activate the ventricles. The sinus impulses are merely taking longer time than expected to reach and activate ventricular depolarization. So, this is a sinus rhythm with a first degree heart block.

That's all it takes to identify a **first degree heart block!**

Because first degree heart block is usually benign (non-life-threatening), it serves only to be watched. However, *an increasing P-R interval should always be reported*. First degree heart block is most frequently associated with coronary artery disease, digitalis administration, and all types of acute myocardial infarction.

On this next strip, notice that the P-R interval measures 0.28 seconds or 7 small squares. (There is other pathology as well, but that will be discussed in later sections).

The above rhythm strip demonstrates a sinus rhythm with a first degree heart block. Most authorities note that a P-R interval may be as long as one second and still conduct!
Now review this next strip.

This strip demonstrates a sinus rhythm, rate approximately 70 per minute, with a prolonged P-R interval. The P-R interval measures *almost* two large squares, or 0.4 seconds! Thus, we have a sinus rhythm with a first degree AV block. It is always important to measure the duration of the P-R interval!

To review then, first degree heart block manifests as a *prolonged P-R interval*. Most usually, the conduction defect or block occurs intranodally, above the bundle of His. **However, if one has only a standard EKG as a tool for interpretation, the location of the block cannot be determined—all one observes is the isoelectric P-R interval**.

Practice Exercise 4

See what you can do with this!

A. Describe all that you see in this rhythm strip!

_____

_____

_____

_____

_____

_____

B. The P-R interval in the above rhythm strip measures approximately _____ small squares or
_____ seconds.

C. First degree heart block is usually benign and serves only_____.

✔ For **Feedback 4**, refer to page 172.

Input Section 5.5: Second Degree AV Block

That brings us to the subject of *Second Degree Heart Block.*

The very *best* description that I've ever heard of second degree AV block went something like this . . .

. . . "Some P's make it and some don't; those that don't, should!"

Very simple and to the point!

To complicate the understanding of second degree heart block, there are two types, Mobitz type I (Wenckebach) and Mobitz type II.

Mobitz Type I—Wenckebach

Mobitz type I, also known as *Wenckebach*, is a fun rhythm . . . **honest!**

In Wenckebach, one finds a *progressive prolongation of the P-R interval until a P wave is finally blocked* or not conducted, as demonstrated in the following strip. Commonly then, the sequential prolongation of the P-R interval repeats until the P wave is again blocked.

In the above strip, notice that the P-R interval gets progressively longer until *finally*, a P wave fails to conduct. Then, the P-R interval progression begins again.

Because the P-R interval progressively becomes longer, the ventricular response is irregular—or, one could say that there is a *varying R-R interval* . . . (the distance between any two R waves varies). In Wenckebach, or Mobitz type I, the **P-R interval lengthens**, while the **R-R interval shortens**.

The Wenckebach rhythm is usually described as a ratio, the number of P waves to QRS complexes per cycle. The following tracing would be described as a "5:4 Wenckebach" (five P waves for four QRS complexes).

A 5:4 Wenckebach pattern

A Wenckebach type of second degree heart block is most frequently associated with acute inferior wall myocardial infarction, and is probably due to ischemic damage of the AV node. The AV junctional artery fills from the right coronary artery—and it is commonly the right coronary artery involved in the inferior wall infarction. Wenckebach may also be a manifestation of digitalis toxicity since digitalis increases block in the AV junction.

Electrophysiologic studies have shown that this conduction disturbance is usually located above the bundle of His. *If associated with acute inferior wall myocardial infarction, Wenckebach will usually develop within the first 24-hours after the infarction, and usually will not persist beyond the third day.* Since we expect it to disappear within 72 hours, we merely observe it. If Wenckebach occurs secondary to digitalis toxicity, the administration of digitalis should be discontinued.

Mobitz type I, or Wenckebach, is thought to occur because of progressive fatigue in the AV junctional tissues. In other words, a sinus beat is conducted normally through the AV junction. The next impulse conducts more slowly because the AV junction is tired. Each additional impulse tends to be conducted progressively slower—until *finally*, the AV junction says, "I'm going to sit this one out boys!" When associated with myocardial infarction, the fatigue occurs secondary to ischemic changes along the conduction pathway. The AV junctional tissues become so fatigued that they are incapable of transmitting the impulse. Thus, an atrial impulse finds the AV junctional tissues *refractory* (unable to receive the next impulse), and the impulse is blocked. This gives the AV junctional conducting tissues a rest! Then, the whole process begins again!

With Wenckebach, the cycle of dropped beats may vary, giving the patient a varying radial pulse—similar to that of atrial fibrillation.

Variable cycle Wenckebach

Another significant feature of the Wenckebach cycle is that it may begin with a junctional escape beat. . . .

L Junctional escape beat

Why does that occur? Well, if the pause following the blocked P wave is prolonged, a lower, more distal pacemaker (with a potential rate of 40–60 per minute) will fire an impulse. Remember, **if the sinus node fails to discharge an impulse—*or* if the SA node discharges so slowly that the heart rate is inadequate—*or* if the sinus impulse fails to be transmitted, a lower (more distal) pacemaker will discharge spontaneously!**

P.S. If you need review of junctional escape beats, refer to page 90.

That about wraps up the subject of Mobitz type I (Wenckebach). So let's explore Mobitz type II.

Mobitz Type II

Most always, Mobitz type II blocks originate below the level of the bundle of His (in the bundle branches or the Purkinje system) and are of organic origin. Frequently, Mobitz type II is associated with acute anterior wall myocardial infarction (extensive myocardial damage).

bundle of His

NON-CONDUCTED P WAVES

On EKG, one sees, without warning, a *suddenly* blocked P wave. The P-R interval of all conducted beats is constant. The P wave that fails to conduct is neither premature nor late . . . *it occurs in rhythmic sequence with the other P waves*. Thus, throughout the rhythm strip, the P-P interval remains unchanged. The ventricular response is irregular owing to the non-conducted P waves. The duration of the QRS complexes are usually within normal limits, though the QRS may be widened depending upon the underlying pathology.

To definitely identify Mobitz II, there must be *two or more consecutively conducted* sinus impulses with a constant P-R interval before the blocked P wave.

Notice the constant P-R interval of the two consecutively conducted sinus beats in the above drawing.

In Mobitz type II, the impulse transmission failure occurs distal to or below the bundle of His. Since the impulse never reaches the ventricles, the problem is due to intermittent bilateral blockage of the bundle branches!

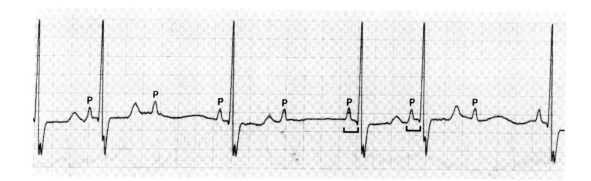

The above strip demonstrates a Mobitz type II block. Notice that the P-R interval of all conducted beats is constant and measures approximately 0.14 seconds. The nonconducted P waves occur in rhythmic sequence with the other P waves. Thus, the P-P interval remains constant. The QRS complexes are widened, measuring almost 0.16 seconds.

Remember: To definitely identify Mobitz type II heart block, one must observe two or more consecutively conducted sinus impulses in order to determine a constant P-R interval.

The patient with Mobitz type II must be monitored closely and constantly. At any point, a Mobitz type II rhythm could progress to complete heart block or ventricular standstill secondary to sustained bilateral bundle branch block.

The above strip demonstrates a Mobitz Type II rhythm that progresses (without warning) to ventricular standstill. In ventricular standstill, none of the P waves conduct. The P waves are *suddenly* blocked resulting in the absence of cardiac output. Ventricular standstill is a medical emergency that requires immediate CPR.

In the presence of a confirmed or suspected Mobitz type II rhythm, a transcutaneous pacemaker will be kept on standby. Depending on the underlying pathology and patient prognosis, consideration may be given to the insertion of a ventricular pacing wire.

You will remember from the first part of this section, the prognosis for a patient with Mobitz type II second degree AV block is usually grave. Mobitz type II is *most usually* associated with extensive myocardial damage. It is the *extent of myocardial damage* that ultimately determines the prognosis or outcome.

To review then, to *definitely* identify Mobitz type II, there must be two or more consecutive sinus impulses with the same P-R interval conducted to the ventricles before a blocked impulse occurs. The blocked sinus impulse is neither premature nor delayed.

Owing to the fact that Mobitz type II is commonly associated with extensive myocardial damage, there is usually evidence of intraventricular conduction defects. In other words, even when the sinus impulses are conducted normally, there may be some delay in ventricular activation. Therefore, the QRSs associated with Mobitz type II rhythms are *commonly* widened, measuring 0.12 seconds or greater.

Mobitz type II second degree AV block with widened QRSs measuring approximately 0.18 seconds.

2:1 AV Conduction

This "cookbook method" of looking at EKGs is not always a sure method. A patient's heart rhythm may appear like the following strip.

The above rhythm strip demonstrates a 2:1 conduction pattern, two P waves for every QRS. One cannot determine whether the P-R interval increases or stays constant because *only* one conducted beat occurs before each blocked beat. In this case, one would simply describe what is observed . . . there are *two* P waves for every QRS (2:1 conduction). The QRS complexes measure 0.12 seconds and the ventricular rate is 38 per minute! Because the P-R interval of the conducted beats is constant, we know that the atrial and ventricular activity are related.

Remember, two consecutively conducted P waves must occur in order to distinguish between Mobitz type I (Wenckebach) or Mobitz type II. Although the above rhythm is a form of second degree heart block, it is *unclear* which type, since there are *never* two consecutive impulses conducted through to the ventricles.

The following rhythm strip also demonstrates a 2:1 conduction pattern. The QRS complexes are widened, measuring 0.12 seconds.

A 2:1 AV conduction pattern associated with *narrow* QRS complexes *usually* represents a form of Wenckebach. A 2:1 AV conduction pattern associated with wide QRS complexes (0.12 seconds or greater) is *commonly* associated with a delay in conduction below the bundle of His—thus, it is *usually* a Mobitz type II block.

If only the 2:1 conduction pattern is observed, further study may be warranted to identify the origin of the block. Oftentimes, if one continues to observe a 2:1 conduction pattern, there may be a point where two sinus impulses are *consecutively conducted* to the ventricles. When this occurs, the P-R of the two consecutively conducted beats can be measured. If the P-R interval *increases*, you are *no doubt* looking at a Wenckebach rhythm! On the other hand, if the P-R interval of the two consecutively conducted beats *remains the same*, the rhythm is *probably* Mobitz type II.

In either instance, a slow ventricular rate may require augmentation. Since the sinus mechanism is healthy, atropine may serve to increase the sinus rate. Although atropine will not reduce the block, it may serve to increase overall rate of those beats which are conducted. Whew!

Practice Exercise 5

It's funny how it **always** seems to be practice time!

A. Study this rhythm strip, then describe what you see!

_____

_____

_____

_____

_____

_____

_____

_____

_____

_____

B. Describe this rhythm strip in detail!

_____

_____

_____

_____

_____

_____

_____

_____

C. What would you say about this rhythm?

_____

_____

_____

_____

_____

_____

_____

✔   For **Feedback 5**, refer to page 173.

Input Section 5.6: Complete Heart Block (CHB)

Now that you have an appreciation for first and second degree heart blocks, it is time to explore third degree, or complete heart block.

Complete heart block (CHB) is a good descriptive term. It simply means that none of the atrial impulses conduct through to ventricles to initiate ventricular depolarization.

In other words, while the sinus pacemaker discharges normally (60–100 per minute) causing atrial depolarization, none of the impulses conduct through to the ventricles.

Thus, the patient's EKG *could* look like this!

However, you will remember . . . if a sinus impulse fails to discharge or *fails to be transmitted*, a lower (more distal) pacemaker will usually take control of heart beat! Hurray for escape pacemakers!

And, that is exactly what happens in complete heart block! Because none of the sinus impulses are conducted through to the ventricles, a more distal pacemaker initiates ventricular activation.

When the AV junction is healthy (uninvolved in the underlying pathology), it will initiate the escape rhythm. Remember at idiojunctional or junction escape rhythms from Section 3?

A junctional escape rhythm with no obvious P waves.

An idiojunctional rhythm is regular with a heart rate usually 40 to 60 beats per minute. A P wave may occur before, during, or after the QRS complex. The QRS complexes are narrow, measuring less than 0.12 seconds!

When the AV junction is diseased or damaged, it may be unable to take over as the escape or safety pacemaker. When this occurs, the next lower (more distal) pacemaker located within the ventricles assumes the ventricular pacing role (ventricular escape rhythm).

Accelerated ventricular escape rhythm.

You will recall that idioventricular or ventricular escape rhythms are usually regular and slow (20–40 beats per minute), though rates may vary from 10–100 beats per minute. Ventricular escape rhythms have no P waves preceding the QRS complexes. However, P waves may be hidden in, or follow, the QRS complexes. Ventricular impulses are *widened*, measuring 0.12 seconds or greater, owing to the fact that ventricular activation is outside the normal conduction pathway.

(If you need review of idioventricular rhythms, turn back to page 131.)

     In complete heart block, none of the sinus impulses are conducted through to the ventricles . . . so, a lower (more distal) pacemaker assumes control of ventricular activation.

There is one thing you need to remember . . . both the sinus P waves and the escape rhythm will be obvious on the EKG recording. There is no failure of the sinus pacemaker or atrial activation, only a failure of impulse transmission to the ventricles. Thus, P waves will be present!

Closely examine this next strip.

First, locate all the P waves and evaluate atrail activation. Atrial activation is occurring at a rate of approximately 107 per minute (count the number of small squares between P waves . . . there are 14 small squares between P waves. So, I looked back to the chart on page 41 and found that 14 small squares yields a rate of 107 per minute).

Next, evaluate ventricular activity. The QRSs are occurring regularly and slowly at a rate of less than 30 per minute. If I wanted to know the exact rate, I could count the number of small squares between the QRS complexes

. . . that comes to 55 small squares. The chart on page 41 does not give the rate for 55 small squares, so I could do the calculation myself! Divide 55 into 1500 . . . there are 1500 small squares in a one minute time interval.

$$55\overline{)1500}^{\,27}$$

So, the ventricular rate in this strip is about 27 beats per minute. *Ugh*!

The QRS complexes measure 0.16 seconds in duration. Thus, we know the escape rhythm is most likely of ventricular origin.

Now comes the important question, *Are atrial and ventricular activity related? No*! The P-R interval is *never* constant in complete heart block.

There are two *independent*, or asynchronous, pacemakers (atrial and ventricular) bearing no relationship to one another! Thus, the two pacemakers are dissociated. Hence, we have a new term . . . *AV dissociation*.

Criteria for Complete Heart Block

- The atrial and ventricular rates are different—the atrial activity is independent of, or dissociated from, ventricular activity (*AV dissociation*).

- The atrial rate (P waves) is faster. No sinus impulses are conducted through to the ventricles.

- The ventricular rate (QRS complexes) is slow and regular.

- The QRS complexes may be narrow (less than 0.12 seconds) or wide (0.12 seconds or greater).

  Junctional escape rhythms have narrow (less than 0.12 seconds) QRS complexes; ventricular escape rhythms have widened QRS complexes (0.12 seconds or greater).

- The P-R interval is never constant.

Important Note: The term *AV dissociation* is a nonspecific generic term that may be applied to any rhythm where the atria and ventricles are activated independently. This independent activation will be evidenced as a varying P-R interval. AV dissociation is never a primary disorder; rather, it is a descriptive term.

Complete heart block with QRS complexes of normal duration (less than 0.12 seconds).

Sometimes, in a complete heart block, the P waves are hidden in other wave forms. We assume they are really there! *P waves are said to be "marching" through the rhythm.* (Personally, I didn't know that P waves marched . . . but I bet John Phillip Sousa would have been happy to know that.)

When QRS complexes measure within normal limits (less than 0.12 seconds), the defect in complete heart block is *usually* in the AV node. In this case, complete heart block usually develops *gradually* as a *progression* from *Wenckebach, Mobitz type I*. Commonly, ischemia resulting from an inferior wall myocardial infarction or digitalis toxicity are the *culprits* responsible for this rhythm! When complete heart block is intranodal in origin, the QRS complexes are narrow and the ventricular rate generally averages 40–60 per minute. Past studies have indicated that complete heart block of intranodal origin has a lower mortality rate than any other form of complete heart block.

Complete heart block associated with widened QRS complexes (0.12 or greater) is usually a manifestation of bilateral bundle branch block (Mobitz type II) and is almost always associated with *extensive* myocardial damage. The ventricular rate in this instance is usually less than 40 per minute. This type of complete heart block can lead to ventricular standstill with dramatic suddenness. The mortality rate has been estimated to be 80%.

Treatment for complete heart block is aimed at managing the underlying condition and supporting or augmenting the ventricular rate.

Complete heart block of intranodal origin (QRSs measuring less than 0.12 seconds) may be observed and not treated if the ventricular rate is adequate for perfusion. This is often the case when associated with inferior wall myocardial infarctions. If necessary, atrophine may be administered to increase the rate of the junctional escape pacemaker. When digitalis toxicity is the causative culprit (as confirmed by a serum digitalis level), digitalis administration is discontinued.

Complete heart block resulting from a blockage below the bundle of His (QRSs measuring 0.12 seconds or greater) poses a greater mortality risk owing to its common association with extensive myocardiam damage. In addition to therapeutic interventions aimed at reducing myocardial workload (to be discussed later in this text), a transvenous pacemaker may be inserted to augment ventricular activation and/or serve as a backup should ventricular activiation fail (ventricular standstill).

The above strip demonstrates complete heart block with a QRS duration of 0.13 seconds. The ventricular rate is 29 beats per minute! Note that the P-R interval is never constant and the P waves *march* through the rhythm. The atrial and ventricular pacemakers are functioning independently.

This next rhythm strip demonstrates ventricular standstill.

Ventricular Standstill (no evidence of ventricular activity).

In ventricular standstill, none of the atrial impulses reach and activate the ventricles, and a lower more distal pacemaker fails to emerge. This is an extreme emergency warranting immediate C.P.R. and the application of a transcutaneous pacemaker (TCP). TCP will be discussed in Section 8.

> **NOTE:** When looking at rhythm strips, a *general rule* to remember is . . . if the P-R interval is *never* constant, the rhythm can only be *Wenckebach* or *complete heart block* (CHB). Wenckebach has a *varying* R-R interval or irregularly occurring QRS complexes. CHB usually has a *regular* R-R interval—the QRSs occur in a regular pattern.

Bonus: Remember atrial fibrillation, the irregularly irregular rhythm with an undulating baseline? (If you need review, turn back to page 73.)

There is *one* instance where one will find an atrial fibrillation with a ***regular*** ventricular response. When a complete heart block exists, all chaotic atrial impulses will be blocked. A lower more distal pacemaker will then assume the role of pacemaker. Thus, the monitor tracing will show undulating atrial activity and a slow, regular ventricular response!

Let's try some practice!

 Practice Exercise 6

A. Complete heart block means that _____

_____

_____

_____

B. When atrial impulses are blocked or fail to conduct to the ventricles, a lower more distal pacemaker will usually take over, initiating ventricular activation. This back-up mechanism for ventricular activation is known as an _____.

C. If an escape rhythm has QRS complexes measuring less than 0.12 seconds and a rate of 40–60 beats per minute, it is probably a/an _____ rhythm. If an escape rhythm has a slow rate (20–40 beats per minute) and widened QRS complexes, it is usually a/an _____ rhythm.

D. Describe this next rhythm strip in detail. Evaluate both atrial and ventricular activity. Then, determine if there is a relationship between the two activities.

_____

_____

_____

_____

✔ For **Feedback 6**, refer to page 173. **Nice work**!

Input Section 5.7: Bundle Branch Block

Blocks, blocks and more blocks!

You will probably be happy to know that this is the last exercise in this section!

We now need to think about **Bundle Branch Blocks** (BBB).

When one speaks of bundle branch blocks, he or she is actually referring to a trifascicular system. You will remember that the left bundle branch has two branches or fascicles. So, the two bundle branches (right and left) have three conducting segments or fascicles (little bundles). That's where we get the term *trifascicular*!

As seen above, the common left bundle branch divides into two separate fascicles early in its course through the ventricles. The anterior fascicle is longer, thinner, and has a single blood supply. In contrast, the posterior fascicle is shorter, thicker, and has a double blood supply.

Using these three fascicles, there are *11* types of block which could exist: bundle branch blocks, hemiblocks, bifascicular blocks, and trifascicular block! To *simplify* this matter, we will concentrate on right bundle branch block (RBBB) and complete left bundle branch block (LBBB)!

Bundle branch block implies that for some reason, conduction through either of the main bundle branches (right or common left) has been delayed or interrupted. This delay causes ventricular activation and depolarization to occur more slowly, causing the QRS to widen, measuring 0.12 seconds or greater.

Bundle branch blocks have a *multitude* of causes. The more *frequent* causative factors include coronary artery disease, myocardial infarction, hypertensive heart disease, excessive potassium intake, rapid tachycardia, and pronestyl or digitalis toxicities. Treatment of either right or left bundle branch block consists of managing the *underlying* disorder.

We will first consider right bundle branch block (RBBB) since it occurs twice as commonly as left bundle branch block.

Right Bundle Branch Block (RBBB)

Right bundle branch block (RBBB) occurs when conduction through the right bundle branch is delayed or interrupted. This delay or interruption may be associated with almost any variety of heart disease, hypertensive cardiovascular disease, right ventricular hypertrophy, or congenital lesions involving the septum. Occasionally, RBBB may be found in an otherwise healthy individual!

In RBBB, an atrial impulse is conducted normally through the atria and through the AV junction. A blockage in the right bundle branch, however, causes right ventricular activation to occur more slowly. And, you now know that slow ventricular depolarization is recorded as a widened QRS, 0.12 seconds or greater.

So, on the monitor, one would see a P wave and a normal P-R interval because the defect is confined only to the right bundle branch. The left ventricle is activated in a normal fashion. The right ventricle is stimulated by an impulse from the left bundle branch which passes to the right side of the septum below the block. This *abnormal* activation of the right ventricle requires a greater duration of time . . . thus, the QRS is widened.

Let's see if we can put that into perspective.

① Septal activation occurs normally, from right to left. If we are monitoring from a right chest lead V_1, the force of septal depolarization moves toward the positive electrode. Thus, the initial part of the QRS is directed upward. You will recall from page 20, the R wave is the first *upward* or *positive* deflection of a QRS complex. If a second positive deflection is observed in the QRS, it is also an R wave (the larger of the R waves is designated as R′; the smaller R wave is designated by a lower case r). ② Next, the free wall of the left ventricle depolarizes. This time, the direction of depolarization is away from the positive electrode, so the next part of the QRS is directed negatively. ③ Last, the right ventricle is stimulated abnormally, with the direction of depolarization moving toward the positive electrode.

Lead V_1 ⊕

So, what does the QRS look like . . . you guessed it! In lead V_1, there are two R waves! And, because of the abnormal right ventricular activation, the QRS is widened! Neat, huh! Remember, when the force of depolarization moves *toward* a positive electrode, the resulting deflection is *upright*, or positive. Likewise, when the force of depolarization moves *away from* a positive electrode (toward a negative electrode) the resulting deflection is *downward*, or negative. If you need a quick review of leads, turn back to page 8! ☺

One can identify a bundle branch block on a monitor tracing by the widened QRS. Everything else about the rhythm is usually normal (at least in "textbook" cases)!

In order to *distinguish* right from left bundle branch block, however, it is necessary to look at the V leads. V leads (V_1–V_6) are the positive chest leads that look directly at the heart (for a refresher, see page 7).

EKG Criteria for RBBB

- QRS measures 0.12 seconds or greater.
- Wide and slurred S waves in lead I, V_5, and V_6
- rsR′ (M pattern) in V_1 and V_2.
- PQRST relationship is normal.
- Secondary ST and T wave changes.

Right Bundle Branch Block Lead Patterns

Lead I   Lead V_1 Lead V_2 Lead V_6

Remember, to distinguish right from left bundle branch block, one must look at the V leads! I have difficulty remembering all of that, so I just remember . . .

In RBBB, the QRS in lead V_1 will appear wide and positive . . . (more or less of an "M" pattern).

No matter which lead one observes, the QRS will be widened, at least 0.12 seconds. This next strip is a lead V_1 monitor trace demonstrating RBBB.

The rhythm is regular at a rate of approximately 80 beats per minute. P waves precede each QRS complex. All P waves are uniform. The P-R interval is of normal duration. The QRS complexes are uniform, occur regularly, and measure approximately 0.16 seconds. The QRS is widened and positive. In lead V_1 a positive, wide QRS characterizes right bundle branch block.

So, this is a sinus rhythm with RBBB!

Right bundle branch block occurs twice as commonly as left bundle branch block and frequently develops with changes in heart rate—especially tachycardias. RBBB is *generally* a consequence of occlusion of the anterior descending coronary artery, and is generally associated with extensive myocardial damage. Most authorities agree it is probably the extent of myocardial damage that determines the patient's prognosis. Treatment is supportive.

Rate Dependent Bundle Branch Block

Now, rate dependent bundle branch blocks will be explored. Conducting tissues that are diseased may only be capable of conducting normally when the heart rate is slow. If that rate is speeded up, there may be delayed conduction or no conduction at all. The involved conducting tissue must have time to recover from its refractory period if it is to conduct normally. If recovery time is insufficient, conduction will be delayed. When conduction through a bundle branch is delayed, the monitor shows a widened QRS complex (a bundle branch block pattern). The delay in a bundle branch is due to unequal refractoriness of the bundle branches.

In a rate dependent bundle branch block, a patient will present with a normal rhythm. If his heart rate increases over a certain point, he will exhibit a bundle branch block pattern. The diseased conducting tissues are unable to recover as quickly at faster rates, so conduction occurs abnormally (wide QRS complexes). When the heart rate slows, conduction will again be normal. This is known as *rate related* or *rate dependent bundle branch block*. Most commonly, the defect in rate related bundle branch blocks occurs in the right bundle branch. That's a mouthful.

Examine this monitor tracing.

The first five complexes demonstrate a sinus rhythm with a heart rate of 75. When the heart rate increases to 80 beats per minute, conduction is *abnormal*. When this patient's heart rate approaches 80 beats per minute, his diseased conducting system requires *more* time for recovery. Notice that at the faster rate, the QRS is widened and positive. Since this is lead V_1, we are looking at a rate related right bundle branch block. Neat huh?

Left Bundle Branch Block (LBBB)

Left bundle branch block (LBBB) occurs when conduction through both segments or both fascicles of the common left bundle is *delayed* or *interrupted* as demonstrated on the next page. This delay or interruption is often associated with coronary artery disease, diseases that produce left ventricular hypertrophy, and congenital lesions involving the septum.

LBBB may be associated with either inferior or anterior wall infarction depending upon the coronary vessel supplying the common left bundle branch.

Common Left Bundle Branch

In LBBB, atrial impulses conduct normally through the atria and through the AV junction. A blockage in the common left bundle branch causes depolarization of the septum and left ventricle to occur *more slowly*. In left bundle branch block, the right ventricle is activated in a normal fashion. The left ventricle is then activated by an impulse from the right bundle branch which passes to the left side of the septum below the block. Thus, activation of the left ventricle is delayed causing a widening of the QRS.

Again, let's put this into perspective as seen from a right chest lead, V_1 ⊕

① Septal activation is abnormal, moving left to right. The force of septal depolarization moves away from the positive V_1 electrode. Thus, the initial part of the QRS is directed negatively. ② The right ventricle depolarizes normally, with the direction of depolarization moving toward the positive electrode. So, the second part of the QRS will be upwardly directed. ③ Left ventricular activation occurs abnormally, moving away from the positive electrode, thus taking additional time.

The "textbook" picture of LBBB in a V_1 lead is that of a *distorted* W. Usually, however, the W is not well defined, appearing more as a V. See for yourself!

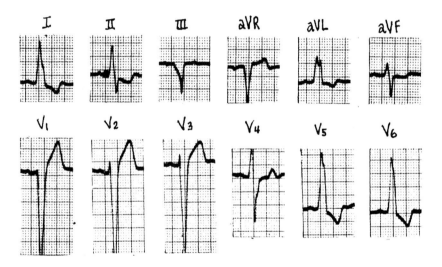

To distinguish left from right bundle branch block, one must look at the V leads.

EKG Criteria for LBBB

• QRS measures 0.12 seconds or greater.

• QRS is wide and may be notched—the T wave is usually inscribed in the opposite direction to the R wave in most leads.

• W or V pattern seen in leads V_1 and V_2.

• M pattern (rsR′) seen in leads V_5 and V_6.

• Secondary ST and T wave changes.

If this is complicated, just remember . . .

In LBBB, the QRS in lead V$_1$ will appear wide and negative.

No matter which lead one observes, the QRS will be widened . . . measuring 0.12 seconds or greater. Here is a V$_1$ monitor tracing showing LBBB. Notice that the widened QRS measures almost 0.16 seconds. Also notice the distortion (elevation) of the ST segment. The ST segment distortion results from the delayed activation of the left ventricle. In other words, altered activation of the left ventricle causes repolarization (ST segment) to be altered, as well.

In the above strip, the rhythm is regular at a rate of 62 beats per minute. P waves precede each QRS complex. All P waves appear uniform. The P-R interval is of normal duration. The QRS complexes are uniform, occur regularly, and measure almost 0.16 seconds. The QRS is wide and negative. In lead V$_1$, a widened and negative QRS characterizes left bundle branch block. So, this is a sinus rhythm with LBBB!

Though *rate dependent* bundle branch block is usually the result of delayed right bundle branch conduction, it occasionally occurs because of delayed left bundle branch conduction! See for yourself! Following is a rate dependent left bundle branch block. The first two complexes demonstrate a LBBB pattern, with a heart rate of approximately 62. When the heart rate slows to approximately 52 (as demonstrated in the remaining complexes), the LBBB pattern disappears.

Rate dependent left bundle branch block.

It is easy to be fooled by widened QRSs . . . always look for preceding P waves! If a single P wave occurs before each widened QRS and the P-R remains constant, a bundle branch block exists. If no P wave is observed before the widened QRS, the beat is likely of ventricular origin!

To clarify any confusion . . . . . . *Remember* . . .

If a rhythm appears normal except for a widened QRS (measuring 0.12 seconds or greater), the patient has a bundle branch block. To distinguish between a right and left bundle branch block, inspect lead V_1.

> LBBB = QRS is wide and negative in lead V_1
> RBBB = QRS is wide and positive in lead V_1

It is the extent of myocardial damage or physiologic concern causing a bundle branch block that determines the patient prognosis. Treatment is aimed at the underlying pathology.

Practice Exercise 7

Are you ready for more practice? **Practice, practice, practice** . . . this is worse than piano lessons!

A. This is lead II patient monitor tracing.

The rhythm is regular with a heart rate of approximately 88 beats per minute. The P-R interval is constant (0.19 seconds). Each QRS complex is preceded by a P wave, and all P waves appear uniform. The QRS complexes, however, are widened, measuring slightly greater than 0.12 seconds.

> Generally speaking . . .
>   There are only two types of rhythm patterns that demonstrate widened QRSs . . . ventricular rhythms and rhythms associated with bundle branch block. Ventricular rhythms **do not have P waves preceding the widened QRSs**.

So, since there are definitive P waves in the above monitor tracing, this must be bundle branch block. **But which type . . . right or left????**
Turn to the next page to solve the mystery.

To determine whether this rhythm is a right or left bundle branch block, one must inspect the V leads—particularly V_1 and V_6. Remember, all V leads (V_1–V_6) are $\oplus$ leads.

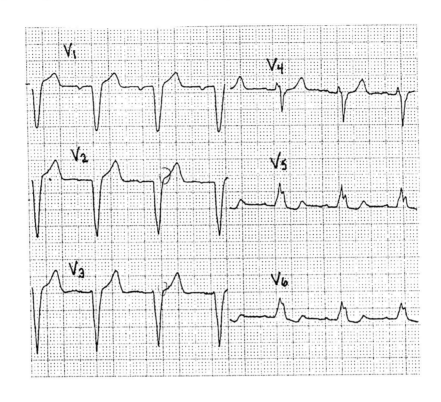

Here are the V leads—all six of them! *Determine whether this rhythm is a right or left bundle branch block and explain your logic.*

_____

_____

_____

_____

_____

_____

_____

_____

_____

_____

_____

_____

_____

_____

_____

_____

_____

_____

B. Another patient has the following lead II monitor tracing.

Everything appears normal—**except** that the QRSs measure 0.14 seconds. To be within normal limits, the QRS duration must be less than 0.12 seconds!

Because you are a *suspicious* creature, you review both the patient's chart and a recent 12-lead EKG. Following are the EKG precordial or V leads! Use the lines provided below to present your analysis and conclusion(s).

_____

_____

_____

_____

C. The following rhythm strip "belongs" to a 78 year old female and demonstrates a rate-related or rate dependent right/left (circle one) bundle branch block.

V_1

Describe the above rhythm strip and justify your conclusion. What do you think might have precipitated the rhythm change?

_____

_____

_____

_____

_____

_____

✔ For **Feedback 7**, refer to page 174.

✔ **Feedback 1**

How did you do? Hope your interpretation resembles mine!

The rhythm is irregular owing to an obvious pause! The rhythm is a sinus rhythm with P waves preceding each QRS and a constant P-R interval, measuring slightly greater than 0.16 seconds. The QRS duration is within normal limits measuring 0.8 seconds. There is a pronounced pause in the sinus mechanism. A P wave fails to occur at the expected time. The pause measures 2.52 seconds!

✔ **Feedback 2**
Good work!

← Atrial tachycardia with 2:1 block

Atrial rate regular between 160-200 per minute. I flattened out T waves so that P waves would be more prominent.
(Don't forget, the P-R is always constant!)

✔ **Feedback 3**

A.

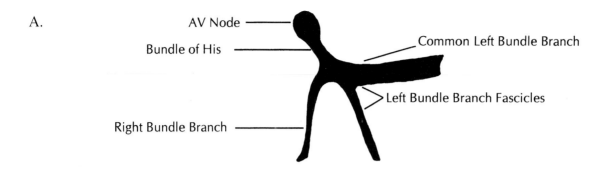

B. Atrial depolarization is represented on the EKG as a P wave. The P-R interval represents <u>the transmission of the pacemaker impulse from the atria to the Purkinje system.</u>

C. The QRS represents <u>ventricular depolarization.</u>

✔ **Feedback 4**

Excellent work!

A. The rhythm is regular with a heart rate of approximately 100 beats per minute. P waves precede each QRS. The P waves are uniform in appearance, sitting on the down slope of the previous T waves. The QRS complexes are narrow, less than 0.12 seconds. But, voila! The P-R interval is prolonged. The P-R interval measures approximately 7½ small squares or approximately 0.30 seconds. The QRS measures 0.08 seconds. So, this is a borderline sinus tachycardia with a first degree heart block!

$$
\begin{array}{r}
0.04 \\
\times\ 7.5 \\
\hline
0.30
\end{array}
$$

B. The P-R interval in this rhythm strip measures approximately <u>6</u> little squares or <u>0.24</u> seconds. The QRS measures approximately 0.08 seconds.

$$
\begin{array}{r}
0.04 \\
\times\ 6 \\
\hline
0.24
\end{array}
$$

C. First degree heart block is usually benign and serves only <u>to be watched</u>. However, if the P-R interval is increasing, digitalis preparations should be withheld.

✔ Feedback 5

Great Job . . .

If your answers look something like mine!

A. The rhythm is irregular. One of the P waves is not followed by a QRS complex. The P-R interval of the conducted beats gradually lengthens until finally a P wave is not conducted. The R-R interval shortens. The cycle then begins to repeat. This is "our friend" **Wenckebach**, usually a <u>benign</u> arrhythmia.

B. This rhythm is irregular and one must become a detective to discover why. There are three cycles that appear identical. The P-R interval of the first beat (first cycle) measures 0.20 seconds. The P-R interval of the second beat (first cycle) measures almost 0.24 seconds. This same pattern is evident in complexes 3 and 4 (the second cycle), and 5 and 6 (third cycle). This is a Wenckebach (Mobitz type I) rhythm. The P wave that fails to conduct (after beats 2, 4 and 6) is somewhat obscured, though it follows the T wave and is "flat" in appearance.

C. The rhythm is regular with a heart rate of approximately 45. There are two P waves for every QRS. Atrial activity is regular. The QRS complexes are widened, measuring approximately 0.12 seconds. This is a 2:1 AV conduction with widened QRS complexes. This may be a Mobitz type II AV block, so it should be observed *closely*! **In order to distinguish between a Mobitz type I and type II, two beats *must* be conducted consecutively so one can determine the constancy or progression of the P-R interval**.

✔ Feedback 6

Nice work.

Awesome!

A. Complete heart block means that <u>none of the sinus impulses are being conducted to the ventricles to initiate ventricular depolarization</u>.

B. When atrial impulses are blocked or fail to conduct to the ventricles, a lower more distal pacemaker will usually initiate ventricular activation. This back-up mechanism for ventricular activation is known as an <u>escape rhythm</u>.

C. If an escape rhythm has QRS complexes measuring less than 0.12 seconds and a rate of 40–60 beats per minute, it is probably an <u>idiojunctional or junctional escape rhythm</u>. If an escape rhythm has a slow rate (20–40 beats per minute) and widened QRS complexes, it is usually an <u>idioventricular or ventricular escape rhythm</u>.

D. P waves are occurring in a regular pattern at a rate of 83 per minute. The P waves appear to be "marching" through the rhythm strip. Two QRSs are apparent at a rate of approximately 28 per minute. The QRS complexes are narrow, measuring less than 0.12 seconds. There is no relationship between the P waves and the QRS complexes. The P-R interval is <u>not</u> constant. The P-R interval of the two conducted beats measures 0.24 and 0.28 seconds, respectively. This is complete heart block with an idiojunctional escape rhythm.

Complete heart block has the following features

• Atrial and ventricular rates are different.

• The atrial rate is faster.

• The ventricular rate is slow and regular.

• The QRS complexes may be narrow or widened.

• The P-R interval is <u>never</u> constant—the P waves appear to be "marching" through the rhythm strip.

✔ **Feedback 7**

A. This is a left bundle branch block. The QRS in V_1 is wide (measuring slightly greater than 0.12 seconds) and negative.

B. This is a sinus rhythm (rate approximately 70 beats per minute) with right bundle branch block! The QRS measures approximately 0.14 seconds and V_1 demonstrate a wide, positively directed QRS.

C. The rhythm strip demonstrates a rate-related (right)/left bundle branch block. The underlying rhythm is a sinus rhythm. The first two complexes occur at a rate of 68 per minute and are conducted normally (QRS measures less than 0.12 seconds). When the heart rate increases to near 100 per minute, a widened QRS is evident. In lead V_1, the widened QRS has a crude M pattern. When the heart rate again slows, normal conduction is evident. An unsuccessful attempt to climb over the side rails precipitated this event!

Notes

Notes

Artifact . . . To Be, or Not To Be . . .

Objectives

When you have completed Section 6, you will be able to describe or identify

1. electrical artifact encountered in monitoring

2. appearances and sources of artifact

   a) 60-cycle interference

   b) motion artifact

   c) signals from therapeutic electrical devices

   d) "off the monitor"

3. concerns associated with artifact

4. principles of artifact recognition

5. steps to reduce or eliminate artifact

Text by:
Delores D. Schultz

Input Section 6.1: Introduction to Artifact

Now that you have been through most of all of the basic dysrhythmias, you may need a change of pace.

Sometimes you will observe "things" on a monitor that have nothing whatsoever to do with electrical conductivity of the heart. These unusual patterns are commonly known as *artifact* or *electrical interference.*Other popular words are "glitches" or "noise." Artifact is an electrical signal which appears on the tracing and which originates from sources other than the heart!

Let's try another simple analogy.

This is a kid watching cartoons on Saturday morning.

Here is the mother in the next room cleaning . . . and . . . she turns on the vacuum.

Instantly, above the noise of the vacuum, the mother hears, **"okay, what's wrong with this picture?"** The picture looks like this:

What is a mother to do???

   a. Kick the television.

   b. Send it off for repair.

   c. Turn off the vacuum.

Fortunately, this mother chose alternative c. The restored picture now looks like this.

And the kid looks like this.

In this case, there was nothing wrong with the television *and* there was nothing wrong with the vacuum. Simply stated, *the impulses generated by one electrical device in operation interfered with the correct operation of a second electrical device*. The precise electrical theory behind all of this is very complicated . . . at least, *I* think so.

If the mother plugs the vacuum into a different outlet, she may discover that the T.V. is working fine and the kid still looks like this . . .

. . . or, she may elect to finish vacuuming at some later time!

A monitoring system attached to a patient acts much like the television. The monitoring system picks up electrical signals from the heart and transmits them to an oscilloscope. If another electrical device is in operation nearby, electrical signals generated from that device may be picked up by the monitoring system as well, thus interfering with the monitor picture. What you see on the monitor might look like this.

Like the T.V. and the vacuum, the patient's heart *and* the electrical device are probably operating correctly . . . it's just that the electrical device is altering the monitor picture. *Whew!*

To expertly monitor a patient, one needs to recognize artifact when it appears, distinguish it from a patient's rhythm, and take appropriate steps to minimize the artifact.

Practice Exercise 1

Now for a short practice session:

Fill in the blank

A. "Glitches" or "noise" on the monitor tracing are known as _____ , or electrical interference.

True or False (Use a T or F to correctly answer Questions B. and C.)

B. ____ The presence of artifact is a signal that there is a disturbance in the heart's electrical activity.

C. ____ The presence of artifact is an indication that an electrical device in proximity to the patient is malfunctioning.

Fill in the blank

D. To monitor a patient's rhythm effectively, one needs to _____ artifact when it appears, _____ it from the patient's rhythm, and take appropriate steps to _____ it.

Not too difficult so far, huh?

✔ For **Feedback 1**, refer to page 194.

Input Section 6.2: Sixty-Cycle Interference

There are several different types of artifact commonly encountered in monitoring. This tracing shows 60-cycle interference.

Sixty-cycle interference is characterized by a *wide, fuzzy baseline* which often makes atrial activity difficult to recognize. A "good" tracing should have a narrow, distinct baseline. Monitors may normally show a few seconds of 60-cycle interference when they are first turned on. If the interference persists, it is usually related to *faulty electrode contact*. Poor electrode contact is usually the result of inadequate skin preparation techniques, dried electrode gel, or defective wires or patient cable. Of course, if the patient is using an electric razor, turning the shaver off may resolve the problem!

The source of 60-cycle interference is the current which supplies power to the electrical wall outlets.

 The 60-cycle energy is given off by the electrical wiring in the patient's room and is picked up by both the lead wires and the patient. This is *normal*, and this radiant energy *cannot be eliminated*. Although monitors are designed to reduce 60-cycle interference, there must still be good contact along the path from the patient skin to the monitor, *and* the electrical path must be well shielded.

Specific interventions (*anti-artifact techniques*) include checking to see that the EKG cable is not draped across, or parallel to, other cables (such as call-light, electric bed, or transducer cables). Also, the EKG cable must not touch the metal parts of other electrical equipment such as side rails of electric beds or metal portions of ventilators. Make certain there are no loose connections in the monitoring system. It may be helpful to apply new electrode patches (using correct skin prep) and/or replacing the cable. If these techniques are unsuccessful, biomedical personnel should be called to evaluate and correct the problem.

Now, it's your turn. You are officially commissioned as a "troubleshooter" or a detective. This is a patient's monitor tracing. Notice the broad baseline.

And, here is the patient.

What should one do?

   a. Nothing.

   b. Notify the *managing* physician regarding a rhythm change.

   c. Try moving the cable away from the call light cable.

If you chose c, the patient's tracing now looks like this:

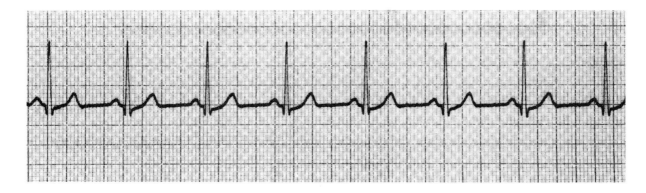

Nice work!

Practice Exercise 2

A. Sixty-cycle interference is characterized by a _____ baseline.

B. Identify at least five ways to reduce 60-cycle interference:

1. _____

2. _____

3. _____

4. _____

5. _____

✔   For **Feedback 2**, refer to page 194.

Input Section 6.3: Motion Artifact

Following is an example of motion artifact.

A Fairy Tale: Long, long ago in a CCU far away, a nurse saw the previous tracing on a monitor. Mr. Jones, the patient, had not been looking too well prior to this "picture." The nurse raced to the room and administered a resounding thump on the patient's chest. Mr. Jones stopped brushing his teeth, leaped from the bed, and was out of the door in a flash, never to be seen again. ☺—The End

The moral of the story . . . *look* (before) *the patient leaps*!

Motion artifact can be the *most troublesome* and *confusing* type of artifact, even for the "so-called" experts! Many patients have undeservedly been thumped on the chest or given antiarrhythmic drugs for this kind of tracing. If the nurse had examined the patient before thumping, (she) would have had the first clue that this was artifact rather than ventricular tachycardia. If the nurse had checked the patient's pulse, (she) would have noted that (his) pulse was regular at a rate of approximately 80.

In the above monitor tracing, you will notice (see arrows) sharp deflections throughout the entire tracing (which just happen to coincide with the patient's pulse). These deflections are QRS complexes. Since ventricular

contraction follows ventricular depolarization (QRS), and ventricular contraction results in a pulse, you can usually verify the presence or absence of QRS complexes by checking the patient's pulse. (Neat trick, huh?)

Believe it or not, the *skin* is the source of the small electrical signals which produce motion artifact. A voltage of several millivolts can be generated by stretching the outer layer of skin, the epidermis. It is the stretching which results in the artifact. *Large baseline shifts* occur when the patient turns over in bed, brushes his teeth, taps an electrode, etc.

The above strip demonstrates an example of a shifting baseline. If an electrode is placed close to the diaphragm, even the skin movement produced by breathing will cause artifact!

Following are some examples of motion artifact.

The notorious toothbrush artifact

In the above strip, the artifact might be mistaken for atrial flutter. Did you notice, though, that the R-R interval (the distance between any two R waves) remains precisely the same when the "supposed flutter" converts to sinus rhythm? In other words, measure the R-R interval at the beginning of the strip and compare that to an R-R interval at the end of the strip. Voila! It's the same! This would *seldom* occur if an actual atrial flutter were converting to a sinus rhythm! There is usually a pause when atrial flutter stops, and then, a different ventricular rate when the sinus node takes over. Makes sense, right?

Following is another patient (like the one in the fairy tale), brushing his teeth. This monitor tracing sent a "rescue squad" rushing to the patient's room in belief that the patient was in ventricular flutter. Can you find the narrow spikes appearing in the tracing at a rate of approximately 95 per minute? Those are the patient's normal QRS complexes . . . and correspond to the patient's pulse. When in doubt, check the patient's pulse. If the patient is alert and in no distress, it is highly unlikely that he or she has a heart rate of 300!

This is the same patient a few seconds later still brushing his teeth, but now his underlying rhythm is more visible! Notice that there is no change in the QRS rate from the previous strip. This constant rate strongly suggests that the underlying rhythm is the same as in the previous strip. If there is any doubt in your mind about a rhythm, always assess the patient. *It is especially important to compare the patient's pulse with the monitor picture.*

Following are two other tracings displaying artifact mimicing ventricular dysrhythmias. In strip A, the patient is swinging his monitor cable. In strip B, an electrode is being tapped. (*Some smart patients learn that if they tap an electrode, someone will appear immediately.*) By now, you can easily discern artifact! The narrow electrical spikes "walk through" the artifact and correspond to the normal QRS complexes.

A.

B.

The next strip is more difficult! See for yourself on the top of page 185.

↑
Baseline shift

The above tracing would send almost anyone running for "the antiarrhythmic drug dujour," *including* me. There are two clues that indicate this might possibly be artifact. The first clue is the shift in the baseline that occurs before the onset of what appears to be "ventricular flutter." This shifting baseline strongly suggests patient movement. The second clue relates to the termination of the "ventricular flutter." When a patient converts from a ventricular tachycardia or flutter to a sinus rhythm, there is *almost always* a *pause* before the sinus pacemaker resumes. It is important to note that in this tracing, the ventricles would not have sufficient time to repolarize before we see the first normal QRS. If this were a true ventricular tachycardia or flutter (rather than artifact), the sinus beat following the termination of the ventricular ectopic rhythm would *usually* be widened since the ventricular recovery period is incomplete.

What should one do if unable to decide between artifact and what might be a run of ventricular tachycardia or flutter? Here are four *possible* actions, although step 3 is most important.

1. Get another opinion. Two or three, or more, heads are often better than one when it comes to deciphering a puzzling strip.

2. If the patient's *managing* physician is present, let him or her diagnose the rhythm and determine the treatment.

3. Check with the patient. He may admit to the fact that he was idly *tapping* his electrode . . . or you might catch him brushing his teeth!

4. If still unable to decide, amiodarone or lidocaine would be the treatment of choice. It is better to treat the rhythm than to risk the consequences of further serious ventricular dysrhythmias.

Following are more examples of motion artifact.

The above monitor pattern demonstrates a *wandering baseline*. It is the result of pronounced, slow patient movements, such as stretching, turning over in bed, and so forth.

The patient above is receiving *chest percussion* and drainage (for respiratory disorders). *Motion* from seizure activity or muscle tremor could also produce this pattern. It is usually impossible to diagnose atrial dysrhythmias with this type of artifact. (Brilliant, right?!)

This next tracing demonstrates one type of respiratory artifact.

Notice the *cyclic* variation in the QRS amplitude and configuration, as well as in the T waves. Chest wall movement during normal respiration can produce cyclic changes in the baseline, the QRS amplitude, and the T wave appearance! When assessing a patient, one can usually correlate (his) respiratory cycle with the changes that appear on the monitor.

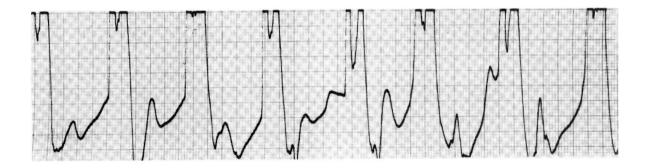

The above tracing is an example of what may be observed when a patient is coding. The artifact is produced by chest compression, or CPR. In order to visualize the underlying rhythm, compression must be stopped momentarily. The underlying rhythm is obvious when chest compression is momentarily interrupted, as evident on the rhythm strip at the top of page 187.

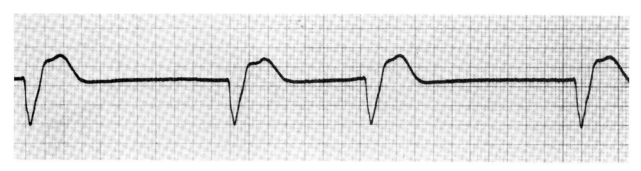

(Just in case your memory has failed, this is an idioventricular rhythm!)

The foremost responsibility in dealing with motion artifact is to *recognize it* as artifact! Accurate analysis will prevent unnecessary patient treatment and will prompt one to take steps to eliminate the artifact. *It is important to eliminate the artifact so that any underlying dysrhythmias will not be masked.*

Some of the same *principles* for eliminating 60-cycle interference also apply to motion artifact. Correct skin preparation and ample gel on the electrode patches can effectively reduce motion artifact. To prevent cable and wire movement, clip the cable to the patient's clothing. Perhaps there is an underlying clinical problem which may need medical treatment. Check to see if the patient is having tremors, seizure activity, or an increase in movement because of discomfort or confusion. Ask the patient to lie quietly or assist (him) in doing so to better analyze the underlying rhythm. Respiratory artifact can be minimized by monitoring on a lead where the positive electrode is *not* directly over the diaphragm, for example, lead I. (Remember the bedside version of lead I? . . . For a quick review, turn back to page 11.) Motion artifact can generally be reduced by *attaching the electrodes over bony areas* rather than over skin folds, large muscle masses, joints, or large amounts of fatty tissue.

Always check the patient before treating any dysrhythmia. Remember, one should . . .

Treat the patient, not the monitor

Practice Exercise 3 . . . Your Turn

A. Motion artifact commonly results from electrical signals produced by the _____.

B. Describe how you can determine this tracing demonstrates motion artifact rather than ventricular tachycardia.

_____

_____

_____

_____

_____

C. List at least three steps one could take to reduce the motion artifact in this tracing.

1. _____

2. _____

3. _____

✔ For **Feedback 3**, refer to page 195.

Input Section 6.4: Artifact Produced by Electrical Devices

More artifact . . . ugh!

The next type of artifact to be discussed originates from *signals* produced by therapeutic *electrical devices*. This artifact appears as little "blips" on the monitor tracing. Two types of electrical devices, *pacemakers* and *pain control devices* (TENS), may produce these little blips!

The above tracing demonstrates pacemaker signals, or spikes, produced whenever a patient's pacemaker fires in an attempt to trigger an electrical impulse in the heart. In this particular strip, the only electrical activity one sees originates from the pacemaker. There is no electrical activity arising in the patient's heart and needless to say, *this patient is in trouble*! The *rhythmic motion* (roller coaster) artifact present is probably the result of chest compressions. Pacemaker spikes may have a positive, negative, or biphasic deflection, and their amplitude will vary depending on the lead. Usually, lead II will demonstrate prominent pacemaker spikes. Section 8 will provide an in-depth overview of pacemakers and paced rhythms.

When the above patient was admitted to a monitored stepdown unit, the artifact present on his tracings caused quite an uproar until the staff became aware that the patient had a *TENS* unit. *TENS* stands for a *transcutaneous electrical nerve stimulator*. People who suffer from various types of chronic pain may experience pain reduction or elimination by wearing this electrical device. Whenever this TENS unit was turned on, the monitor tracing appeared like the one above. In order to obtain a meaningful 12 lead EKG and monitor tracing, the TENS unit had to be turned off periodically.

How about a simple practice exercise?

Practice Exercise 4

A. Little "blips" or spikes occurring on a monitor tracing usually originate from adjacent electrical

equipment. Two of the *most*-frequent electrical equipment culprits are _____

and _____.

B. Pacemaker spikes may be nearly invisible or they may have a larger amplitude than the patient's QRS complexes. This variation in amplitude often depends on the _____.

✔ For **Feedback 4**, refer to page 195.

Input Section 6.5: "Off the Monitor"

The following tracing is from a patient who is "off the monitor." The straight line, indicating the absence of rhythm, may be mistaken for asystole. If you have experience with monitors, you already know that the most common cause of an "asystole-appearing" tracing is a loose electrode. Rarely do patients go directly from a normal rhythm to the complete absence of any rhythm! Reattaching the wire or electrode will restore the normal rhythm to the scope.

"Off the monitor"

At this point, however, I am reminded of a little lady who, in fact, did go into asystole (the absence of rhythm) from her normal rhythm. The "rescue squad" went to her room immediately to reattach the electrode and found themselves calling a code. Here the maxim is, *"look at the patient—immediately."*

In most monitoring systems, all of the electrodes must be attached to the patient in order for a tracing to be present. If the wires come loose at either end, if an electrode patch comes loose, or if a wire is broken internally, the tracing will disappear.

In the above strip, the amplitude setting (gain) was decreased causing the tracing to nearly disappear. When a monitor can no longer "sense" the QRS complexes, a rate alarm may be activated.

When a patient looks like this . . .

and her tracing looks like this . . .

there are several steps one may take to solve the problem.

Steps for correcting "Off the Monitor"

- Reattach any disconnected wires.

- Check to see that the cable is attached to the monitor.

- Check electrode patches for intactness and replace any loose patches, making certain than an ample amount of gel is present.

- Replace lead wires.

- Check for a defective cable by replacing the cable.

- Check the amplitude setting to see if the amplitude is set correctly.

Sometimes a patient intermittently goes "off the monitor" and the tracing looks like this!

This type of tracing is produced by intermittent interruption of the continuous path from the patient to the monitor. It may be remedied by all the same actions that one might take if the patient were completely "off the monitor."

Practice Exercise 5

Make a run at this one!

A. Describe what has happened in this tracing:

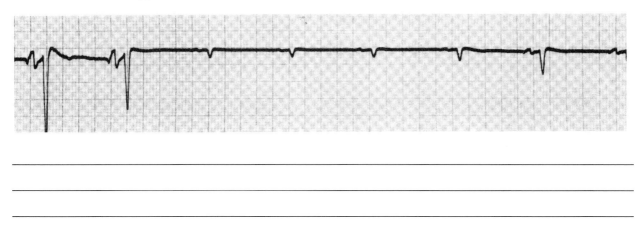

_____
_____
_____
_____

B. Name at least three steps one can take to correct "off the monitor."

"Off the monitor"

_____
_____
_____
_____
_____
_____

✔ For **Feedback 5**, refer to page 195.

Input Section 6.6: Concerns Associated with Artifact

There are two major concerns associated with artifact. The **first** is that artifact may *mimic* atrial or ventricular dysrhythmias and cause treatment to be initiated unnecessarily. (Even if one does not treat the patient, it may cause you unnecessary worry.) With a little practice you will be able to look at a tracing and recognize that something is "wrong with the picture," rather than the patient.

Here is a list of *clues* that may assist you in *determining* the presence of artifact.

Clues for Identifying Artifact

- Baseline should be fine, narrow lines.

- QRS complexes *must* be followed by T waves. Whenever ventricular depolarization occurs, ventricular repolarization must follow. A T wave is always preceded by a QRS complex. If one observes a T wave in the middle of nowhere, chances are, this is an artifact.

- A change in supraventricular rhythm, e.g., atrial flutter to sinus rhythm or vice versa, is usually accompanied by a change in ventricular rate.

- Cells in the heart cannot be depolarized by two impulses simultaneously. They must repolarize after the first impulse before they can be depolarized by a second. If one observes portions of normal QRS complexes superimposed on a run of "ventricular tachycardia," the "V tach" is probably artifact. Whew! ☺

- P waves should have an established rhythm and a logical configuration. P waves do not usually appear out of nowhere, except sometimes in digitalis toxicity or sick sinus syndrome. If P waves occur prematurely in the cardiac cycle, there should be a pause before the next P wave is observed.

- Patients rarely go from a normal rhythm to a straight line rhythm. Usually, "off the monitor" relates to a disconnected electrode or patch. However, **always** check the patient.

If you are still uncertain after considering all of the above points, obtain a second opinion, and remember—look at the patient!

The **second** major concern is that artifact may *mask* underlying dysrhythmias which deserve or warrant treatment. With experience, you will be able to determine the cause of the artifact and then proceed with appropriate measures to reduce or eliminate it. For troubleshooting steps, refer back to the specific type of artifact covered in this section.

Prevention

There are two simple actions one can take to prevent or reduce artifact and the associated problems. The *first* is assuring the presence of conductive gel. (If electrode gel is partially dry, problems with 60-cycle interference and motion artifact will be magnified and intermittent loss of tracing may occur. Completely dry gel will result in the *absence* of any tracing.) To prevent drying, store the electrodes in their original foil package until ready for use. Keep the package tightly closed and avoid storing the container in warm areas. Use the electrodes prior to the expiration date on the package and check each one for adequate gel before applying it to the patient.

A *second action* to help prevent artifact is correct skin preparation before electrode application or reapplication. To defat the skin, that is, to remove oils, rub the skin with an alcohol gauze pad prior to electrode application. Avoid using acetone which is more irritating, produces less contact, and is a fire hazard!

Preventing, recognizing and coping with the various kinds of artifact is an ongoing function of cardiac monitoring. The ability to recognize and eliminate artifact is a skill which will assist one in monitoring patients safely, effectively, and efficiently. However, *recognizing artifact is a function of monitoring experience*! *I* do not expect you to remember all the details in this section, though a periodic review of this material may be helpful. (Personal note from the management!)

Practice Exercise 6

A. QRS complexes must be followed by_____, and T waves must be preceded by _____.

B. When you see QRS complexes superimposed on a "run of ventricular tachycardia," the "V tach" is probably _____.

C. Describe three methods for storing electrodes to prevent drying of the gel.

    1. _____

    2. _____

    3. _____

D. _____ is the best compound for defatting the skin.

✔ For **Feedback 6**, refer to page 196.

✔ Feedback 1

You probably have answered all the practice exercises correctly. If so ... ***Hooray!***

A. "Glitches" or "noise" on the monitor tracing are known as <u>artifact</u>, or electrical interference.

B. False. (The presence of artifact is *NOT* a signal that there is a disturbance in the heart's electrical activity.)

C. False. (The presence of artifact is *NOT* an indication that an electrical device in proximity to the patient is malfunctioning.)

D. To monitor a patient's rhythm effectively, one needs to <u>recognize</u> artifact when it appears, <u>distinguish</u> it from the patient's rhythm, and take appropriate steps to <u>minimize</u> it.

✔ Feedback 2

You are quickly becoming an expert! ⭐ (color this gold)

A. Sixty-cycle interference is characterized by a <u>wide</u>, <u>fuzzy</u> baseline.

B. Any of these are acceptable answers:

    1. Make certain that the EKG cable is not draped across, or parallel to, other cables such as call-light, electric bed, or transducer cables.

    2. Make certain that the EKG cable is not touching the metal parts of other electrical equipment.

    3. If possible, try momentarily pulling the plug of any other electrical equipment in contact with the patient to see if the artifact disappears.

4. Tighten any loose connections in the monitoring system.

5. Apply new electrode patches using correct skin preparation.

6. Check for the presence of sufficient gel on the electrode patches.

7. Replace any defective wires.

8. Try a different monitor cable.

✔ Feedback 3

You are becoming more skillful at coping with artifact!

A. Motion artifact commonly results from electrical signals produced by the <u>skin</u>.

B. This is a bit more difficult!

1. The beginning of the strip demonstrates motion artifact that is fairly obvious and does not look like ventricular tachycardia. This gives one a clue that the patient is moving.

2. During the portion that looks like "V tach," one can still walk the normal QRS complexes through the strip, and in most cases, one can see portions of the normal QRS.

3. A QRS complex occurs immediately after the cessation of "V tach." In true ventricular tachycardia, there is usually a pause before a normal QRS appears.

C. Any of the following responses are correct.

1. Check with the patient to see if you can help reduce excessive patient motion.

2. Make certain all the electrode patches are secure and that sufficient gel is present.

3. Secure loose wires.

4. Replace defective wires.

5. The wandering baseline could be due to respirations. Try changing the location of the positive electrode slightly or try switching to a lead I.

(Perhaps you can think of others that I neglected to mention!)

✔ Feedback 4

You're doing super!

A. Little "blips" or spikes occurring on a monitor tracing usually originate from electrical equipment. Two of the *most* frequent electrical equipment culprits are <u>pacemakers</u> and <u>pain control devices</u>.

B. The variation in amplitude often depends on the <u>lead</u>.

✔ Feedback 5

You know almost everything there is to know about artifact!

A. Someone has decreased and then increased the amplitude setting. (Sometimes your *tricky* cohorts may try to fool you.)

B. Any three of these actions can be considered:

   1. Make certain that all electrodes are intact.

   2. Make certain that the monitor cable is plugged in.

   3. Check for defective wires and replace if necessary.

   4. Check for a defective cable by replacing the cable.

   5. Check the amplitude setting and adjust if necessary.

✔ Feedback 6

You are truly an expert! (If you have not *absolutely* mastered this material, do not panic.) You may wish to refer back to this chapter for future help when problems with artifact develop.

A. QRS complexes must be followed by T waves and T waves must be preceded by QRS complexes.

B. When you see QRS complexes superimposed on a "run of ventricular tachycardia," the "V tach" is probably artifact.

C. Methods for storing electrodes to prevent drying of the gel include:

   1. Keeping the electrodes in their original foil package.

   2. Closing the package tightly.

   3. Avoiding storage in warm areas.

   4. Using the electrodes prior to their expiration date.

D. Alcohol is the best compound for defatting the skin.

Notes

Notes

Cardioversion and Defibrillation

Objectives

When you have completed Section 7, you will be able to describe or identify

1. refractory and vulnerable phases of the cardiac cycle
2. synchronized precordial shock or cardioversion
3. nonsynchronized precordial shock or defibrillation
4. automatic external defibrillator (AED) functioning

Input Section 7.1: Refractory and Vulnerable Phases of the Cardiac Cycle

In previous sections, reference was made to *precordial shock* as a treatment option for uncontrolled rapid dysrhythmias producing hemodynamic imbalance. To appreciate precordial shock treatment, one must have an understanding of the cardiac cycle.

Each cardiac cycle has an **absolute refractory period** during which time the tissues are immune or resistant to further electrical stimulation. A brief **vulnerable period**, essentially encompassing the T wave, follows the refractory period. It is during the vulnerable period that an electrical stimulus (a shock from a live electrical source, lightening, a P.V.C. occurring in an ischemic heart, etc.) can induce ventricular fibrillation.

The vulnerable period, the T wave, can actually be thought of as having two parts. The first half of the T wave is relatively refractory to electrical stimulation, meaning that a sufficiently strong electrical current would be necessary to stimulate action. The middle and latter half of the T wave is truly the vulnerable period, requiring only a minimal electrical stimulus to initiate a response.

Thus, when electrical stimulation (precordial shock) is used as a therapeutic intervention to disrupt rapid dysrhythmias, a method of delivery must prevent the shock from occurring during the vulnerable period (the T wave) to avoid the risk of ventricular fibrillation. Avoiding the vulnerable period is achieved by synchronizing the timing of the electrical shock to the patient's rhythm, specifically to the R wave of the QRS (the refractory period). Precordial shock introduced during the refractory period will avoid the risk of ventricular fibrillation.

Synchronization of the defibrillator unit to the patient's rhythm is achieved by connecting a cable from the patient's EKG recording device (EKG machine or monitor) to the defibrillator unit. Once connected, a *synchronization option* (or button) is selected on the defibrillator unit. The defibrillator unit is then able to *sense* the tall R wave of the QRS cycle. Occasionally, the gain or amplitude setting will need to be increased for the R waves to be sensed.

R

The defibrillator unit will have an indicator (usually a blinking light) that signals the sensing of R waves. Each time the light blinks, it's saying "I see an R wave, I see an R wave" . . . etc.

Artifact

In addition, the monitoring device will show an artifact above each R wave. The artifact also indicates that the defibrillator unit is reading or sensing the R wave of each QRS complex. Now, no matter when in the cardiac cycle the buttons for releasing the electrical energy are pressed, the defibrillator unit will not deliver the energy until it senses the R wave! The synchronized defibrillator does *all* the work.

In essence then, this synchronization prevents the electrical shock from occurring during the vulnerable period (T wave).

The following rhythm strip illustrates a rapid supraventricular tachyarrhythmia. Because the patient's clinical condition was rapidly deteriorating, the treatment objective was to terminate the rapid rhythm as quickly as possible. Though the location of T waves or vulnerable periods are difficult to discern, we *know* that each time the heart muscle depolarizes, there is a rest or recovery period (T wave).

Often, the fastest and most effective way for terminating such a rhythm is synchronized cardioversion (through intravenous drug intervention may be the initial choice of treatment). When electrical shock is initiated as the primary or secondary treatment, the defibrillator unit must be synchronized with the patient's heart rhythm—because the accidental induction of ventricular fibrillation is non-therapeutic!! Delivering synchronized precordial shock to the patient's chest wall causes a critical mass of myocardial cells to depolarize or discharge. This momentarily stops or interrupts all myocardial activity. Hopefully, the patient's sinus pacemaker will then resume as the controlling pacemaker, restoring a normal rhythm! (Of course, the patient may need ectopic-suppressing drugs to prevent any abnormal rhythm from breaking through again. Other treatment options might include ablation, discussed on page 67.)

Usually, a *minimal* current setting is all that is required to disrupt a rapid supraventricular rhythm. Commonly, the current setting ranges from 10–250 watt/seconds or joules. However, it is good to remember that the current setting will vary with patient size and the dysrhythmia being treated, considering whether or not the patient has been receiving digitalis or other drugs.

There are two types of precordial shock, *synchronized* and *nonsynchronized*. Synchronized precordial shock is most usually referred to as **cardioversion**. Nonsynchronized precordial shock is referred to as **defibrillation**.

Defibrillation is the treatment of choice for ventricular fibrillation, the chaotic, uncoordinated, ineffective depolarization of the ventricles (for review, refer to page 128) and for pulseless ventricular tachycardia. Remember, CPR must be instituted immediately upon the recognition of ventricular fibrillation or the determination of pulselessness.

Earlier it was noted that QRS completes must be present (are required) to achieve synchronization and deliver synchronized precordial shock. When QRS complexes are *absent, defibrillation* or *non-synchronized* precordial shock is used.

Both synchronized cardioversion and defibrillation work on the same principle. Electrical energy of brief duration is delivered through the chest wall. This shock causes depolarization (release of energy) of a critical mass of myocardial cells, thus halting or disrupting the chaotic or ectopic activity, and hopefully allowing the sinus pacemaker to resume control of the rhythm.

Review the following rhythm strips demonstrating ventricular fibrillation.

1.

2.

The first strip depicts a *coarse* ventricular fibrillation; the second strip displays a *fine* ventricular fibrillation. (The second tracing resembles atrial fibrillation *without* the QRSs!) To interrupt the chaotic ectopic activity, precordial shock must be instituted. . . .

. . . but which kind?

synchronized, or non-synchronized?
cardioversion, or defibrillation?

Ah-ha! Since no QRSs are present, it is *impossible* to use synchronized precordial shock! As a matter of fact, if one set or programmed the defibrillator unit to deliver synchronized shock, the machine would **never** release the energy through the paddles. It would hold the energy until it "sensed" an *R wave* . . . which would never appear! Thus, because QRS complexes are absent, non-synchronized precordial shock or defibrillation would be used.

With non-synchronized precordial shock or defibrillation, the energy is delivered through the paddles at any point during the chaotic rhythm, as soon as the "energy delivery" button(s) is pressed. Usually, a high current setting is used—between 200 and 400 watt/seconds or joules of energy (depending upon the patient's size and chest wall thickness).

It should be noted that there are two *general* types of defibrillators. The hospital type (referenced on the previous pages) is a manual device requiring the clinician to determine the underlying cardiac dysrhythmia, make treatment decisions, and program the defibrillator accordingly. Hospital defibrillator units have three capabilities: defibrillation; synchronized cardioversion; and, external pacing.

A second type of defibrillator unit, an **automatic external defibrillator (AED)** is a "grab and go" unit used by fire departments, airlines, rescue squads and certain large businesses for the treatment of cardiac emergencies. An AED is a battery-powered portable unit equipped with adhesive electrodes, electrical circuitry, and an internal microprocessor for interpreting rhythms. The AED unit includes diagrams for guiding the placement of electrodes and usually has both visual and audio prompts. Essentially, the AED senses and analyzes the underlying cardiac rhythm, then advises (prompts) the operator whether electric shock is needed (shock/no shock). When electrical shock is needed (ventricular fibrillation/ventricular tachycardia), the AED automatically calculates and delivers a predetermined amount of energy (joules), though most units allow a manual override for alternate current settings. In the presence of ventricular tachycardia, the AED senses the QRS configuration and synchronizes the timing of energy release to avoid current delivery during the vulnerable phase of a cardiac cycle. AED units come with treatment algorithms and can both record and print monitor tracings.

As this text goes to press, the FDA is evaluating a foreign AED (FRED easyport) that is small enough to be worn on the belt. The unit is light weight and uses a pulsed biphasic waveform, allowing the same efficiency using less energy.

Additionally, the FDA approved *over-the-counter* sales of an in-home defibrillator with programmed audio directions.

CRITICAL NOTE: Owing to variation in defibrillator equipment (both portable and manual models), the practitioner is strongly cautioned to become familiar with devices available for use. Initial training and periodic "hands-on" reviews are required to maintain competency. In cardiac emergencies, speed is critical. In the face of ventricular fibrillation (pulselessness), chances of survival decrease approximately 7–10% each passing minute. Defibrillation within the first 3–4 minutes affords the best chance for survival. Immediate CPR is required for any pulseless event and should be continued until the "all standback for defibrillation" command is given. If defibrillation is unsuccessful, CPR should be reinstituted immediately. Clinicians and *field-warriors*, alike, should stay abreast of current resuscitation guidelines published by the American Heart Association (ACLS Guidelines).

Practice Exercise 1

Let's see how much you remember!

A. Here is a QRS complex. Draw and label the refractory and vulnerable periods.

B. Refractory means that _____

_____

_____

_____

C. Vulnerable implies that _____

_____

_____

D. In synchronized precordial shock, or _____ the defibrillator unit

will deliver its energy *only* on _____ of the EKG cycle.

E. When defibrillation or non-synchronized precordial shock is used, the defibrillator unit will deliver its

energy

_____

_____

_____

F. Following is a rhythm strip of a patient experiencing severe chest pain and a falling blood pressure.

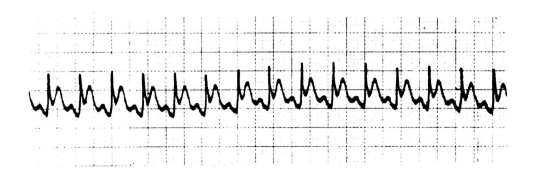

This rhythm is an _____. Because the clinical condition is deteriorating rapidly, it has been decided to administer precordial shock to terminate the ectopic rhythm. Cardioversion / defibrillation (circle one) would be used because _____

_____

_____

_____

G.

The rhythm strip above is that of a code arrest victim. _____ precordial shock would be administered because there are no _____ complexes present!

H. The abbreviation AED stands for _____.

✔   For **Feedback 1**, see page 206.

✔ Feedback 1

A.

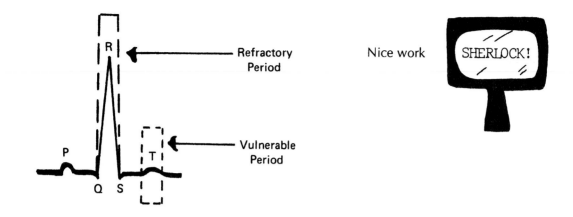

B. Refractory means that <u>this phase in the cardiac cycle (the QRS) is immune to any additional electrical stimulation</u>.

C. Vulnerable implies that <u>this phase in the cardiac cycle (the T wave) is extremely sensitive to any electrical stimulation. Electrical stimulation during the vulnerable period may induce ventricular fibrillation</u>.

D. In synchronized precordial shock, or **cardioversion**, the defibrillator unit will deliver its energy <u>only</u> on the **R Wave** of the EKG cycle.

E. When defibrillation or non-synchronized precordial shock is used, the defibrillator unit will deliver its energy <u>as soon as the energy delivery buttons are pressed anywhere in the chaotic rhythm</u>.

F. This rhythm is <u>atrial tachycardia</u>. (For a quick review of atrial tachycardia, see page 67.)

<u>Cardioversion</u> would be used because <u>QRS complexes are present and principally to avoid the risk of inducing ventricular fibrillation</u>.

G. <u>Non-synchronized</u> precordial shock or defibrillation would be administered because there are no <u>QRS</u> complexes present!

H. The abbreviation AED stands for <u>automatic external defibrillator</u>.

Notes

Notes

Pacemaker Basics

Objectives

When you have completed Section 8, you will be able to describe, identify or define

1. the purpose of pacemaking

2. indications for pacemaker support

3. pacemaker generated heart rhythms

4. pacemaker sensing and capture

5. pacemaker identification codes

6. common pacemaker modes

Text by
Stephanie L. Woods, Ph.D., R.N.

Section 8 is included to provide a *basic* overview of cardiac pacemakers. Pacemakers can be used temporarily or permanently to pace the heart when the normal conduction tissue is unable to generate a normal or adequate rhythm. Pacemaker technology has become very sophisticated over the past many years. Pacers have evolved from simple ventricular demand mode to multi-programmability. This chapter will briefly overview the principles of pacemaking. Further study will be required to understand the many different types of pacemakers.

Input Section 8.1: Pacemaker Fundamentals

Cardiac pacemakers, often called pacers, are small battery powered generators used to deliver electrical stimulation to the myocardial muscle when the normal conduction tissue of the heart fails to generate adequate beats per minute. The functions of the pacer depend upon the type of pacemaker inserted and the programmability of the generator.

General Purposes for Pacemakers

- To provide electrical stimulation when the SA node has failed and the AV node or Purkinje fibers cannot provide an adequate back-up rhythm

- To generate a heart rate that creates an adequate cardiac output and stable blood pressure

- To generate atrial contractability in lower generated pacer rhythms (junctional and ventricular), improving ventricular filling

- To override (outpace) ectopic tachycardic rhythms

Types of Pacemakers

There are two basic types of pacemakers: temporary and permanent.

Temporary pacemaker generator

Permanent pacemaker generator

<u>**Temporary pacing**</u> **can be accomplished by:**

➤ Inserting a pacing wire (pacing catheter) into the right atrium and into the right ventricle via the subclavian vein. The end of the pacing catheter is visible outside of the patient's body and is attached to an external generator. **This is called <u>transvenous pacemaking</u>.**

Temporary pacemaker

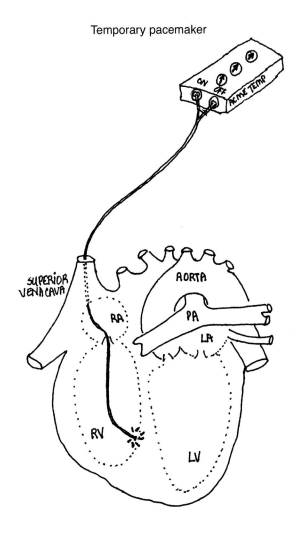

➤ Applying a large electrode patch to the anterior and the posterior chest surfaces over the heart. Pacing wires are attached to each patch and a pacing module that is part of a defibrillator unit acts as the generator. An electrical impulse is applied directly to the skin over the heart and conducts from the anterior to the posterior patch, thereby stimulating contraction of the heart muscle. **This is called transcutaneous pacing. This type of pacing is used for minutes to hours until a transvenous or permanent pacemaker is inserted.**

➤ During heart surgery, temporary pacing wires can be applied directly to the epicardium (the outer surface of the heart). One wire can be placed directly onto the right atrium, and another wire directly onto the right ventricle. These wires are brought out through the skin and usually coiled up and taped to the patient's chest. They can be attached to an external pacing generator if the need arises. **This is called epicardial pacing**.

Permanent pacing is accomplished by inserting a pacing wire into the right atrium and into the right ventricle via the subclavian vein, as well. However, the permanent pacing wire is much shorter than the temporary wire and is not visible outside the patient's body. The permanent pacing wire is attached to a small generator that is implanted underneath the patient's skin, usually below the clavicle, near the shoulder.

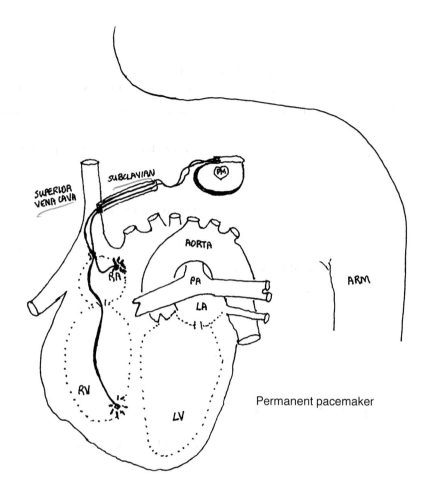

Permanent pacemaker

Special Note: In both temporary and permanently implanted pacemakers, the pacemaker wire(s) is placed in the right heart muscle wall. This is because the pacer wires are inserted transvenously, via the superior vena cava which enters the right atrium.

Temporary Pacemaker Lead Placement

• Right ventricular muscle wall

Permanent Pacemaker Lead Placement

• Right ventricular muscle wall (ventricular pacer only)

or

• Right atrial and right ventricular muscle wall (atrio-ventricular)

Pacemaker stimulation induces cell depolarization in the placed chamber(s). Electrical impulse (mA) is delivered at the point of lead implant. That wave of depolarization then spreads outward, activating all myocardial muscle cells . . . more or less of a domino effect!

Anatomy of a Pacemaker

Both tempoorary and permanent pacemakers have the following standard parts:

➤ Generator—The generator is the power source for the pacer. Electrical energy or output is measured in milliamperes (mA). Electrical output can be varied from 0.1 to 20 mA. Pacemakers are powered by batteries. Temporary pacers can use simple 9 volt mercury zinc batteries where permanent pacemakers usually use lithium batteries. Lithium batteries can have a life span of ten years or greater.

➤ Wires/Electrodes—All pacemakers must have pacing wires with electrodes. Wires attach to a generator. The generator provides the electrical energy that flows down the pacer wire. The pacer wire is inserted into the heart until the pacer wire comes in contact with the myocardium. When energy flows down the pacer wire, the myocardial muscle should contract in response.

➤ Rate setting—Rates can be widely varied in pacers, depending upon the pacer's intended use. If the pacer is to be used to create an adequate ventricular rhythm the rates may be set between 40 and 80 beats per minute. If the pacer is to be used to overrride an etopic rhythm such as atrial tachycardia, the rate may vary between 150 and 350 beats per minute.

➤ Mode—The mode describes the primary function of the pacer. Most modern pacers are programmable, allowing for varying functions. The mode may be as simple as single chamber pacing or as complex as atrial and ventricular pacing with several programmed responses.

➤ Sensivity—Sensivity refers to the ability of the pacer to "sense" or know when the patient is having his own heart beat. When the patient is having his own beat, the pacer should not deliver a stimulus at the same time.

Indications for Pacing: Short-Term and Long-Term

Pacemakers can be used temporarily or permanently, depending upon the clinical problem or patient condition.

Temporary pacemakers are used for crisis intervention and anticipated short-term support.

➤ Examples of crisis intervention:

• Third degree AV block

• Symptomatic bradycardia

• Cardiac arrest

➤ Examples of short-term support:

• Second-degree AV block following cardiac surgery

• Insertion of a temporary atrial pacing wire to override a patient's atrial tachycardia

Permanent pacemakers are inserted for long-term rhythm disturbances such as sinus bradycardia, sinus arrest, heart blocks, sick sinus (brady-tachy) syndrome, tachyarrythmias such as P.A.T., and atrial fibrillation with a slow ventricular rate.

Recognizing Pacemaker Rhythms

Pacemaker generated rhythms have three characteristics that distinguish them from normal rhythms. These characteristics are: ① the presence of pacemaker artifact; ② larger than normal atrial and ventricular wave formations; and ③ a rate not lower than the pacemaker "set" rate. Read on for detail!

① **When a pacemaker fires an electrical impulse, one will typically see what is known as pacer spikes or pacer artifact on the EKG.** These spikes are usually about five boxes tall (5mm).

- If the pacemaker is an atrial pacer (single lead), one will see this spike just prior to the P wave (these are very rarely used!)

- If the pacemaker is a ventricular pacemaker (single lead), one will see this spike just prior to the QRS.

A Demand Ventricular Pacemaker

A demand pacemaker generates beats when the patient's heart rate falls below a set (programmed) number.

In the above strip, the pacemaker senses a patient's own ventricular activity (beats 1, 2, and 3). Thus, the pacemaker does not discharge a stimulus. When a ventricular beat fails to occur at the expected time (pause following premature beat 3), the pacemaker begins firing. Note the pacemaker spikes occurring before beats 4–7.

- If the pacemaker is an atrio-ventricular (AV sequential, dual lead) pacer, one will see spikes before both the P wave and the QRS.

When a patient requires atrial depolarization and contraction to increase ventricular filling in addition to ventricular pacing, an AV sequential pacer is inserted. The AV sequential pacemaker achieves synchronized atrial and ventricular functioning.

Dual Lead AV Sequential Pacing

In the above schematic, note both the atrial spike prior to the P wave and the ventricular spike prior to the QRS. An AV sequential pacer requires the placement of two leads.

An AV Sequential Pacemaker

The above strip is an example of an AV (atrial/ventricular) sequential pacemaker. Here the generator paces both the atrium and the ventricle, in sequence, and upon demand. In other words, when patient-generated atrial and ventricular activation fails to occur, the pacemaker initiates first an atrial, and then a ventricular (sequenced) stimulus. This dual sensing and pacing requires a two lead pacemaker system! The advantage of an A-V sequential pacemaker is that it allows complete atrial emptying and improved ventricular filling (a.k.a. **"atrial kick"**) and therefore increases cardial output.

The interval between the atrial and ventricular spikes simulates a P-R interval, but in *pacer language* is called the *automatic interval*. A normal PR is 0.12–0.20 seconds. A normal automatic interval is approximately the same, but is measured in milliseconds. To convert seconds to milliseconds move the decimal point 3 places to the right. The normal automatic interval is usually 120ms.–160ms.

> **Important Terminology:** You will often hear people refer to pacer spikes as pacer artifact. **Pacer artifact** always means that a waveform is created by an outside or artificial source rather than by normal heart depolarization. Pacer artifact tells us that the pacer is discharging electrical impulses.

2. **A pacemaker spike is followed by a *larger than normal* P wave in atrial pacing, or a wider than normal QRS in ventricular pacing.** These larger or wider waveforms occur because the pacemaker is depolarizing the heart in an abnormal fashion.

> **Important Information:** This larger than normal P wave or QRS following the pacer spike is referred to as **capture.** Capture means that the pacer has discharged an adequate electrical impulse (mA) and depolarization has occurred.

3. **The heart rate of the paced rhythm should not be lower than the lower rate limit set on the pacemaker.** A lower rate limit means, that the pacer is set to fire when the patient's heart rate falls below a set rate or limit. For instance, if the pacer is set to fire at 60 beats per minute, once the patient's heart rate falls below 60, the pacer should begin to pace the heart at 60 beats per minute. This is referred to as **demand pacing.**

IMPORTANT NOTE: A **demand** type pacemaker setting is sometimes referred to as *synchronous* pacing meaning that the pacemaker generated impulse occurs on an *as needed* basis only. The demand pacemaker works in synchrony with the underlying rhythm. In contrast, a *triggered* or **non-demand** pacemaker setting programs the pacemaker to fire continuously at a fixed or set rate, regardless of the underlying rhythm. A triggered pacemaker response is often referred to as *asynchronous* pacing. It is the underlying rhythm pathology that determines the synchronous or asynchronous setting.

Practice Exercise 1

A. List two indications for instituting pacemaker therapy.

1. _increase slow or inadequate ventricular heart rates_
   –stimulate atrial activity in the absence of a sinus pacemaker
2. _–stimulate ventricular activity in the absence of a ventricular_
   or higher order pacemaker

B. Temporary pacemakers are used to support *anticipated* short-term pathology or to correct crisis situations. List three underlying rhythm disturbances that may warrant temporary pacemaker insertion.

1. _Symptomatic bradycardia_
2. _third degree AV (complete) block_
3. _bradyarrhythmias assoc. w/ drug therapy_

C. List the three characteristics of paced rhythms.

1. _pacer artifact or "spike"_
2. _Capture_
3. _actual pacer rate = pacer rate setting_

D. A demand pacemaker generator response means that
   that the pacemaker fires only when the patient's own rate falls
   below the pacemaker setting

✔ For **Feedback 1**, refer to page 222.

Input Section 8.2: Determining Pacemaker Rate

Determining the pacemaker rate on an EKG strip is a function of measuring the interval (small squares) between two consecutive pacer spikes. The trusty rate guide on page 41 can then be consulted, or one can divide 1500 (the number of small squares in one minute) by the number of small squares between the two pacer spikes.

Note the rate calculations on the following two strips.

A ventricular pacemaker rhythm

$$\frac{79}{19)\overline{1500}} = \text{ventricular rate}$$

An atrio-ventricular (AV sequential) pacemaker

$$17\overline{)1500} \; \begin{array}{c}88\end{array} = \text{atrial rate}$$

$$17\overline{)1500} \; \begin{array}{c}88\end{array} = \text{ventricular rate}$$

Practice Exercise 2

Calculate the heart rate in the following AV sequential pacemaker rhythm.

Atrial rate = _____58_____.

Ventricular rate = _____58_____.

✔ For **Feedback 2**, refer to page 223.

Input Section 8.3: More about Capture

Earlier, the term *capture* was introduced. Capture is the term used to describe depolarization occurring secondary to a pacemaker stimulus. Capture occurs when a pacemaker spike is followed by the appropriate cardiac complex (P wave or QRS). *Non-capture* is present when a pacemaker spike fails to produce the desired effect (atrial depolarization or ventricular depolarization). Non-capture may result from: pacemaker malfunction, too low an mA setting; lead placement in electrically inactive scar tissue; or, drifting of the lead wire(s) away from the muscle wall. When non-capture occurs, any of the following *medical* actions may be appropriate.

Methods for "Fixing" Pacemaker Non-Capture

- Increase energy output of generator (mA)
- Check battery
- Reposition the pacer wire (medical intervention)
- Evaluate lead wire for fracture (by x-ray)

The significance of sustained non-capture is dependent upon the presence of an underlying rhythm and patient signs and symptoms.

The following strip demonstrates both pacemaker non-capture and failure to sense.

Failure to capture (pacer stimulus fails to produce ventricular depolarization)

Failure to sense (pacemaker fails to recognize patient's intrinsic electrical activity)

A quick "eyeball" analysis of the above strip reveals pacemaker spikes occurring regularly throughout the tracing. However, the pacemaker is not sensing the patient's underlying feeble rhythm and the pacemaker spikes are failing to capture. (This patient was scheduled for a "pacemaker replacement"!)

Practice Exercise 3

A. Pacemaker capture means

depolarization occuring secondary to pacemaker stimulus

B. Pacemaker non-capture *may* be corrected by any of these three methods: (If uncertain, look above!) 🙂

1. _increased energy output of generator (mA)_
2. _Check battery_
3. _reposition the pacer wire (medical intervention)_

✔ For **Feedback 3**, refer to page 223.   _- Evaluate lead wire for fracture (by x-ray)_

Input Section 8.4: Failure to Sense

When a pacemaker is programmed to *sense* electrical activity, it means that the pacer is "set" to detect a patient's *own* heart rhythm. Sensing can be programmed to recognize ventricular activity as well as atrial activity (in the case of dual leads.) In most cases, when the pacer senses the patient's own electrical activity, the pacer is inhibited from generating a pacer impulse. If the pacemaker fails to sense the patient's own cardiac rhythm and initiates an electrical impulse, the problem is referred to as *failure to sense*. The strips below are examples of failure to sense.

A.

B.

In the first strip (A), note the pacer spike that falls on the first part of the T wave following the second QRS. The pacer did not sense the patient's own beat and generated a paced beat. Luckily, the heart muscle was still in a refractory state; thus, the myocardium did not respond to the pacer impulse.

In the second strip (B), note the fourth QRS complex. Again, the pacer fired on the first part of the T wave. The pacer did not sense the patient's beat and generated a paced beat. This is much like the R on T phenomenon discussed earlier. There is a potential for the patient to experience ventricular tachycardia as a result. The pacer should be reprogrammed and sensitivity increased.

Another interesting phenomenon is observable in the above two strips. Notice the fourth QRS complex in strip A. Just prior to that complex, you will see a pacer spike. And, if you look very closely, you will see the beginnings of a P wave, just before the pacer spike. This particular set of waveforms and pacer spike is called a **fusion beat.** In this case, the patient generated a beat just as the pacer was generating a beat and the two fused together. This occurs again on strip B just before the second QRS, and again before the sixth QRS. When a patient is having frequent fusion beats, it is not a sensing problem, but rather a competition problem. When the patient's sinus node is firing at, or near, the same rate as the pacer, there will be competition for pacing the heart. In this case, the pacer should be reprogrammed or rate adjusted to a lower rate.

☆ **Note:** This brief section is informational with no associated practice exercise!

Input Section 8.5: The Pacemaker Rhythm

The pacemaker generator (temporary or permanent) generates a small electrical current (mA) intended to stimulate the cells at the point of pacemaker wire or lead contact with the muscle. This causes cellular depolarization which spreads across the myocardium, outside the normal conduction pathway. Again, if the mA is adequate, one will see capture. Sound familiar?

The exact functioning of the pacemaker is dependent upon the programming sequence or settings. There are five programming sequences:

➤ Rate

➤ Chamber(s) paced

➤ Response

➤ Programmability

➤ Anti-tachyarrhythmic

These programming sequences have been established by the North American Society of Pacing and Electrophysiology (NASPE) as indicated on the following table.

North American Society of Pacing and Electrophysiology (NASPE) Permanent Pacemaker Codes

Position	I	II	III	IV	V
Category	Chamber(s) paced	Chamber(s) sensed	Response to sensing	Programmability	Anti-tachyarrhythmic functions
	O = None A = Atrium V = Ventricle D = Dual (A-V)	O = None A = Atrium V = Ventricle D = Dual (A-V)	O = None T = Triggered I = Inhibited D = Dual (A-V)	O = None P = Simple Program. M = Multiprogram. C = Communicating R = Rate modulation	O = None P = Pacing (anti-tachyarrhythmia) S = Shock D = Dual (P + S)

Permanent pacemakers are identified by letter codes. The first letter in the code identifies the chamber(s) being paced. The second letter identifies chambers in which the pacer can sense the patient's electrical activity. The third letter tells one what the pacer does in response to sensing the patient's own electrical activity.

The fourth letter of the NASPE permanent pacemaker code tells one the sophistication of the pacer. Programmability refers to the ability of the pacemaker to have its functions changed. Some permanent pacers have only simple programmability for one or two functions, while other pacers have highly sophisticated multi-programmability, allowing virtually all functions to be programmed. These sophisticated programs and functions will be discussed in Section 9. Specially trained physicians, nurses, and technicians can use a pacemaker programmer (a hand-held device) held over the pacemaker to reprogram various functions. Additionally a programmer can "interrogate" the pacemaker. Interrogation asks the pacer to identify current settings and functions. A printout is obtained listing the various settings and functions (see next page). This is very helpful when a patient cannot find his or her pacer ID card with the original functions and settings listed, or if the medical records are not immediately accessible. Permanent pacemakers manufactured in the past ten years will have four letter codes like DDDR and VVIR. Permanent pacemakers used to override tachydysrhythmias (Anti-tachyarrhythmic functions) will have a five letter code such as DDDRD.

Pacer interrogation strip

Most implanted (permanent) pacemakers are of the ***AV sequential variety (dual lead)*** and are programmed on a ⅅ ⅅ ⅅ setting. However, when implanted in patients with chronic atrial fibrillation, AV sequential pacemakers are programmed to a Ⅴ Ⅴ Ⅰ setting. Because of the erratic firing of the atria in atrial fibrillation, a DDD pacer would be inhibited by sensed atrial activity. Anti-arrhythmic pacing will be discussed in detail in Section 9!

Less complicated temporary pacemakers are identified by a three letter code like VVI, AAI, DDD, as demonstrated in the following examples.

Temporary Pacemaker Codes

1 2 3	
Ⅴ Ⅴ Ⅰ :	Paced = Ventricle
	Sensed = Ventricle
	Response = Inhibited

1 2 3	
ⅅ ⅅ ⅅ :	Paced = Dual (Atrium and Ventricle)
	Sensed = Dual (Atrium and Ventricle)
	Response = Dual (Atrium and Ventricle)

Practice Exercise 4

A. When assessing a pacemaker rhythm strip, one must know the pacemaker programming sequence which includes ___Chambers paced___ , ___chambers sensed___ , _response to sensing_ , _programmability_ and _anti-tachyarrhythmic functions_

B. Identify (circle) the atrial and ventricular spikes in the following strip and measure the automatic interval in milliseconds.

automatic interval = ms.

✔ For **Feedback 5**, refer to page 223.

Message from Management

In order to determine correct pacemaker functioning, one must first know what the pacemaker is programmed to do! ALWAYS ask to see the patient's "PACEMAKER ID CARD" that details information about the pacemaker.

In summary, the indications for the various types and modes of pacing vary greatly depending upon the type and severity of the underlying dysrhythmia, the etiology of the dysrhythmia, and the extent of hemodynamic embarrassment.

This section was intended to be an *introduction* to pacemakers and a *warm-up* for Section 9!

Hope we captured your attention!

✔ **Feedback 1**

A. Pacemaker therapy may be instituted for any of the following indications:

 1. to increase slow or inadequate ventricular heart rates.

 2. to stimulate atrial activity in the absence of a sinus pacemaker.

 3. to stimulate ventricular activity in the absence of a ventricular or higher order pacemaker.

B. Any of the following rhythm disturbances may warrant temporary pacemaker insertion:

1. second degree AV block associated with acute myocardial infarction.

2. bradyarrhythmias associated with drug therapy.

3. third degree AV (complete) block.

4. symptomatic bradycardia.

C. Characteristics of a paced rhythm:

1. Pacer artifact or "spike"

2. Capture

3. Actual pacer rate equals pacer rate setting

D. A demand pacemaker generator response means that the pacemaker fires only when the patient's own rate falls below the pacemaker setting.

✔ Feedback 2

The AV sequential paced heart rate is 60 per minute.

Atrial rate = 60 (Approximately)

Ventricular rate = 60 (Approximately)

✔ Feedback 3

A. Pacemaker capture means that muscle depolarization is caused by the pacemaker stimulus. On the EKG strip, capture occurs when a pacemaker spike is followed by the appropriate cardiac complex (P wave or QRS).

B. Pacemaker non-capture *may* be corrected by

1. increasing the energy output of the pacemaker generator.

2. changing the generator (battery).

3. repositioning or replacing the pacer wire.

✔ Feedback 4

There is no practice exercise associated with input 8.4.

✔ Feedback 5

A. When assessing a pacemaker rhythm strip, one must know the pacemaker programming sequence which includes: *rate; chamber(s) paced; response (demand* or *synchronous); programmability;* and, *anti-tachyarrhythmic.*

B.

Atrial spike
Ventricular spike

Automatic interval = 140 milliseconds

Need review? Please see page 216.

Bonus Points!

If you think the above symptomatic patient may need a pacemaker . . . You are doing GREAT!

Now that you have *captured* pacemaker basics, move on to the "Not So Basics" of pacemaker functioning in Section 9!

BASICS ➤ NOT SO BASICS
(completed)   (upcoming)

Notes

Notes

Advanced Pacemaker Features and Interventions (The *Not so Basics* of Pacemaker Function!)

Objectives

When you have completed Section 9, you will be able to describe or define

1. The **Who, What, When, Where and How** of common programmable pacing parameters:

    a. rate modulation

    b. hysteresis

    c. mode switching

    d. auto capture

    e. atrial arrhythmia suppression

    f. pacemaker mediated tachycardia

2. implantable devices for anti-tachy pacing, cardioversion and defibrillation

3. bi-ventricular pacing

Text by:
Victoria A. Paparelli, MSN, RN, CCNS-AC
NASPE Testamur in Pacing and Defibrillation

> **NOTE: This section is intended to augment basic understanding and is not meant to be an in depth study of these options!**

Introduction

The *Not-So-Basic* pacemaker functions presented in this Section represent programmable options now considered part of *basic* dual-lead (or soon to be discussed bi-ventricular) pacemaker functioning. These topics build upon concepts presented in Section 8.

Review and Introduction of Some New Uses of Terms

A *"lead"* may represent a surface ECG lead or a portion of the permanent pacemaker that carries the electronic signals to and from the generator to the heart.

Surface ECG
leads

Permanent
pacemaker lead

Many pacemaker options are programmed "**ON**" at the time of device implant. Other options may be added or changed in a *pacemaker follow up clinic*, as required by the patient. Options are selected or adjusted using a *manufacturer specific programmer* that communicates by telemetry with each device.

Input Section 9.1: Rate Responsive or Rate Modulated Pacing

Chronotropic incompetence is the inability of the heart to increase heart rate in response to increased oxygen demands. Chronotropic incompetence may occur in the following clinical conditions or situations.

Who

➤ Persons with sinus node and conduction pathway disease

➤ Individuals requiring medications that decrease the ability of the sinus node to respond to increased physiologic requirements.

When a healthy person exercises, is under psychologic stress, or is exposed to physiologic stressors (such as infection), heart rate increases in response. A person with chronotropic incompetence may have a slow heart rate, and lack the inherent ability to increase heart rate as required. Thus, activity tolerance is diminished.

Rate responsive pacing or rate modulated pacing is frequently the treatment option of choice for individuals with chronotropic incompetence. Rate responsive pacing is a dual lead pacemaker option that paces the heart at a rate faster than the base programmed pacemaker rate.

Rate responsive pacing is designated with a "**R**" (see NBG code below) as part of coding, i.e.

DDDR

Rate response is programmable—**ON** or **OFF,** and varies in degree.

Following are NBG pacemaker codes. (For a review of *code interpretation*, refer back to Section 8, page 220)

NBG Pacemaker Code				
I	II	III	IV	V
Chamber(s) Paced	Chamber(s) Sensed	Response to Sensing	Programmability Rate modulation	Antitachy Function
O = None	O = None	O = None	O = None	O = None
A = Atrium	A = Atrium	T = Triggered	P = Simple Prog.	P = Antitachy Pacing
V = Ventricle	V = Ventricle	I = Inhibited	M = Multiprog	
D = Dual	D = Dual	D = Dual	C = Communicating	S = Shock
			R = Rate Modulation	D = Dual

Bernstein AD, Camm AJ, Fletcher RD, et al. The **NASPE/BPEG** Defibrillator Generic Pacemaker Code for Antibradycardia and Adaptive-Rate Pacing and Antitachyarrhythmic Devices. PACE 1987; 10:794–799, Appendix II.

NASPE / BPEG

North American Society
for
Pacing and Electrophysiology
(now
known as The
Heart Rhythm Society
hrsonline.org)

British Pacing
and
Electrophysiology Group
(Part of the
British Cardiac
Society)

Collaborative Agreement on Terms

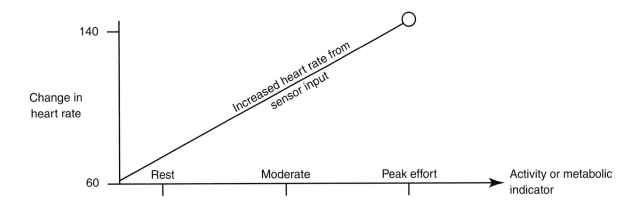

What

Sensors built into the pacemaker device identify and respond to changes in heart rate.

➤ The *sensor* information is transmitted to the pacemaker to elicit the response of *change in rate*.

➤ The most common sensors are the piezoelectric (PE) crystal (**A**) and the accelerometer (**B**), which are inside the pacemaker and respond to movement, muscle motion and vibration.

➤ The response to movement is transformed into electrical signals. These signals are then transmitted to the pacemaker which increases or decreases the paced rate in accord with the pacemaker programming.

NOTE: Manufacturers have designed different methods for modulating or changing the paced rate.

Two Most Common Sensors

Thoracic impedance and minute ventilation sensors are also available but require a specific lead. The sensors are programmable and may be used alone and or in combination.

Concept of Blended Sensors

Exercise stops here

- - - PE crystal

——— Dual (both types together)

• • • • • MV (minute ventilation)

Heart rate

Immediate response

Sensor input continues until respirations slow down, even though movement ceased.

Time

Sensors for catecholamine levels, temperature, right ventricular pressure changes, and oxygen saturation are also available, but limited in use. These sensors require special leads and/or complicated algorithms. Further scientific development is needed to increase *user friendliness* for both the patient and clinician.

When

Rate responsive sensors are most commonly used for *sinus bradycardia* with *chronotropic incompetence* or *drug induced rate suppression*. (Beta-blockers are the most commonly used drug producing this effect.) A sensor is indicated when the patient's ability to increase heart rate and meet metabolic requirements for physical activity is impaired (and there are no contraindications to rate response therapy.) If a patient has severe coronary disease, the demands of increased heart rate on the myocardium may be a *relative* contraindication for rate responsive pacing.

Pacing above the base programmed rate of the pacemaker is known as **sensor input** or **rate modulated** pacing.

A pacemaker programmed to DDDR at a set rate of 60, paces the atrium at a rate higher than 60 if there is *sensor input*. Pacing occurs in the ventricle only if the A-V delay is shorter than the patient's intrinsic P-R delay (P-R interval). In other words, the pacer senses the activity and increases the heart rate appropriately based on sensor input.

A *channel* is part of the programmer's monitoring system. Information is displayed on *channels* of the programmer. These *channels* may be selected to monitor different information (for example, the surface EKG, the atrial and ventricular recordings and the markers).

The diagram at the top of page 233 demonstrates a pacemaker functioning at a rate *above* the programmed rate.

Device programmed DDDR at a rate of 60, A-V delay 150 msec

An atrial rate of 97 bpm is the result of sensor input

Marker channels

$$\text{Calculating Rate} = \frac{60,000 \text{ milliseconds/minute}}{\text{interval in milliseconds/beat}}$$

or

$$\frac{60,000 \text{ msec/min}}{620 \text{ msec/beat}} = 96.7 \text{ bpm}$$

Markers are a built-in *identity* mechanism. The pacemaker communicates to the operator the activity it senses, *identifying* and *labeling* activity as demonstrated in the graphics on the next page.

It should be noted that markers are *manufacturer specific*, differing from one manufacturer to another. Following are example markers.

➤ The **P-R** designation identifies intrinsic (patient-generated) activity.

➤ **AP** indicates atrial pacing.

➤ **AS** refers to atrial *sensing*.

➤ **VP** indicates ventricular pacing.

➤ **VS** refers to ventricular *sensing*.

Marker Channel Connotations

A Side Bar here (AKA a Special Note!):

Electrograms (abbreviated EGM) display internally recorded activity from the leads of the implantable device. The recording of the cardiac waveforms is taken at the lead tip as viewed from an electrode inside the heart. The waveforms are transmitted to the programmer by telemetry and can be visualized and printed. Atrial and ventricular electrograms appear on the next page.

Atrial and Ventricular Electrograms

Why

Rate modulated pacing helps to increase a patient's activity tolerance by augmenting heart rate, as necessary. However, providing for an increased heart rate *will not replace* conditioning and proper exercise regimes to improve cardiovascular health! Patients with extensive coronary artery disease *may* tolerate only limited rate modulation. These persons may experience episodes of angina or anginal equivalent associated with rate modulation.

Practice Exercise 1

A. Two common indications for rate modulated pacing are:

　1. _____

　2. _____.

B. Electrograms (EGMs) are _____

_____.

C. Intrinsic atrial and ventricular activity are represented on the

_____.

✔ For **Feedback 1**, refer to page 259.

Input Section 9.2: Hysteresis, Mode-Switch and Auto Capture

Hysteresis, mode-switch and auto capture represent additional programmable options in permanent pacemakers.

Hysteresis

Hysteresis is a programmed option that allows a patient's heart rate to drop to a specific rate, lagging behind the base pacemaker set rate, before pacing is initiated.

Who

Hysteresis is indicated for a patient with bradycardic episodes who occasionally needs to "catch-up." Stated differently, a patient who experiences a few episodes of bradycardia may require temporary help (a temporary boost) to recover. The patient feels better when the pacemaker is sensing and pacing only for support of a few bradycardic episodes.

> A pacemaker functions something like a clock. The programming instructs the *clock* how long to observe for specific electrical events. The pacemaker response is based only on what it *senses or doesn't sense* in the programmed interval.

What

The hysteresis program directs electrical pacing to *lag behind* the base pacemaker set rate. This *lag behind* function allows a patient's intrinsic activity to be maintained at a rate slower than the base pacing rate.

For example: Base pacing rate is 70 bpm (beats per minute)
Hysteresis rate is 60 bpm (beats per minute)

In this example, the pacemaker will not initiate pacing until the patient's heart rate falls below 60 beats per minute. The pacing is then initiated at a rate of 70 beats per minute. When the pacemaker *searches* and *senses* the patient's intrinsic activity occurring above 60 beats per minute, it will cease pacing until the intrinsic rate again falls below 60 beats per minute. In addition to preserving intrinsic activity and AV synchrony, the hysteresis function preserves pacemaker battery life.

The **thinking** definition of hysteresis is the *facilitation of a longer escape interval following a sensed beat* (intrinsic beat).

Example of a longer escape interval following a sensed beat

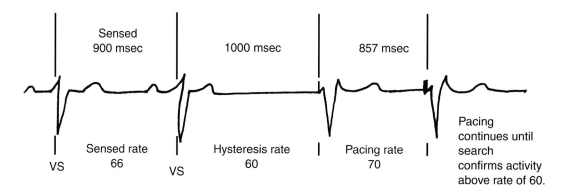

| Sensed 900 msec | 1000 msec | 857 msec |

VS   Sensed rate 66   VS   Hysteresis rate 60   Pacing rate 70   Pacing continues until search confirms activity above rate of 60.

When

Patients uncomfortable with the pacing sensation and those with certain types of syncope are candidates for this *lagging behind* option.

How

Hysteresis is a programmable option in most pacemakers.

Mode-Switch or Atrial Tachy Response

Mode switch or **atrial tachycardia (tachy) response** is a programmable option in a dual chamber pacemaker that allows the pacemaker to respond to an abnormally fast rhythm. Mode switch or atrial tachy response (**ATR**) is a specific program designed to change the pacemaker mode of function in response to a change in the patient's intrinsic rhythm.

Who

Persons with paroxysmal supraventricular tachyarrhythmias including supraventricular tachycardia (SVT), atrial flutter and atrial fibrillation are candidates for the mode switching option.

(For a quick review of rapid atrial dysrhythmias, turn back to Section 2!)

What

When a pacemaker senses no tachycardic or fast rhythm, the dual chamber pacing mode functions. However, when a rapid atrial rhythm occurs, the pacemaker will attempt to sense the rapid atrial activation and pace the ventricle accordingly. This may precipitate a rapid ventricular heart rate. Programming the *mode switch* or *atrial tachy response* function prevents rapid ventricular pacing, thus preventing a rapid heart rate. In essence, the mode switch option deactivates ventricular pacing during rapid atrial dysrhythmias.

For example:

➤ Dual chamber pacing in the **DDD** mode at a rate of 70.

➤ Mode switch or ATR is turned **ON** for atrial rates >170

➤ The patient has an episode of atrial fibrillation (atrial rate >170).

➤ *Switch* occurs when atrial rates are >170 (this is a programmed selected rate).

➤ After a *device specific* time period, the atrial channel is activated to search for atrial activity. If the atrial arrhythmia has terminated, the pacemaker *switches back* to the DDD mode.

Side Bar, Again (AKA Another Special Note)

Device specific refers to pacemaker generator responses *specific to the device manufacturer*. These responses may or may not be programmable. For example, in the *switched mode*, the number of ventricular beats sensed or paced by the pacemaker before it begins searching for atrial activity is device specific. This feature differs by manufacturer, depending on the designed algorithm.

> **An algorithm is a set of precise rules.**

In *pacemaker thinking*, an algorithm directs the pacemaker to respond in a certain way to a specific physiologic event.

When

If the atrial channel senses activity above the *trigger rate* (as in atrial fibrillation) the pacemaker is programmed to **CHANGE** its mode.

Mode Switch or ATR

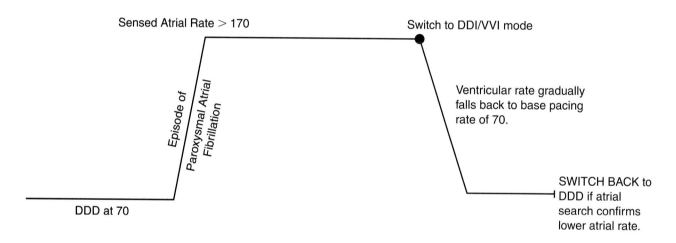

The specifics of this option are dependent on the manufacturer's design. All manufacturers include a method for selecting the sensed rate that will trigger the *switch*. Some devices have options allowing the selection of *mode switch* (for example: to **DVI** or **VVI**). The amount of time and manner of return to dual chamber pacing mode also varies by manufacturer and generation of device.

Auto-Capture

Auto-capture is another programmable option of permanent ventricular pacemakers, *more or less of* a safety feature to assure adequacy of the pacing stimulus.

What

Auto-capture refers to the pacemaker's beat by beat analysis of the pacing threshold, and adjustment of outputs according to the analysis. An interval algorithm provides for increased energy output if a pacemaker stimulus fails to elicit a paced response (failed capture).

Auto Capture Algorithm

When

The auto capture function is continuous and automatic if programmed "**ON**".

Where

The function is programmable and optional in some devices.

Auto-capture advantages include a beat by beat analysis of the paced rhythm and a preserved pacemaker battery life. The disadvantages are: the option is limited to certain manufacturers; and, from a patient's perspective, some persons may feel an uncomfortable difference associated with higher energy outputs.

Practice Exercise 2

A. Hysteresis is defined as _____

_____.

B. Mode switch or ATR is defined as _____

_____

_____.

C. Mode Switch or ATR is recommended for the treatment of _____

_____

_____.

D. An advantage to having mode switch turned on is _____

_____

_____.

E. The #1 advantage for auto-capture is _____

_____.

✔ For **Feedback 2**, refer to page 259.

Input Section 9.3: Atrial Arrhythmia Suppression/Atrial Rate Stabilization (AKA Overdrive Pacing for Atrial Dysrhythmias)

Atrial fibrillation is defined by *rapid, irregular atrial impulses occurring at a rate of 300–600 per minute.* Prevalence of atrial fibrillation in the general population is about 1%. This prevalence increases with age, up to 10% in those 80 years and older. Persons with cardiovascular disease, such as coronary artery disease and congestive heart failure, have an increased incidence of atrial fibrillation.

Atrial Fibrillation

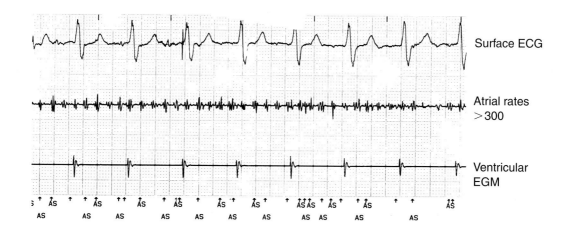

Atrial flutter is defined by regular atrial contractions occurring at a rate of 250–350 times per minute. A consistent degree of physiologic block (2:1, 3:1, 4:1, etc.) will result in a regular, slower ventricular response. Varying degrees of physiologic block produces an irregular ventricular response. Atrial flutter is less common than atrial fibrillation and, at the outset, is not usually associated with structural heart disease. Without treatment, atrial flutter may deteriorate to atrial fibrillation.

Atrial Flutter

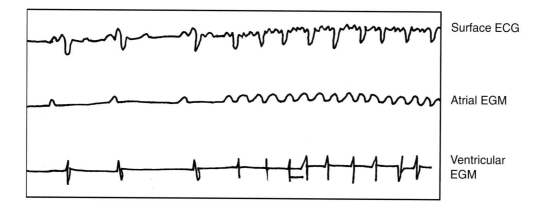

Overdrive suppression is a therapeutic intervention for both rapid atrial and ventricular arrhythmias. As the name implies, the treatment overdrives the arrhythmia by attempting to *capture* the myocardium with a faster, stronger impulse than that of the existing arrhythmia. Here, the discussion focuses on atrial dysrhythmias.

As an example, a patient with atrial flutter (atrial rate of *250* beats per minute) is paced with a temporary atrial pacemaker. The action involves pacing the atria at a rate of *275* impulses per minute (slightly faster than the flutter rate) for 5 seconds with a high voltage stimulus, 5 mA (milliamphere). The atria is *captured* with the higher energy stimulus, *overdriving* the existing rate of 250. This is known as **entrainment** of the atria. In this situation, entrainment means the pacemaker is now controlling the rhythm rather than the intrinsic atrial flutter stimulus. Once the atria are captured, the quick termination of the pacing stimulus (275 bpm) results in the return to sinus rhythm.

Rapid Atrial Pacing

Rapid atrial pacing is now a programmable option in some permanent pacemaker devices.

A variation of this *atrial arrhythmia suppression* can sense isolated premature atrial contractions. These premature contractions or P.A.C.s are often the precursor to atrial tachyarrhythmias, such as atrial flutter and fibrillation. When the pacemaker senses a premature atrial contraction, an *overdrive (faster)* stimulus is emitted by the pacemaker to suppress other early beats. The faster pacemaker rate is short in duration, returning to the base pacing rate when early (premature) beats are no longer sensed on the atrial channel.

Overdrive Suppression

Practice Exercise 3

A. Another name for rapid pacing is _____.

B. Overdrive suppression is used to treat _____
_____.

✔   For **Feedback 3**, refer to page 260.

Input Section 9.4: Pacemaker Mediated Tachycardia (PMT)

As its name implies, a pacemaker mediated tachycardia results when paced impulses create an anomalous conducting circuit. (You will recall, anomalous circuitry is responsible for most rapid, sustained ectopic rhythms!) Pacemaker mediated tachycardia (PMT) is a form of reentrant tachycardia that can occur in patients with dual-chamber pacemakers. When PMT occurs, the pacemaker serves as one leg (the antegrade leg) of the abnormal conducting circuit. The AV node serves as the other leg (the retrograde limb). PMT can be precipitated by electrical events which result in retrograde P waves.

The most common events than can precipitate PMT are: (1) P.V.C.s; or, (2) failure of atrial capture. These events produce retrograde P waves (indicating that ventricular activation precedes atrial activation) which can trigger pacemaker mediated tachycardia. A retrograde P wave may follow a P.V.C. owing to the timing of the backward activation of the atria. When an atrial pacemaker spike is not followed by atrial capture, the ventricular pacemaker fires (following the set AV delay). The paced ventricular stimulus initiates ventricular depolarization, followed by retrograde depolarization of the atria. This backward activation of the atria produces a retrograde P wave.

A pacemaker senses retrograde P waves as atrial events. When a pacemaker senses an atrial event, the AV delay clock starts. If no intrinsic (patient generated) ventricular activity occurs by the time the AV delay times out, a ventricular stimulus is emitted by the pacemaker. The paced ventricular stimulus produces ventricular depolarization and a backward activation of the atria, (retrograde P wave).

This backward activation of the atria (retrograde P) again starts the AV delay clock. When the AV clock times out, the pacemaker (once again) emits a ventricular pacing stimulus. This repeating process (retrograde P followed by a pacing ventricular stimulus) results in PMT. The PMT can continue until the atria becomes refractory or until the retrograde conduction is lost.

Following are examples to aid understanding.

A Retrograde P Wave Following a P.V.C.

DDD pace with induction of PMT following a PVC with retrograde P wave

P.M.T. Initiated by a P.V.C.: Sequence of Events

P.V.C. Fires → Depolarization of ventricles → Retrograde depolarization of atria producing a retrograde P wave → AV delay clock starts → AV delay clock times out → Paced ventricular beat

Repeating loop (Reentrant Tachycardia)

Loss of Atrial Capture

Atrial capture present

A retrograde P wave is sensed which starts the AV delay clock. When the delay clock times out, ventricular pacing begins

P.M.T. Initiated by Failed Atrial Capture: Sequence of Events

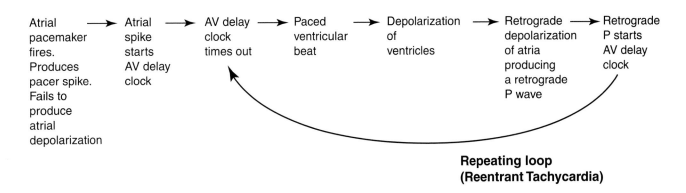

Atrial pacemaker fires. Produces pacer spike. Fails to produce atrial depolarization → Atrial spike starts AV delay clock → AV delay clock times out → Paced ventricular beat → Depolarization of ventricles → Retrograde depolarization of atria producing a retrograde P wave → Retrograde P starts AV delay clock

Repeating loop (Reentrant Tachycardia)

Pacemaker Mediated Tachycardia (PMT)

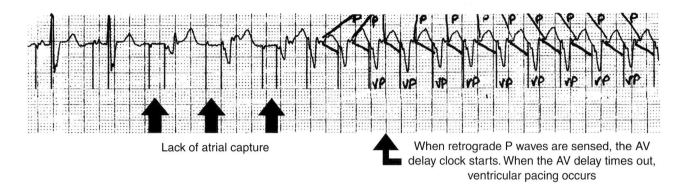

Lack of atrial capture

When retrograde P waves are sensed, the AV delay clock starts. When the AV delay times out, ventricular pacing occurs

NOTE: When a tachycardia occurs at the upper rate limit (**URL**) of the pacemaker, it suggests PMT!

Since the mid-1990s, most pacemakers have an algorithm to identify, record and terminate PMT. Older pacemakers do not have algorithms; thus, PMT may be encountered. There are, however, methods to prevent PMT by programming adjustments to **PVARP** (Post-Ventricular Atrial Refractory Period). In the following illustration, notice that PVARP programming prevents the sensing of retrograde P waves.

PVARP is the interval following ventricular activity when the pacemaker is "blind" to atrial activity.

"AR"–The P wave occurring during PVARP is marked "atrial" during refractory or "AR". This P wave does NOT start the AV delay clock. No ventricular pacing is initiated.

Practice Exercise 4

A. Two causes of PMT are:

1. _____

2. _____.

✔ For **Feedback 4**, refer to page 260.

Input·Section 9.5: Implantable Devices for Overdrive Pacing and Defibrillation

Implantable devices for overdrive pacing *and* internal cardioversion or defibrillation are relatively young and *rapidly* changing technologies. Sophisticated capabilities now include

➤ Anti-tachycardia Pacing

➤ Automatic Internal Cardioversion

➤ Automatic Internal Defibrillation

➤ Criteria-based detection and treatment

Before moving on, several key terms and conditions deserve attention!

Some Key Terms and Conditions

> An **AICD** is an implantable Automatic Implantable Cardioverter, Defibrillator device
>
> A **PCD** is an older generation implantable Pacemaker, Cardioverter, Defibrillator device
>
> An **ICD** is an Implantable Cardioverter, Defibrillator Device

Originally both AICDs and PCDs were company proprietary terms for competing devices with similar functions. Now the *generic* ICD term is most often used.

For review, *defibrillation* is defined as the termination of an unsynchronized quivering of the ventricular muscle, using a high energy, asynchronous electrical stimulus delivered to the cardiac tissue. *Cardioversion* is defined as the termination of a tachyarrhythmia using a moderate electrical stimulus synchronized to the cardiac depolarization phase of a cardiac cycle (the R wave).

Here, it is helpful to again review NBG and NBD pacemaker codes and to consider the differences between *older* and *current* devices.

NBG Pacemaker Code

I	II	III	IV	V
Chamber(s) Paced	Chamber(s) Sensed	Response to Sensing	Programmability Rate modulation	Antitachy Function
O = None	O = None	O = None	O = None	O = None
A = Atrium	A = Atrium	T = Triggered	P = Simple Program	P = Antitachy Pacing
V = Ventricle	V = Ventricle	I = Inhibited	M = Multiprogram	
D = Dual	D = Dual	D = Dual	C = Communicating	S = Shock
			R = Rate Modulation	D = Dual

Bernstein AD, Camm AJ, Fletcher RD, et al. The NASPE/BPEG Defibrillator Generic Pacemaker **Code for Antibradycardia and Adaptive-Rate Pacing and Antitachyarrhythmic Devices.** PACE **1987**; 10:794–799, Appendix II.

NBD Pacemaker Code			
I	**II**	**III**	**IV**
Shock Chamber	Antitachycardia Pacing Chamber	Tachycardia Detection	Antibradycardia Pacing Chamber
O = None A = Atrium V = Ventricle D = Dual (A+V)	O = None A = Atrium V = Ventricle D = Dual (A+V)	E = Electrogram H = Hemodynamics	O = None A = Atrium V = Ventricle D = Dual (A+V)

Bernstein AD, Camm AJ, Fisher JD, et al. The NASPE/BPEG Defibrillator Code PACE **1993**; 16:1776–1780, Appendix III.

The Similarities and Differences between *Older* and *Current* Implanted Defibrillator Devices

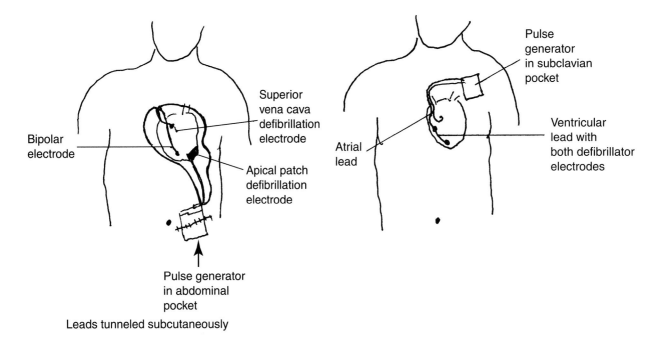

Bipolar electrode

Superior vena cava defibrillation electrode

Apical patch defibrillation electrode

Pulse generator in abdominal pocket

Leads tunneled subcutaneously

Pulse generator in subclavian pocket

Atrial lead

Ventricular lead with both defibrillator electrodes

Older devices (1980's)

- Generator the size of a pack of cigarettes
- Implanted in the abdomen, due to weight and size
- Implanted with transthoracic approach
- Leads placed **epicardially**
- Recovery from open chest procedure
- Prolonged hospitalization

Newer devices (1990's)

- Generator the size of a pacemaker
- Implanted in subclavian region
- Percutaneous, transvenous approach
- Leads placed **transvenously**
- IV sedation and minimal recovery
- 24–48 hours for initial implant

Anti-Tachycardia (Overdrive) Pacing

Anti-tachycardia or overdrive pacing is a treatment option for rapid, re-entry dysrhythmias. Anti-tachycardia pacing involves rapid electrical stimulation in attempt to entrain and interrupt a re-entrant tachycardia mechanism, as demonstrated below.

Markers

ⓣ – tachy interval

Trigger – tachy detection interval number has been met, so
     therapy begins

"ATP" – anti-tachy pacing therapy

Complex Arrhythmia Intervention
Implantable Defibrillators (ICDs)

An implantable defibrillator (ICD) is the therapy of choice for patients with lethal ectopic ventricular disorders and certain high risk conditions. It should be emphasized, however, clinical studies are ongoing to determine the specific clinical criteria warranting an implantable defibrillator.

Who

Candidates for implantable defibrillator therapy include patients with the following disorders:

➤ documented episodes of *Sudden Cardiac Death*

➤ documented *inducible ventricular arrhythmias*

➤ high-risk conditions such as ischemic heart disease and low ejection fractions

➤ congenital cardiomyopathies and/or arrhythmogenic syndromes (such as long QT syndrome)

What

Implantable defibrillators (ICDs) are multi-functional devices with the following capabilities.

➤ *Monitoring* constantly for both bradycardic and tachycardic rhythms.

➤ *Recording* information about the rhythm.

➤ *Pacing* for bradycardia.

➤ *Overdrive pacing* for tachyarrhythmias.

➤ *Cardioversion and defibrillation* for the interruption of tachyarrhythmias when specific criteria are met.

NOTE: All implantable defibrillators have some pacemaker capability. The specific functions are dependent upon the device model and programming.

Counters

Implantable defibrillators (ICDs) have **Counters** which identify and document rhythm events as demonstrated below.

Counters		

Recent Data Includes:	Episodes:	to		
	Dates:	06-MAR-2003	to	04-JUN-2003

	Since Last Cleared 06-MAR-2003	Device Totals	
Episode Counters			
Treated			
VF Therapy	0	③	← 3 therapies delivered for the lifetime of device.
VT Therapy	0	0	
VT-1 Therapy	0	0	
Commanded Therapy	0	0	
Nontreated			
No Therapy Programmed	0	0	
Nonsustained Episodes	0	②	← Non-sustained episodes are counted.
Total Episodes	0	5	
A-Tachy Response	0	0	
Therapy Counters			
Shocks Attempted	⓪	3	← No shock therapy this INTERVAL since 06-Mar-2003.
Delivered-Detection Met	0	3	
-Physician Commanded	0	0	
Diverted -Reconfirm	0	0	
-Physician Commanded	0	0	
ATP Schemes Attempted	0	0	
Delivered-Detection Met	0	0	
-Physician Commanded	0	0	

First-attempt Success Rate:

	Delivered	Converted	Accelerated	% Success	
VF Zone	0	0	—	0	Electrogram are recorded for treatment purpose.
VT Zone	0	0	0	0	
VT-1 Zone	0	0	0	0	

Parameters

describe the range of arrhythmia for this patient.
Defines the treatable rhythm

This patient's VF detection parameter is set to >200 bpm for a duration of 4.0 seconds. Redetect carried out in 1.0 second.

Pacing Parameters – ☆
Brady and Post Shock Brady

VF Zone	
Initial Detection	
Rate	≥ 200 bpm
Interval	≤ 300 ms
Duration	4.0 sec
Redetection	
Redetect Duration	1.0 sec
Post-shock Duration	1.0 sec
Shock Therapy	
Shock 1	17 J ☆
Shock 2	31 J
Max Shocks	31 J

Brady Pacing	
Normal Brady Pacing ☆	
Mode	DDDR
Lower Rate Limit	85 ppm
Maximum Tracking Rate	120 ppm
Adaptive Rate	
Maximum Sensor Rate	120 ppm
• Activity Threshold	Medium
• Reaction Time	30 sec
• Response Factor	8
• Recovery Time	5 min
Dynamic A-V Delay	OFF
A-V Delay	80 ms
Minimum Delay	— ms
Sensed A-V Offset	OFF ms
Hysteresis Rate	— ppm
Rate Smoothing	
Smoothing Up	OFF %
Smoothing Down	OFF %
Post-Shock Brady Pacing ☆	
Mode	DDD
Lower Rate Limit	85 ppm
Maximum Tracking Rate	120 ppm
Adaptive Rate	
Maximum Sensor Rate	— ppm
• Activity Threshold	—
• Reaction Time	— sec
• Response Factor	—
• Recovery Time	— min
Dynamic A-V Delay	OFF
A-V Delay	100 ms
Minimum Delay	— ms
Sensed A-V Offset	OFF ms
Hysteresis Rate	— pm
Rate Smoothing	
Smoothing up	OFF %
Smoothing Down	OFF %

Therapy Features	
Shock	
Waveform	Biphasic
Polarity	INITIAL
Committed Shock	NO
ATP	
Atrial ATP Amplitude	5.0 V
• Atrial ATP Pulse Width	1.0 ms
Ventricular ATP Amplitude	7.5 V
Ventricular ATP Pulse Width	1.0 ms
• Only available during EP test	

Therapy

describes the treatment regimen to be followed for a particular arrhythmia, defined by the parameters set in the device.
Shock Therapy set at 17 J once VF detect is met.

When and How

Automatic-Implantable-Pacer-Cardioverter-Defibrillators (ICDs) can *"think through"* rhythm analysis and therapy selection based on sophisticated algorithms and program selections.

➤ The ICD analyzes rhythms based on rate and morphology.
  Rate is a programmed detection number
        (i.e.-ventricular tachycardia detect rate 160 bpm)
  Morphology analyzes width, shape and size of the sensed electrogram.
        (This is a device specific algorithm and differs among manufacturers.)

➤ Therapy is delivered based on meeting programmed requirements for
  1. rate and/or morphology
  2. duration of the arrhythmia
  3. continuing rhythm disturbance (after the device charges and re-evaluates the rhythm)

Rate Identification with Marker Channels and Intervals of VT

Therapy Initiated

Confirmation Post Charge

Therapy delivered

A Bit More About ICDs

The therapy delivered by an ICD is based on programmed criteria. For example, the treatment for monomorphic (originating in one site) ventricular tachycardia (VT) is often overdrive or anti-tachycardia pacing (ATP). If ATP is unsuccessful, cardioversion (CV) is initiated. If CV is unsuccessful, defibrillation (DF) is used. In other words, when the least aggressive therapy (ATP) is unsuccessful, the more aggressive therapy (CV or DF) will be initiated as evidenced in the following diagram.

An Artist's Rendering of Unsuccessful Anti-tachycardia Pacing (ATP) Progressing to Cardioversion (CV)

The ICD device can discriminate between a supraventricular tachycardia (SVT) and ventricular tachycardia (VT) by comparing data from each lead and other discriminators as discussed on page 254.

Atrial and Ventricular Electrograms with AF

253

Supraventricular Discrimination Options

Supraventricular discriminator options assist the ICD device in *deciding* if the arrhythmia is atrial or ventricular in origin based on criteria other than rate and morphology. Discriminator options are *device specific* (differing by manufacturer) and are designed to prevent the patient from receiving unnecessary ventricular therapy for atrial arrhythmias. The supraventricular discriminators include the following comparative criteria.

The Discriminators

➤ *A to V comparison* – the number of atrial events compared to ventricular events.

➤ *Onset* – how fast the rate has changed. (Exercise may produce a high heart rate, but the increase in rate is gradual.)

➤ Stability – the measured intervals vary by < or > in a number of milliseconds. Atrial arrhythmias, such as atrial fibrillation, have inconsistent R-R (ventricular) intervals (owing to variable A-V conduction) compared to ventricular tachycardia.

☆ In the event that the ICD device cannot discriminate between an atrial and ventricular dysrhythmia, it treats the rhythm as ventricular, delivering the ventricular arrhythmia therapy.

An Example of Onset Enabled Discriminators

From *Guidant, Vitality 2 ICD Systems.* Copyright © 2004 by Guidant Corporation. Reprinted by permission.

Two discriminators are in effect:

1. Onset (VT onset is usually fast. If the atrial rate increases with exercise, the increase is gradual; thus, it is not VT).
2. Ventricular rate > Atrial rate (If the rhythm is atrial or sinus tachycardia, the A to V rate is equal.)

To complexify things just a bit 🎵, there are devices which treat rapid atrial dysrhythmias with atrial anti-tachycardia pacing (ATP) or suppression. Other clinically available devices treat atrial arrhythmias with cardioversion.

Practice Exercise 5

A. Two indications for ICD therapy are:

1. _____

2. _____

B. Two criteria necessary for initiating defibrillation therapy are:

1. _____

2. _____

✔ For **Feedback 5**, refer to page 260.

Input Section 9.6: Bi-Ventricular Pacing

You have previously *learned* that AV or dual lead pacemakers are used to achieve synchronized atrial and ventricular functioning. As the name "biventricular" implies, pacemakers can now stimulate both the right and left ventricle. Bi-ventricular pacing is the newest of pacing applications and, there is still *much* to learn about selecting treatment groups and evaluating (and increasing) efficacy.

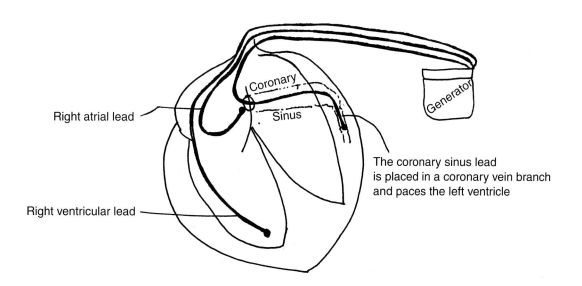

Right atrial lead

Coronary Sinus

Generator

The coronary sinus lead is placed in a coronary vein branch and paces the left ventricle

Right ventricular lead

As demonstrated in the above diagram, the bi-ventricular pacemaker has three lead wires. The bi-ventricular (bi-V) pacemaker incorporates dual chamber AV pacing (a right atrial and a right ventricular lead) and (a third lead, positioned in a vein in the coronary sinus) (in the same device). These features are combined in a device with defibrillator capability, as well. A bi-ventricular pacemaker sends a stimulus to the atria, followed by a programmed AV delay. The stimulus is then simultaneously sent to both ventricles.

Normal HF/Brady Parameters		
	INITIAL VALUE	PRESENT VALUE
Basic Pacing		
Mode		DDD
A-Tachy Response		On
Lower Rate Limit		90 ppm
Max Tracking Rate		130 ppm
Max Sensor Rate		120 ppm
AV Delay (Paced)		120 ms
Pacing Chamber		BiV
Atrial		
Pulse Width		0.4 ms
Amplitude		3.5 V
Right Ventricular		
Pulse Width		0.4ms
Amplitude		2.4 V
Left Ventricular		
Pulse Width		0.5 ms
Amplitude		3.5 V
Post-shock Delay		1.5 sec
Sensor		
Accelerometer		ATR Only
Activity Threshold		Med-Lo
Reaction Time		30 sec
Slope		11
Recovery		5 min

Individually programmable parameters for pacing

Atrial ——— (Atrial)

Right Ventricle ——— (Right Ventricular)

Left Ventricle ——— (Left Ventricular)

A bi-ventricular programming strip demonstrating programmed parameters

Next, it is helpful to think briefly about characteristic EKG patterns and cardiac muscle pathology. When a pacemaker is used in the right ventricle as in *AV* or *dual chamber* pacing, a conduction abnormality is created. On EKG, this abnormality resembles a left bundle branch block pattern. Pacemaker activation of the right ventricle causes the wave of ventricular depolarization to spread from right to left, outside the normal conduction pathway. This anomalous route of depolarization requires more time and delays left ventricular activation.

A characteristic LBBB pattern associated with right ventricular pacing

A left bundle branch pattern may also be observed in patients with muscle scarring associated with coronary artery disease, as demonstrated at the top of the next page. In both groups, the ventricles no longer work synchronously (together) as they would if normal conduction occurred from the SA to AV node and through the bundle branches and the His-Purkinje system.

EKG demonstrating a LBBB conduction defect

Long-standing congestive heart failure often results in structural changes within the heart. The heart may become globally dilated (the entire heart takes the shape of a globe) as in a patient with dilated cardiomyopathy.

Large areas of cardiac muscle scarring may follow large scale myocardial infarction. In areas where infarction has occurred, the heart muscle becomes *dyskinetic* or *dysynchronous* (does not move together) as a result of scarring. *Re-synchronization therapy*, another name for bi-V pacing may be employed to achieve synchronized ventricular muscle functioning.

The following patient clinical conditions warrant consideration for bi-V pacing or re-synchronization therapy.

Eligibility for Bi-ventricular Pacing or Re-synchronization Therapy

Who

➤ Patients with congestive heart failure continuing to experience moderate to severe symptoms despite maximum medical therapy

➤ Patients with delay in electrical conduction evident on the EKG (widened QRS)

➤ Patients with congestive heart failure, continuing to experience symptoms despite maximum medical therapy, and echocardiographic evidence of mitral regurgitation (backflow across the mitral valve when the left ventricle contracts)

What

Bi-ventricular pacing affords an **improved** quality of life!

➤ *Functionally*, bi-V pacing improves exercise tolerance and decreases symptoms of shortness of breath and fatigue associated with activities of daily living.

➤ *Electrically*, bi-V pacing produces electrocardiographic (EKG) evidence of improved conduction (decreased QRS duration).

Quality of Life Changes

CHAIR BOUND

Versus

WALKING

When

The results associated with bi-ventricular pacing or re-synchronization therapy vary by patient.

➤ It *may* take months to see improvement in symptoms.

➤ Electrical (EKG) evidence may improve first.

➤ Improvement will vary among patients regardless of selection for device therapy.

Where and How

As demonstrated in the next diagram, lead wires are positioned in the right atrium, the right ventricle, and in a branch of the coronary sinus (the large venous system of the coronary arterial system.)

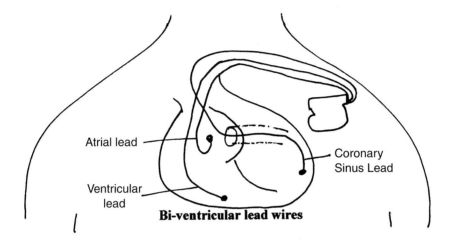

Atrial lead

Coronary Sinus Lead

Ventricular lead

Bi-ventricular lead wires

Atrial pacing occurs if necessary, when the sinus rate falls below the programmed atrial rate. Pacing of the right and left ventricles occurs simultaneously. Remodeling or reshaping of the ventricles occurs over time, secondary to electrical (bi-V) re-synchronization. In other words, over time the improved electrical conduction is *expected* to produce a positive change in the mechanical functioning of the ventricles. The expected positive change includes improved septal and ventricular contractions and decreased mitral regurgitation.

 Practice Exercise 6

A. Two differences between AV pacing and bi-V pacing are:

    1. _____

    2. _____

B. The third lead in a bi-V pacemaker is positioned in _____

_____

C. The goal of bi-ventricular pacing is _____

_____

_____

D. Electrical improvement may precede _____

_____

_____

✔ For **Feedback 6**, refer to page 260.

Now, a new generation of pacing has combined bi-ventricular pacing with anti-Tachy pacing and defibrillation! Therapies are now combined in many different ways. For example, bradycardic pacing therapies may be used alone or in combination with optional treatments for tachyarrhythmias. Combination therapies represent an *evolv ing* science and have likely changed since you began this Section! Stay tuned to the written and *virtual* resources available from all pacemaker manufacturers!

SPECIAL NOTE: The left ventricular (or coronary sinus) lead is inserted transvenously through the right atrium and coronary sinus into a branch of the coronary vein. The coronary sinus lead is situated in a branch of the coronary vein rather than against the muscle wall of the heart. (You will recall that other leads rest on the muscle wall.) Owing to positioning, this lead behaves differently. If the position of the lead does not change, the impedance remains stable. The energy required to stimulate the heart muscle through a vein is often higher than direct muscle stimulation. As a result, the battery drain is greater (battery requirements and battery size may differ from a standard pacemaker).

✔ Feedback 1

A. Two common indications for rate modulated pacing are:
1. Sinus bradycardia with chronotropic incompetence
2. Drug induced rate suppression

B. Electrograms (EMGs) are displays of internally recorded activity from the leads of implantable devices.

C. Intrinsic atrial and ventricular activity are represented on the markers.

✔ Feedback 2

A. Hysteresis is defined as a programmed option that allows the heart rate to lag behind the base pacemaker set rate.

B. Mode switch or ATR is defined as a programmable option in a dual chamber pacemaker that changes the pacemaker mode of function in response to a change in the patient's own rhythm. The mode switch stops ventricular pacing during rapid atrial dysrhythmias.

C. Mode switch or ATR is recommended for the treatment of supraventricular tachycardia, atrial flutter and atrial fibrillation.

D. An advantage to having mode switch turned on is to prevent rapid ventricular pacing during rapid atrial dysrhythmias.

E. The #1 advantage for auto-capture is that it provides for increased energy output if a pacemaker stimulus fails to elicit a paced response. It corrects a failure to capture.

✔ Feedback 3

A. Another name for rapid pacing is overdrive suppression.

B. Overdrive suppression is used to treat rapid atrial and ventricular arrhythmias.

✔ Feedback 4

A. Two causes of PMT are:

    1. P.V.C.s

    2. Failure of atrial capture

✔ Feedback 5

A. Indications for ICD therapy are

    1. Documented episodes of sudden cardiac death

    2. Documented inducible ventricular arrhythmias

    3. High-risk conditions (ischemic heart disease, low ejection fractions)

    4. Congenital cardiomyopathies or arrhythmogenic syndromes

B. Two criteria necessary for initiating defibrillation therapy are

    1. Rate of onset (VT onset is usually fast)

    2. Ventricular rate greater than the atrial rate

✔ Feedback 6

A. Two differences between AV pacing and bi-V pacing are

    1. An AV pacemaker (2 leads) paces the right atrium and right ventricle; a bi-V pacemaker (3 leads) paces the right atrium and the right and left ventricles

    2. Bi-V pacing re-synchronizes ventricular functioning

B. The third lead in a bi-V pacemaker is positioned in the coronary sinus.

C. The goal of bi-ventricular pacing is synchronized ventricular muscle function.

D. Electrical improvement may precede the improvement in symptoms.

Notes

_____

_____

_____

_____

Electrolyte Changes

Objectives

When you have completed Section 10, you will be able to describe or identify clinical conditions and EKG manifestations associated with

1. hypokalemia

2. hyperkalemia

3. hypocalcemia

4. hypercalcemia

5. hypomagnesemia

6. hypermagnesemia

7. prolonged QTc interval

Input Section 10.1: Ions, Electrolytes, and Potassium

Section 10 deals with certain electrolyte imbalances as reflected on the EKG. Even though that sounds less than intriguing, there are some unique and interesting things you should know. 😊 **Honest!**

The author is making the assumption that you have a reasonable understanding of electrolytes . . . but if you are uncertain, a *brief* overview follows.

Remember **ions**? They are the electrically charged particles contained in the various fluid compartments of the body—the intracellular fluid (ICF) compartment and the extracellular fluid (ECF) compartment. If your long-term memory is operative, you will recall that the ECF includes *both* the fluid in the blood vessels (intravascular fluid) and the fluid located between the cells (interstitial fluid).

Anions are negatively charged particles—like bicarbonate (HCO_3^-) and chloride (Cl^-).

Cations are positively charged particles—like potassium (K^+), sodium (Na^+), calcium (Ca^{++}), and magnesium (Mg^{++}).

Cat-ion

Electrolytes are combinations of anions and cations in solution.

It is interesting to consider what happens to all the ions or charges in the processes of heart contraction and relaxation and in the processes of cellular depolarization and repolarization.

All cells in the body, including the myocardial cells, have an electrical charge which is a result of all the ions (cations and anions) in the body. These ions are found both inside and outside of the cells—some in greater concentrations than others.

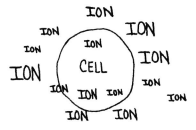

When a cell is at rest (polarized state), the inside of the cell has a net negative charge, while the cell membrane has a net positive charge. Sodium (Na^+) tends to be mainly outside the cell, and potassium (K^+) tends to be mainly inside the cell during this polarized state.

CELL "AT REST"

When a cell is electrically stimulated, sodium (Na$^+$) rushes into the cell, while potassium (K$^+$) moves out. Sodium and potassium basically change places for awhile.

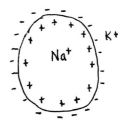

This movement of K$^+$ and Na$^+$ upsets the charge on the inside of the cell—giving it a net positive charge. This reversal of charges is ***depolarization.*** Depolarization causes calcium (Ca^{++}) move into the cell. Calcium then causes the mechanical activity of **contraction**. Following depolarization, the ions move back to their "resting state" or repolarized positions in order to receive the next impulse.

It is important to recognize clinical conditions causing electrolyte imbalances and anticipate changes associated with depolarization, repolarization, and contractility of the myocardial cells.

Serum Potassium

We will begin by examining potassium (K$^+$), a major intracellular cation. **A normal serum potassium ranges between 3.6–5.2 mEq. per liter.** Potassium is the cation that influences myocardial cell **repolarization**.

Hypokalemia

Hypokalemia is the term used to describe a **serum potassium (K$^+$) level below 3.6 mEq/liter**. Because the potassium ions play an important role in repolarization activities of myocardial cells, certain changes occur in the EKG pattern when the potassium level is unbalanced. Those changes may be subtle or pronounced.

For instance, *hypokalemia* may cause any or all of the following EKG changes.

A. *Depressed ST segment*

B. *Prominent U wave**

C. *Prolonged QT or QU interval*

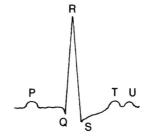

The QT interval (depicted on the following page) is measured from the beginning of the QRS complex to the end of the T wave. The QT interval simply represents the total time for ventricular depolarization and repolarization.

* The U wave is thought to represent the prolonged repolarization of the Purkinje fibers.

A U wave superimposed upon or near the T wave (more or less of a camel back presentation) gives the appearance of a prolonged QT interval. In effect, it is the U wave that makes the interval prolonged.

Just for the record, QT intervals vary with age, gender and heart rate, though, a normal QT interval should be no greater than half of the R-R interval. The QT interval is best measured in leads V_2 and V_3.

| | Normal EKG | Hypokalemia |

In a healthy state, the normal male QT interval averages 0.39 seconds; the normal female QT interval averages 0.41 seconds. Because the QT interval varies with heart rate, a formula (Bazet's formula) was derived to correct for heart rate variation.

$$\text{Bazet's formula} \qquad \textbf{QTc} = \frac{\text{QT interval in seconds}}{\sqrt{\text{R} - \text{R interval in seconds}}}$$

QTc is the abbreviation utilized for a heart-rate corrected QT interval. Fortunately, QTc calculators are programmed into 12 lead EKG machines! See more detail on page 273.

Oftentimes it is difficult to visualize U waves or determine where a T wave stops and the U wave begins. It may help to view those leads where the T waves tend to be flat.

Here is a 12 lead EKG demonstrating hypokalemia (and demonstrating the difficulty of U wave identification!).

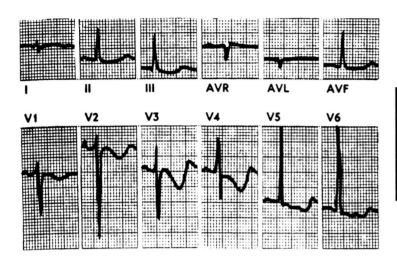

IMPORTANT NOTICE: One can never diagnose hypokalemia from an EKG—it can only be suspected. Hypokalemia must be confirmed by a serum potassium level.

Hypokalemia may be associated with any of the following conditions or therapies.

➤ starvation

➤ vomiting

➤ diarrhea

➤ diuretic therapy

➤ intermittent gastric suction

➤ excessive digitalis therapy

➤ excessive use of steroids

Because hypokalemia *increases electrical instability,* the following dysrhythmias may be associated with low serum potassium levels.

➤ **P.V.C.s**

➤ **Atrial tachycardia**

➤ **Junctional tachycardia**

➤ **Ventricular tachycardia**

➤ **Ventricular fibrillation**

If this is *confusing, just remember that **potassium mainly affects the repolarization** period of cardiac activity. Since the T wave represents repolarization, **look for EKG changes near the T wave.** Probably the most common EKG feature associated with pronounced hypokalemia is the prominent *U wave.*

Here's a Poem for U . . .

Roses are Red
Violets are Blue
Potassiums that are *Low*
Will give you a U (wave)!

Hyperkalemia

Of course, there are EKG effects and electrical considerations associated with elevated potassium (K^+) levels, as well. **A serum potassium (K^+) level greater than 5.2 mEq. per liter** is termed *hyperkalemia*.

The most characteristic EKG features associated with *hyperkalemia* include

➤ Tall, peaked, narrow, tent-like T waves that are symmetrical in appearance.

➤ Diminished height or amplitude of the R wave.

➤ Small or low amplitude P waves.

➤ A widened QRS (intraventricular block) in severe hyperkalemia.

Normal

Hyperkalemia
(Mild)

Hyperkalemia
(Severe)

Here is a rather impressive rhythm strip demonstrating a serum potassium level near 7.0 mEq. per liter.

(It is difficult to miss the tall, peaked, tent-like T waves!)

IMPORTANT NOTICE: One can never diagnose hyperkalemia from an EKG—it can only be suspected. Hyperkalemia must be confirmed by a serum potassium level.

Hyperkalemia *may* be associated with any of the following clinical conditions or therapies.

➤ infusions of excessive amounts of potassium solutions (**most common cause!**)

➤ burns

➤ crushing injuries

➤ adrenal insufficiency

➤ oliguria

➤ kidney damage

Hyperkalemia *depresses* **the normal electrical activity of the myocardial cells** and may result in any of the following dysrhythmias.

➤ **Sinus bradycardia**   ➤ **Idioventricular rhythm**

➤ **Sinus arrhythmia**   ➤ **Ventricular tachycardia**

➤ **First degree AV block**   ➤ **Ventricular fibrillation**

➤ **Junctional rhythm**   ➤ **Asystole** (the absence of rhythm)

Hint: Tall, peaked (tent-like), symmetrical T waves should lead one to suspect *hyperkalemia*.

Review Guide

Hypokalemia	Hyperkalemia
$K^+ < 3.6$ mEq./L.	$K^+ > 5.2$ mEq./L.
Depressed ST segment	Tall peaked T waves
Prominent U wave	Small P waves
Prolonged (QU interval)	Widened QRS, when severe

. . . I suppose we should try a bit of practice. . . . **right?**

Practice Exercise 1

A. Potassium plays an important role in the (circle one) repolarization / depolarization activity of the myocardial cells.

B. During a normal cardiac cycle, the _____ wave represents repolarization activity.

C. This one is easy!

Match the terms with the EKG complexes at the right.

Hypokalemia

Normal Conduction

Hyperkalemia

D.   Briefly describe your observations and note any appropriate actions.

_____

_____

_____

_____

E.   Describe this rhythm strip and actions you might take.

_____

_____

_____

_____

_____

✔ For **Feedback 1,** refer to page 273.

Input Section 10.2: Serum Calcium

That brings us to calcium. Remember calcium? Calcium is the cation (-ION) that moves into the cells following depolarization, causing mechanical activity or contraction. In other words, calcium (Ca^{++}) is a cardiac *stimulant* whose **main function is *contractility*.**

Normal serum calcium levels range between 9–11 mg.%. EKG changes associated with hypocalcemia are seen in the ST segment of the cardiac cycle.

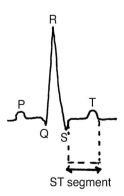

ST segment

Hypocalcemia

Hypocalcemia refers to a **serum calcium (Ca^{++}) level below 9 mg.%** and causes *decreased contractility of the heart.*

On EKG, a low serum calcium presents as a *lengthening* or prolongation of the ST segment, without changing the appearance of the QRS or the T wave. There is no change in the QRS or T wave because calcium does its work between depolarization and repolarization.

> **Always remember to observe for hypocalcemia when there is an upset in acid base balance and in the presence of hypoparathyroid disease.**

In a hypocalcemic state, the ST segment appears flat (*isoelectric*) and *prolonged*, as illustrated in the above drawing. If you recall the earlier discussion of QT intervals, you will remember that the *QT interval is prolonged.* The other significant feature is the low amplitude T waves, squatty in appearance. (I'm not certain that *squatty* is a real word . . . but you get the idea!)

Here are two EKG leads demonstrating hypocalcemia.

> **IMPORTANT NOTICE:** One can never diagnose hypocalcemia from an EKG—it can only be suspected. Hypocalcemia must be confirmed by a serum calcium level!

Hypercalcemia

Hypercalcemia, on the other hand, refers to a **serum calcium level greater than 11 mg.%.** A high serum calcium will cause *increased contractility of the heart.*

The EKG changes associated with hypercalcemia appear opposite to those of hypocalcemia (brilliant deduction, right ?).

As seen in the above drawing, hypercalcemia causes a shortening of the ST segment (without changing the appearance of the QRS or T wave (because calcium does its work *between* depolarization and repolarization).

As a matter of fact, the ST segment is *commonly* absent! Often one observes an abruptly ascending T wave immediately following the QRS, as illustrated below.

Always remember to watch for hypercalcemia in the presence of acidosis.

Following is a 12 lead EKG demonstrating a high serum calcium level.

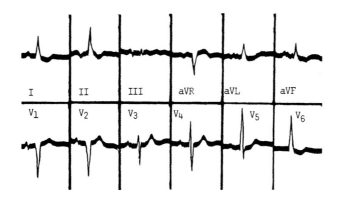

IMPORTANT NOTICE: One can never diagnose hypercalcemia from an EKG—it can only be suspected. Hypercalcemia must be confirmed by a serum calcium level!

Review Guide

Hypocalcemia	Hypercalcemia
$Ca^{++} < 9$ mg.%	$Ca^{++} > 11$ mg. %
↓ contractility	↑ contractility
prolonged ST segment	shortened ST segment

Practice Exercise 2

Surprise . . . it's practice time again!

A. Calcium is a cardiac _____, so its main function is contractility.

B. Hypocalcemia refers to a serum calcium level (circle one) above / below 9 mg.%.

C. Hypocalcemia can be suspected when one sees a _____ ST segment.

D. Draw a cardiac cycle (PQRST) that demonstrates a low calcium effect.

E. Hypercalcemia refers to a serum calcium level above _____ mg.%.

F. Hypercalcemia can be suspected when one sees a _____ ST segment.

G. Draw a cardiac cycle (PQRST) that demonstrates a high calcium effect.

H. Hypocalcemia causes _____ cardiac contractility.

I. Hypercalcemia causes _____ cardiac contractility.

✔ For **Feedback 2,** refer to page 274.

Input Section 10.3: Magnesium

Magnesium (Mg^{++}) is the second most frequently occurring intercellular cation. The normal serum magnesium level ranges between 1.8–3.0 mg/dL. However, serum magnesium levels are rarely diagnostic since 60% of magnesium resides in the bones, 40% resides in cells, and only 1% resides in the interstitial compartment and serum! Magnesium plays a number of important roles including mediating neural transmission and influencing the transport of ions regulating cardiac action potential.

Magnesium is particularly important in that a low magnesium level (hypomagnesemia ... often suspected, rather than confirmed by lab values) causes an increase in the QTc interval (refer to page 264). An abnormal QTc interval suggests that ventricular repolarization is delayed, and that delay poses a risk for dysrhythmias. **Quite frequently, hypomagnesemia occurs in tandem with hypokalemia and should be suspected when hypokalemia is present.** You will recall that a prolonged QT interval is associated with hypokalemia, as well.

When therapeutically administered, magnesium has both antiarrhythmic (similar to calcium channel blockers) and anti-platelet properties. It also has coronary vasodilator effects, reducing contractility. **Magnesium slows cardiac conduction and ventricular refractoriness.** Magnesium is often used to treat unresponsive lethal ventricular dysrhythmias (ventricular tachycardia, torsades de pointes) and may be given to acute myocardial infarct patients for its antiarrhythmic, anti-platelet and vasodilator effects. Clinical research is ongoing to determine the efficacy of magnesium in treating rapid, re-entry atrial dysrhythmias.

Hypomagnesemia may result from diarrhea, hypoparathyroid disease, pancreatitis, ulcerative colitis and alcoholism. Hypermagnesemia may be associated with chronic renal failure, dehydration, diabetic acidosis and oliguria.

Hypermagnesemia may be associated with chronic renal failure, dehydration, diabetic acidosis and oliguria.

There is no accompanying practice exercise! Instead, together we will evaluate a rhythm strip demonstrating a prolonged QT interval. Then, just for fun, we will calculate the QTc using Bazet's formula! You will recall (from Section 1), the QT interval is measured from the beginning of the QRS to the end of the T wave. Often times, the QT interval is most easily measured in leads V_2 and V_3.

The above rhythm is a sinus bradycardia (approximate rate 55 beats per minute). The QRS is borderline, measuring just slightly less than 0.12 seconds. The QT interval measures 13 small squares or 0.52 seconds ($13 \times 0.04 = 0.52$). The R-R interval measures 27 small squares or 1.08 seconds ($27 \times 0.04 = 1.08$).

The QTc is a measure of the total time for depolarization and repolarization, corrected for heart rate. EKG machines automatically calculate the QTc rate, though a manual calculation can be performed using Bazet's formula.

$$\text{Bazet's formula} \qquad QTc = \frac{QT \text{ interval in seconds}}{\sqrt{R\text{-}R \text{ interval in seconds}}}$$

$$QTc = \frac{0.52 \ (QT \text{ in seconds})}{\sqrt{1.08 \ (R\text{-}R \text{ in seconds})}}$$

$$\sqrt{1.08} = 1.039$$

$$QTc = \frac{0.52}{1.039}$$

$$QTc = 0.50$$

The normal male QTc interval averages 0.39 seconds; the normal female QT interval averages 0.41 seconds. For both sexes, a normal QTc is less than 0.44 seconds. Thus, the above QTc interval is significantly prolonged at 0.50 seconds.

BREAK TIME! ☺

✔ Feedback 1

How did you do? If your answers are similar to mine, you deserve a banana! (Bananas are packed full of potassium)

A. Potassium plays an important role in the (repolarization)/depolarization activity of the myocardial cells.

B. During a normal cardiac cycle, the <u>T</u> wave represents repolarization activity.

C. If your matching does <u>not</u> match mine, the Great Banana suggests that you reread Input 9.1.

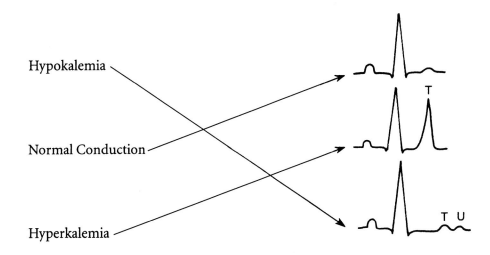

D. The rhythm appears to be a sinus bradycardia with a rate between 50–60 beats per minute. The ST segment is slightly depressed and there is a prominent U wave. I suspect hypokalemia, but would need to verify with a serum potassium level.

E. The rhythm is a borderline sinus bradycardia with a heart rate of 60. The P waves are small. The T waves are tall and peaked (tent-like). I suspect hyperkalemia, but would need to verify with a serum potassium level.

✔ Feedback 2

You're Doing Super . . .

. . . especially if you answered all the questions correctly!!

A. Calcium is a cardiac **stimulant,** so its main function is **contractility.**

B. Hypocalcemia refers to a serum calcium level (below) 9 mg.%.

C. Hypocalcemia can be suspected when one sees a <u>lengthened or prolonged</u> ST segment.

D.

E. Hypercalcemia refers to a serum calcium level above <u>11</u> mg.%.

F. Hypercalcemia can be suspected when one sees a <u>shortened</u> ST segment.

G.

H. Hypocalcemia causes <u>decreased</u> cardiac contractility.

I. Hypercalcemia causes <u>increased</u> cardiac contractility.

A Final Refresher

Hypokalemia	Hyperkalemia
$K^+ < 3.6$ mEq./L.	$K^+ > 5.2$ mEq./L.
Depressed ST segment	Tall peaked T waves
Prominent U wave	Small P waves
Prolonged (QU interval)	Widened QRS, when severe

Hypocalcemia	Hypercalcemia
$Ca^{++} < 9$ mg.%	$Ca^{++} > 11$ mg. %
↓ contractility	↑ contractility
prolonged ST segment	shortened ST segment

IMPORTANT NOTICE: Electrolyte effects on EKG are often subtle, and many times missed. When laboratory studies identify abnormal serum electrolyte levels, review a current 12 lead EKG to see if you can *spot* the subtle changes. ☺

Notes

Notes

The Identification of Ischemia, Injury, and Infarct

Objectives

When you have completed Section 11, you will be able to describe or identify

1. The classification scheme for myocardial infarction
2. The relationship between coronary blood supply and EKG patterns
3. the normal 12 lead EKG
4. the orientation of EKG leads to the left ventricular surfaces
5. EKG changes associated with ischemia
6. muscle layers in the heart
7. criteria for diagnosing or suspecting myocardial infarction
8. injury pattern in leads overlying an infarct
9. the hallmark of large scale myocardial infarction or necrosis
10. anteroseptal wall myocardial infarction
11. inferior wall myocardial infarction
12. criteria suggesting a posterior wall myocardial infarction
13. serum markers

☆ **Reread "LEADing into Section 1" (pages 1–12) before progressing!**

A Brief Introduction

by Stephanie Woods, Ph.D., R.N.

The Relationship between Coronary Blood Supply and the EKG

The conduction tissues generate electrical energy which is observable on the EKG as it travels through and activates cardiac muscle. Both the muscle and the conducting tissues require oxygen which is extracted from blood perfusing through the coronary arteries. When the blood supply is inadequate, both muscle and conducting tissues suffer secondary to the inadequate oxygenation. A diminished blood supply to the muscle typically results in pain (*angina*). The inadequate blood flow to conduction tissue results in characteristic changes on the EKG.

Decreased coronary blood flow sufficient to interfere with oxygen (O^2) and carbon dioxide (CO^2) exchange is referred to as *ischemia*. If the ischemia is transient or episodic in nature, it is usually unassociated with permanent damage, serving more as a warning. If ischemia persists, it can lead to varying degrees of cardiac muscle and conduction tissue damage. This damage, known as *injury,* may result in changes in both muscle and conduction tissue functioning. When marked ischemia persists over time, or in the face of complete vessel occlusion, the muscle and conduction tissue will actually die, thus ceasing both electrical and mechanical activity. Muscle and conduction tissue cellular death is termed *myocardial infarction*. Once cardiac cells die, there is an immediate loss of muscle activity (*contraction*) and electrical activity (*conduction*) in the involved tissues.

Ischemia Has the Following Classical Presentations

➤ Intermittent or sustained ischemia typically produces chest pain known as *angina pectoris*. Anginal pain may also radiate to the neck, jaw, arms, and back. Some patients will describe feelings of pressure, and may experience nausea, vomiting, and diaphoresis (sweating). Intermittent or *transient* ischemia produces characteristic T wave inversion and ST segment depression patterns on the EKG.

IMPORTANT NOTES:

(1) While most patients will experience anginal pain during ischemia, some will not. Smokers and patients with certain neurological disorders may be unable to sense pain in the chest wall. When coronary blood flow is diminished but unassociated with pain, this is referred to as *silent ischemia*. This is a dangerous situation because, without pain, the patient is unaware of danger and may not seek help.

(2) Chest pain can be associated with various types of illnesses. One must be able to correctly determine the cause of pain in order to institute the appropriate treatment. To *rule out* ischemia (verses other causative factors of chest pain), one must correlate chest pain with changes in the EKG pattern and the presence of serum markers in the blood.

➤ Persistent ischemia causes cell injury. In the *injury phase,* cell membranes break down (lysis) causing leakage of the cell contents into the blood stream. This leakage contains proteins and biomarkers which can be measured by specific lab tests. During injury, some degree of dysfunction occurs. Conduction tissue injury may manifest as changes in heart rate, ectopic activity or life-threatening rhythms. Injury to muscle tissue may present as pump failure or congestive heart failure. The EKG demonstrates a classic ST elevation pattern during the injury phase. Ischemia is frequently associated with ventricular dysrhythmias.

➤ Continuous and prolonged ischemia produces cellular necrosis and death (*acute myocardial infarction*). Large scale myocardial infarction or complete vessel occlusion is evidenced on the EKG as a *pathologic Q wave* pattern.

☆ It is important to recognize that the classifications for myocardial insult are evolving as the intricacies of pathology are better understood. In past years, myocardial infarction was classified as *Q wave* or *non-Q wave* infarction, the Q-wave infarct representing more extensive myocardial muscle involvement or damage. That classification scheme focused more on the outcome of the myocardial event. **Today's classification scheme for myocardial insult is oriented toward *early recognition and intervention* rather than outcome.** The newest classification scheme is as follows and will be discussed in greater detail in Section 12.

ST-Elevation MI (STEMI) (myocardial infarction)

ST elevation > or equal to 1 mm in 2 or more contiguous leads

☆ Anterior leads
☆ Inferior leads
☆ Lateral leads
☆ Antero-lateral leads
☆ Posterior leads

New (or presumably new) LBBB

Non-ST-Elevation MI (NSTEMI) (myocardial infraction): Includes high-risk or unstable angina

---

ST depression < or equal to 0.5 mm in two or more contiguous leads
Marked symmetrical T wave inversion in multiple precordial leads
ST-T wave changes with chest pain

Indeterminate/Low Risk Unstable Angina: Includes normal or non-diagnostic changes in ST segment or T waves

---

ST depression < 0.5 mm
T wave inversion or flattening in leads with dominate R waves
Normal EKG

Before advancing further, it is helpful to preview a normal 12 lead EKG and review the leads representing the various surfaces of the left ventricle.

The Standard 12 Lead Electrocardiogram

The standard 12 lead electrocardiogram allows one to view electrical activity on the surfaces of the heart—or, to look at the electrical activity from various angles or from various points of reference.

The left ventricle is the most important chamber of the heart in that it functions as *the pump* or as the *driving force* for systemic circulation. Because the left ventricle is such an important structure, the 12 lead system is designed to view the various surfaces of the left ventricle!

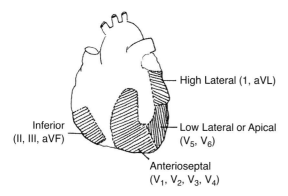

Leads I and aVL look at the lateral surface of the left ventricle (high lateral).

Leads II, III, and aVF look at the inferior or diaphragmatic surface of the left ventricle.

Leads V_1, V_2, V_3, and V_4 look at the anteroseptal surface of the left ventricle.

Leads V_5 and V_6 look at the low lateral surface or apical surface of the left ventricle.

You will recall from page 9, there are no leads designated to look directly at the posterior surface of the left ventricle.

Up until now, this "lead business" may have seemed to be of little importance to you . . . but your thinking is about to be transformed!

Serious coronary artery events are typically reflected on the EKG as ischemic changes, patterns of injury, and/or areas of myocardial infarction or cellular death. That of course, is nothing new . . . but depending upon the extent of the cardiac embarrassment and the location of the insult, a patient's hospital course and prognosis can be anticipated. And you know what tells us the location of the insult? . . . **The leads!**

For both treatment and patient management purposes, one must also have an appreciation for myocardial blood supply.

Myocardial Blood Supply

The heart muscle is supplied by two main coronary arteries—the right coronary artery (RCA) and the left coronary artery (LCA). Please see the diagram at the top of page 283. Both the RCA and the LCA arise from the base of the aorta, traveling on the outer surface of the heart muscle. Smaller branches of these major arteries penetrate into the deeper muscle layers, thus nourishing the inner muscle with an adequate blood supply. You will notice that the left coronary artery divides into the left anterior descending artery (LAD) and the left circumflex (Cx) artery. The table on the following page maps the *common* supplying coronary artery branch with the various surfaces of the left ventricle.

Myocardial Blood Supply

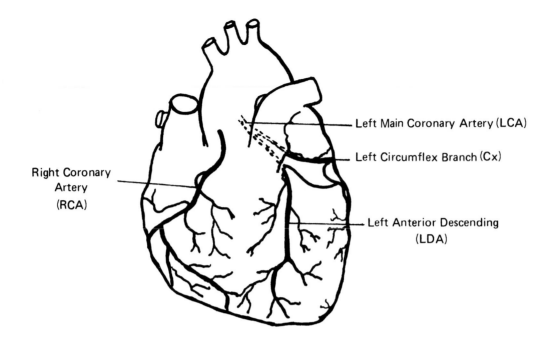

Artery	Tissue Supplied
Left Anterior Descending (LAD)	Anterior surface of the left ventricle Anterior surface of the septum The middle portion of the anterior surface of the right ventricle The lower portion of the posterior surface of the right ventricle
Right Coronary Artery (RCA)	The remainder of the right ventricle The upper portion of the posterior wall of the left ventricle (The SA node is supplied by the RCA in approximately 75% of the population, and the AV node is supplied by a branch of the RCA in about 90% of the population.)
Left Circumflex (Cx)	Lateral wall of the left ventricle Lower half of the posterior wall of the left ventricle

Note: This table, will be referenced throughout this Section.

By understanding which vessels commonly supply certain portions of the left ventricle and by viewing EKG leads that reflect the electrical activity of the various left ventricular surfaces, one can assess ischemia, tissue injury, and infarction changes in a noninvasive manner.

Input Section 11.1: Myocardial Ischemia

Myocardial ischemia is sometimes referred to as angina or coronary insufficiency. As noted in the introduction to this section, *ischemia* is the change that results in the myocardial cells from a *temporary, insufficient* blood supply. Most usually, ischemia is due to atherosclerosis of the coronary arteries. Atherosclerosis is characterized by narrowing of the lumen (diameter) of the coronary arteries due to atheroma deposits, fibrosis, and calcification in the intima of the artery.

Following are schematics demonstrating first, the lumen of a healthy patent coronary artery and next,

the lumen of a coronary artery compromised by severe atherosclerotic changes.

The dark arrows represent blood flow, normal and compromised.

A situational example demonstrating the temporary nature of myocardial ischemia begins with an elderly lady with known atherosclerotic disease.

← This is a stray cat.

When rocking peacefully in her chair she experiences no symptoms because at rest, her myocardial cells receive an adequate blood supply. However, when she chases the stray cat from her garden, she experiences severe chest pain. Temporarily, the blood supply through her atherosclerotic coronary vessels is inadequate to meet tissue oxygenation needs. When she sits down to rest again, the pain subsides. This is *ischemia*. Typically, myocardial ischemia or coronary insufficiency is precipitated by exertion and relieved by rest.

The oxygen requirements of the myocardium are approximately three times that of other body tissue. Normally, in a resting state, the myocardium extracts 70–75% of the oxygen from the blood flowing through the coronary arteries. When the oxygen demand increases with exertion, the myocardium cannot significantly increase its oxygen extraction rate. Rather, increased oxygen is realized through increased blood flow or perfusion. The heart rate increases and healthy coronary arteries dilate in response to increased myocardial oxygen demand. Healthy coronary arteries can increase perfusion five times that of normal. In the presence of coronary artery disease, the ability to increase blood perfusion is limited. A coronary artery can be as much as 90% or greater obstructed before mechanical hindrance to blood flow results in symptoms.

EKG Wave Form Changes Associated With Myocardial Ischemia

Characteristic EKG patterns are commonly associated with ischemia episodes. Typically, myocardial ischemia presents on the EKG as ST segment and T wave changes in *leads looking at the ischemic surface*. Frequently, the T waves are inverted or upside down and tend to have an arrow appearance as demonstrated in the following strip.

T waves may also present as slightly flat or depressed in appearance as shown below. Because the precordial chest leads (V_1–V_6) are nearest to the ventricles, the T wave changes may be most obvious in these leads.

Notice the flat and slightly depressed T waves

Coronary insufficiency or ischemia may also be reflected on EKG by ST segment changes. Instead of the characteristic smooth joining of the ST segment and the T wave, there may a be sharp angle at the ST-T junction.

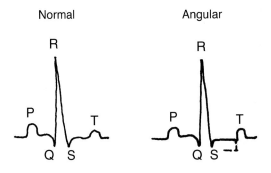

Or, as more commonly observed, the ST segment will be depressed.

Note the depression of the ST segment below the isoelectric (. . .) line.

If you think these ST-T wave changes resemble changes associated with certain electrolyte and drug effects, you are correct!! That is precisely why one never diagnoses any condition based solely on EKG findings!
   . . . Okay, now back to the elderly lady chasing the stray cat out of her garden!
Following is the 12 lead EKG taken while she was experiencing chest pain. Notice the ST-T wave changes. For comparison, please refer to the example 12 lead EKG, page 280.

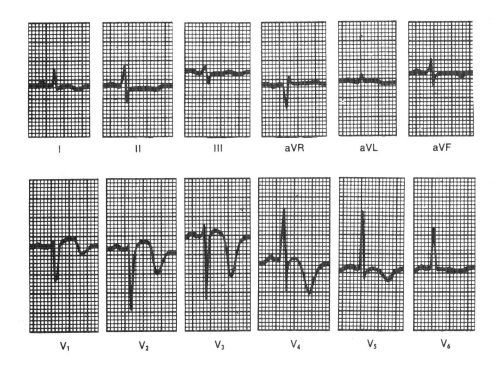

It is safe to say that our "rocking chair friend" has generalized ST-T wave changes throughout the 12 leads. Thus, it is likely that her myocardial blood flow is significantly compromised during exertion.

Remember:

Leads I and aVL look at the high lateral surface of the left ventricle (LV);
Leads II, III, and aVF look at the inferior surface of the LV;
Leads V_1, V_2, V_3, and V_4 look at the anteroseptal surface of the LV;
and
Leads V_5 and V_6 look at the low lateral or apical surface of the LV.

IMPORTANT NOTE: Coronary artery disease is a more dynamic process than once thought. Just as clots or thrombi may form, they may be subsequently altered or influenced by normal fibrinolysis processes. The net effect of these two opposing processes is an unstable or changing clinical situation. Thus, some clinical presentations may remain *steady state* while others may progress, or even diminish in intensity. Myocardial ischemia maybe temporary or *transient* in nature (less than 20 minutes) or sustained (*unstable*). When ischemia persists, myocardial injury begins.

Practice Exercise 1

Are you ready for some practice?

Practice will be kept simple since this material has a tendency to be somewhat difficult!

A. The 12 lead EKG allows one to look at the electrical activity of the heart from various _____

_____

_____

B. The most important chamber of the heart is the left ventricle because _____

_____

_____

_____

C. Match the leads with the correct surfaces of the left ventricle.

(If in doubt, refer to the bottom of page 281!)

Leads I and aVL	High lateral surface of the LV
Leads II, III, and aVF	Low lateral surface of the LV
Leads V_1, V_2, V_3, and V_4	Inferior surface of the LV
Leads V_5 and V_6	Anteroseptal surface of the LV

D. By definition, *ischemia* is the myocardial change that results from _____
   blood supply.

E. Myocardial ischemia presents on the EKG as _____ and _____ changes in
   leads looking at the ischemic surface.

F. Here is a 12 lead EKG. Describe the ST-T wave changes that you see.

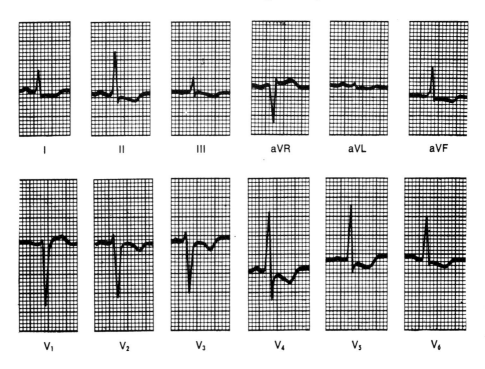

_____
_____
_____
_____
_____
_____
_____
_____
_____

G. Describe the differences between an "ST-elevation myocardial infarction" (STEMI) and a "non-ST elevation myocardial infarction" (NSTEMI).

_____
_____
_____

✔ For **Feedback 1,** refer to page 314.

Input Section 11.2: Myocardial Injury and Infarction

Before delving into the subject of myocardial infarction, it is helpful to review the muscle layers of the heart.

The *endocardium* is the muscle lining on the inside of the heart, while the *epicardium* is the outer muscle covering. The muscle layer between the endocardium and the epicardium is the *myocardium.*

Myocardial infarction is the term used to describe actual necrosis and death of a portion of heart muscle resulting from an insufficient blood supply to keep the muscle viable. In other words, the heart muscle is deprived of an adequate blood supply over a period of time, thus causing *cellular destruction and death.* In most cases, a fatty arterial wall plaque ruptures, allowing red blood cells and platelets to aggregate, forming a clot which occludes (in part, or total) the lumen of a coronary artery.

A myocardial infarction may be limited to any one of the muscle layers, or may extend through all muscle layers. The extent of muscle damage is related to the duration or stability of the occlusion and the presence or absence of collateral circulation.

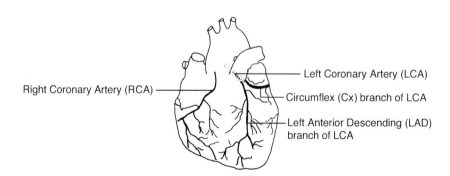

Because the two main coronary arteries, the right coronary artery (RCA) and the left coronary artery (LAD), and the circumflex (Cx) and descending (LAD) branches of the LCA supplying the heart muscle run along the epicardium, the inner muscle layers are more prone to injury in the face of coronary artery disease. The inner muscle layers receive their blood supply from smaller branches of the LCA and RCA that penetrate into the muscle. If these small branches are occluded, muscle destruction is inevitable. In fact, infarction may result from incomplete occlusion of a coronary artery if the blood supply is significantly limited to a portion of the heart muscle!

On the other hand, if coronary artery disease is slow progressing (over many years), sufficient collateral circulation may develop to supply the heart muscle with adequate blood and oxygen despite progressive occlusion of a supplying vessel. In this case, complete occlusion of a coronary artery branch *could* occur without significant muscle destruction. Complicated, right!

Before discussing the EKG findings associated with acute myocardial infarction, one must first memorize the following caution.

CAUTION

The diagnosis of acute myocardial infarction is NEVER based solely on EKG findings.

The diagnosis of a acute myocardial infarction or acute coronary syndromes is based on:

➤ **Positive patient history** (chest pain, radiating pain, indigestion, jaw pain, elbow pain, sweating, nausea, vomiting, etc.)

➤ **Elevated serum markers** (indicating cellular membrane destruction . . . serum markers will be discussed on page 313).

➤ **Positive or suggestive EKG findings**

It should be noted that the EKG *may* remain normal in acute myocardial infarction . . . or show nonspecific changes that are not diagnostic. *Usually,* however, the following electrocardiographic findings are associated with large scale ST-elevation myocardial infarction (STEMI).

Generally, the *first* electrocardiographic finding associated with acute myocardial infarction (STEMI) is *ST segment elevation* in two or more contiguous leads *overlying the area of injury.* The ST elevation measures 1 mm or greater in amplitude and represents current *injury.* ST elevation simply means that the ST segment rises above the isoelectric line. Usually, ST elevation is observable 30–40 minutes post vessel occlusion.

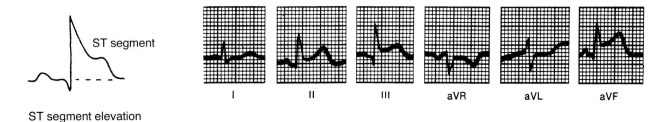

ST segment

ST segment elevation

I   II   III   aVR   aVL   aVF

Observe the ST elevation evident in leads II, III and aVF above.

Note: An injury pattern (ST elevation) cannot be determined in the presence of left bundle branch block! Look back to page 166. ST segment distortion (altered recovery or repolarization) occurs secondary to delayed activation of the left ventricle.

If monitoring is initiated at the very onset of acute myocardial infarction (STEMI), tall, peaked, "tent-like" T waves may be evident in leads overlying the infarct (see the illustration at the top of the next page). It has been suggested that this is a result of intracellular potassium leaking from the damaged muscle cells into the extracellular space. Within several hours post infarct, however, the tall peaked T waves evolve. The ST elevation persists in leads overlying the infarct during the acute phase of the infarct.

Tall peaked T waves may be observed at the very
onset of myocardial cellular damage.

What is meant by *leads overlying the infarct?*
Remember this chart?

> Leads I and aVL look at the lateral surface of the LV (high lateral).
> Leads II, III, and aVF look at the inferior surface of the LV.
> Leads V_1, V_2, V_3, V_4, look at the anteroseptal surface of the LV.
> Leads V_5 and V_6 look at the low lateral surface of the LV (apical).

If ST elevation is observed in leads I and aVL, one can assume there is current injury of the high lateral wall of the left ventricle . . . or, if ST elevation is seen in leads II, III, and aVF, one can assume there is injury of the inferior wall of the left ventricle, etc. (One can only *assume* there is injury because other conditions such as pulmonary embolus and pericarditis result in ST elevation!)

That's fairly easy, huh?

So, in STEMI, ST elevation will be observed in the leads overlying the injured myocardial surface. Additionally, *reciprocal ST segment depression* often occurs in the leads oriented toward the *uninjured* myocardial surfaces. Look at the illustration on the previous page. Notice the slight ST segment depression in leads I and aVL.

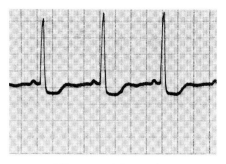

ST segment depression

Note: When ST elevation is evident in most all leads, one should suspect pericarditis.

The EKG *hallmark* of extensive myocardial necrosis (complete occlusion) in *upright leads* (leads I, II, III, aVL, aVF, V_5, and V_6) is the presence of pathologic *Q waves,* observed in leads oriented toward the necrotic area. To qualify as abnormal, Q waves must be wide and deep in appearance, measuring at least **0.04 seconds in width** (one small EKG square) and measuring **deeper than ¼ of the R wave amplitude.** You will note there is a loss of R wave amplitude as well (see illustration at the top of page 291).

Normal

Pathologic Q Wave

The appearance of pathologic Q waves follows the appearance of the ST-T wave changes in many cases. The appearance of pathologic Q waves is an evolutionary phase of an extensive acute myocardial infarct process and is usually evident several hours post occlusion.

(**P.S.** *Small* Q waves, nonpathologic, may normally be seen in leads I, II, V_4, and V_5.)

The EKG *hallmark* of large scale myocardial necrosis in *negatively oriented leads* (V_1, V_2, V_3, and V_4) is the loss of the positive R wave (loss of R wave progression) found in leads oriented toward the necrotic area. Thus, the resulting wave pattern is a QS configuration.

Loss of R wave

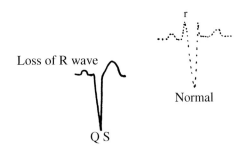

Normal

Q S

The loss of the R wave in negatively oriented leads follows after the appearance of the ST-T wave changes (just as the pathologic Q wave appears in upright leads following the appearance of ST-T wave changes). The loss of R waves is an evolutionary phase of an extensive acute myocardial infarct process.

Understanding pathologic Q waves or the loss of R waves requires first knowing a bit about normal or healthy ventricular depolarization.

Depolarization of the ventricles begins in the left side of the intraventricular septum . . . and spreads to the right, through the septum.

Next, ventricular depolarization spreads outward through the free walls of both the left and right ventricles.

Because the left ventricle has greater muscle mass, the left ventricular depolarization forces are greater than the right ventricular forces. Thus, the net general direction of ventricular depolarization is leftward.

In summary, ventricular depolarization can be thought of as first ①, a left to right activation of the septum, followed by a large net force of activation moving from ② right to left through the free wall of the left ventricle.

To lend clarity, let's explore the spread of ventricular depolarization, using the precordial leads V_6 and V_1 as examples. Remember, the V leads . . . V_1, V_2, V_3, V_4, V_5, and V_6 . . . are all positive leads. (For a quick refresher on V leads, refer to page 00.)

This is the left ventricle . . .

. . . And this is an electrode . . . lead V_6 ⊕ (oriented toward the left heart)

The V_6 electrode will first see the left to right depolarization of the septum. Since the depolarization wave is moving away from the positive electrode, the first part of the QRS deflection will be negative.

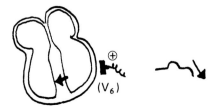

Next, the larger (net) force of depolarization moves from right to left through the free wall of the left ventricle toward the positive electrode. So, a large upward deflection is then seen on EKG. Note the positive R wave in the QRS below.

Thus, in a lead oriented toward the left ventricle (like V$_6$), the entire picture of ventricular depolarization will look like this.

Depolarization of the right and left ventricle muscle

Septal depolarization

Next, let's consider the ventricular depolarization process from a lead oriented toward the right ventricle (like V$_1$). Remember, all V leads are positive leads!

The first phase of ventricular depolarization is always septal activation, and you will remember that the interventricular septum is activated from left to right. That means that the initial depolarization force is moving toward the positive electrode.

> **When the depolarization force moves toward a positive electrode, the EKG deflection will be positive or upright.**

Thus, the initial phase of the QRS deflection observed in this lead (V$_1$) is positive or upward.

Next, the wave (net force) of depolarization moves from right to left through the free wall of the left ventricle, away from the positive electrode.

(V₁)
⊕

> **When the depolarization force moves away from a positive electrode, the EKG deflection will be negative.**

The entire picture of ventricular depolarization as seen from a right chest electrode looks like this (lead V_1 or V_2).

Septal depolarization

r

s — Depolarization of the right and left ventricle muscle

Here are leads V_1 through V_6 as recorded from a healthy individual.

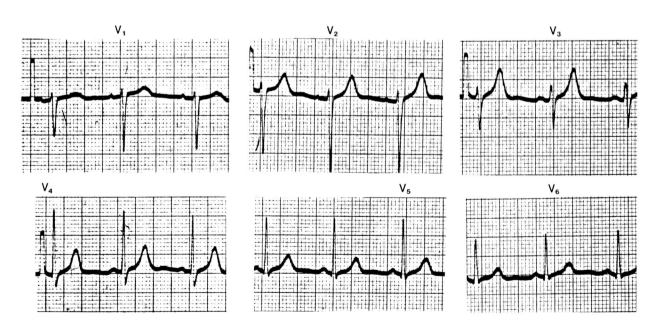

Knowing how the forces of depolarization move normally through the ventricular muscle, it's easy to understand why each of the V leads appear as they do!

In the previous strip (bottom of page 294) notice how the R waves gets progressively larger in each lead until the complexes are upright in leads V_4, V_5, and V_6. This is known as *normal R wave progression.*

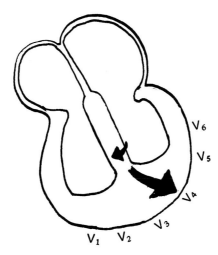

Leads V_1 and V_2 are oriented toward the right heart, while leads V_3 and V_4 are oriented toward the septum. Since the septal force of depolarization moves toward the right, these leads usually record a small initial R wave, a positive wave that progresses in size. Following septal depolarization, the net force (direction) of ventricular depolarization is leftward, moving away from the right V leads. Thus, the positive R wave is followed by a negative wave, a QS pattern.

Leads V_5 and V_6 are oriented toward the left heart. Since the septal force of depolarization moves away from these electrodes, a small negative Q wave is the first EKG deflection observed. The remainder of the QRS complex in these leads is positive, as the major ventricular wave of depolarization is moving toward the left chest electrodes.

Sounds relatively simple . . . right?

Pathologic Q waves (in positive leads) and loss of R waves (in negative leads resulting in a QS pattern) represent *electrical death!* In other words, the area of muscle, represented by the leads demonstrating abnormal Q waves or loss of R waves, has lost its ability to transmit electrical impulses.

That is sometimes a difficult idea to grasp . . . so we will use a window analogy to add clarity. Tissue that is dead cannot repolarize or depolarize . . . it is electrically inactive. If all the muscle layers are involved in the infarct (transmural infarct), then electrically speaking, there is a "hole" or a "window" in the muscle.

The Window Analogy Graphically Illustrated

Okay . . . this is you.

Suppose you are standing in a room looking at a wall . . . what will you see?

Naturally, you see the wall.

But, if instead of a solid wall, there is a window . . . what will you see?

Naturally, you will see through the window, viewing the activity outside or beyond the window.

A similar phenomenon occurs in the case of an electrical "hole," or "window." If an electrode is placed over this window (over the electrically dead muscle tissue), the electrode will see the healthy electrical activity beyond the window!

Here are the precordial (chest leads) of a normal healthy individual. Note the normal progression of R waves, beginning small and progressing until the QRS is upright.

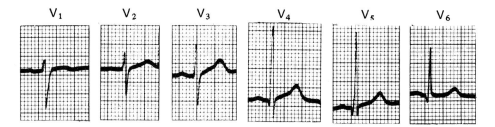

Example

When a large scale infarct (STEMI) occurs in the anteroseptal wall of the left ventricle, the necrotic region becomes an "electrical" window. Since leads V_1–V_4 view the anteroseptal region of the left ventricle, they will look through the window at distant heart activity. Compare this example to the one directly above.

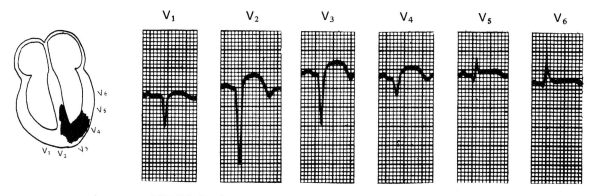

Anteroseptal Wall Infarction: Note the loss of R wave in leads V_1, V_2, V_3, and V_4 and the ST segment elevation in those same leads.

Remember, necrotic tissue has no ability to transmit electrical impulses! One would normally expect septal depolarization (the first phase of ventricular depolarization) to move toward the positive V_1–V_4 electrode producing a positive, upward stroke (R wave). In the presence of an anteroseptal infarct, the V_1–V_4 electrode captures only the second phase of ventricular depolarization, moving away from the electrode. Thus, there is no initial positive upstroke (loss of R wave). Rather, only a large negative wave (QS) is observed. The ST elevation signifies that the injury is current.

To review then, the positive R forces in these leads are completely lost. There are no initial positive R forces. The first deflection is a downward wave , a Q wave. When the deflection is negative (without an R wave), the complex is referred to as a QS—as opposed to a QRS.

Important Note of Elevated Significance

ST segment elevation is not predictive of the development of Q waves or the loss of R waves. Tissue necrosis may occur when only ST depression is present. Myocardial infarctions are now classified as ST elevation myocardial infarction (SIEMI) or non-ST elevation myocardial infraction (NSTEMI). STEMI's are associated with a 1 mm or greater rise in ST amplitude in two or more contiguous leads. NSTEMI's are defined by a 0.5 mm or greater ST depression in two or more contiguous leads and marked symmetrical T wave in version in multiple precordial leads.

Before progressing further, a brief summary is in order!

➤ The right and left coronary arteries and their branches supply the heart muscle with nutrients.

➤ If the blood supply to a portion of the heart muscle is only temporarily interrupted, ischemic changes can be seen in those leads that look at the ischemic heart surface.

➤ Ischemic changes include inverted or upside down T waves and ST depression, as noted in the strip at the top of page 298.

Summary, continued:

Pronounced inverted T waves

➤ When ischemia persists or when a coronary artery or a branch of an artery becomes occluded, myocardial tissue damage will rapidly ensue.

➤ Myocardial injury is generally seen on the EKG as ST segment elevation in the leads overlying the injured tissue.

ST elevation in an upright lead

ST elevation in a negative lead

➤ As myocardial cells die and the infarct evolves, abnormal (pathologic) Q waves may become evident (depending on the duration of the occlusion and the presence of collateral circulation) in leads overlying the infarct. Pathologic Q waves (measuring at least 0.04 seconds in width and deeper then ¼ of the R wave amplitude) in upright leads represent electrical death!

Abnormal Q wave

➤ When a complete occlusion (Q wave infarct) occurs in areas of the heart reflected in the right precordial leads (V_1, V_2, V_3, and V_4), the initial R wave is lost, so that only a QS configuration is seen, as demonstrated in the drawing on the top of page 299.

Loss of R wave

QS

Basically, that covers the critical points discussed thus far . . .

Whew! (I'm just long-winded!!)

Before looking at some actual electrocardiograms, there is another phase of myocardial infarct (STEMI) evolution to consider. As the infarct begins to resolve, the abnormal ST segments gradually return to the baseline. In this stage, the T waves will commonly be inverted, denoting *resolution.*

Evolutionary Phases of Myocardial Infarction

Injury   Cellular Necrosis   Resolution

ST segment elevation   The appearance of the   T wave inversion
                              pathologic Q wave or the loss
                              of R wave is almost always
                              evident with complete occlusion.

> **Note:** ST elevation that persists following the evolutionary phase is suggestive of a ventricular aneurism.

The only residual (long-term) EKG evidence of myocardial infarction (Q-wave infarct) will be the persistent Q waves or the absence of R waves. *Almost* all patients retain the Q waves or maintain the loss of R waves in the leads representing the affected muscle tissue.

. . . So when a patient comes back to see you—a hundred years from now . . . you can very intelligently ask him or her, "When was it you had your heart attack?" (You will know the infarct occurred because the pathologic Q waves or the absence of R waves will be evident on the EKG!)

On the next page, a **chart** is provided to assist you as you analyze upcoming 12 lead EKGs.

* *RESEARCH NOTE*: Clinical research is ongoing to determine if autologous skeletal myoblasts (skeletal muscle cells) transplanted to an injured left ventricle (post infarct with left heart failure) can partially restore left ventricular function (J.American College of Cardiology 2003:42 [12]).

CHART DEPICTING CHANGES TYPICALLY ASSOCIATED WITH EXTENSIVE MYOCARDIAL DAMAGE (MUSCLE NECROSIS AND DEATH)

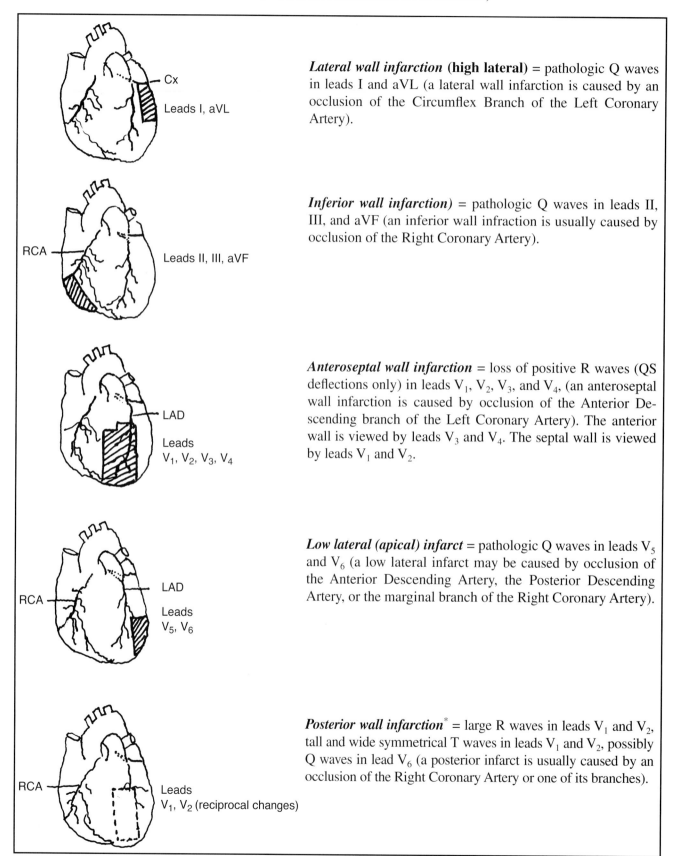

Lateral wall infarction (high lateral) = pathologic Q waves in leads I and aVL (a lateral wall infarction is caused by an occlusion of the Circumflex Branch of the Left Coronary Artery).

Cx
Leads I, aVL

Inferior wall infarction) = pathologic Q waves in leads II, III, and aVF (an inferior wall infraction is usually caused by occlusion of the Right Coronary Artery).

RCA
Leads II, III, aVF

Anteroseptal wall infarction = loss of positive R waves (QS deflections only) in leads V_1, V_2, V_3, and V_4, (an anteroseptal wall infarction is caused by occlusion of the Anterior Descending branch of the Left Coronary Artery). The anterior wall is viewed by leads V_3 and V_4. The septal wall is viewed by leads V_1 and V_2.

LAD
Leads V_1, V_2, V_3, V_4

Low lateral (apical) infarct = pathologic Q waves in leads V_5 and V_6 (a low lateral infarct may be caused by occlusion of the Anterior Descending Artery, the Posterior Descending Artery, or the marginal branch of the Right Coronary Artery).

LAD
RCA
Leads V_5, V_6

Posterior wall infarction* = large R waves in leads V_1 and V_2, tall and wide symmetrical T waves in leads V_1 and V_2, possibly Q waves in lead V_6 (a posterior infarct is usually caused by an occlusion of the Right Coronary Artery or one of its branches).

RCA
Leads V_1, V_2 (reciprocal changes)

*Posterior infarcts will be addressed on page 310.

There is only one more item to remember. *Ignore* lead aVR when looking for infarcts . . . Q waves appearing in this lead are *not* significant. Rather than being oriented to the left ventricular surface, lead aVR is oriented to the cavity of the left ventricle.

If you need to compare the following electrocardiograms to a normal EKG, reference page 280.

Okay! Following is a patient that has been experiencing severe chest pain for 24 hours. He has experienced nausea and vomiting since the onset of chest pain.

Observe each lead . . . look for evidence of current injury (ST elevation), and look for pathologic Q waves or loss of R waves (indicating cellular death or necrosis).

How about me helping you?

Lead I looks okay to me—there is a normal P, QRS, and T wave. The ST segment is "just a tad" below the isoelectric line.

Except . . . you know what . . . the P-R interval measures 6 small squares or 0.24 seconds! That is grounds for a first degree heart block! (First degree heart block can be reviewed on page 147.)

In *Lead II,* I see several abnormalities . . . there is a prominent Q wave and the ST segment is elevated above the isoelectric line.

Lead III also has a large Q wave and ST elevation. You will remember that *lead aVR* is the lead we are going to *ignore!*

Lead aVL shows slight ST segment depression—dipping below the isoelectric line.

Lead aVF also has a large Q wave and slight ST elevation.

All the V leads (V_1–V_6) look fairly normal.

So, in summary, there are pathologic Q waves and ST elevation in leads II, III, and aVF and slight ST depression in leads I and aVL.

What Does All of That Mean?

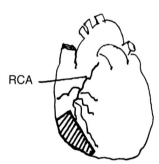

Well, review the summary chart on page 300. Elevated serum markers (see page 313) and pathologic Q waves in leads II, III, and aVF mean that there is an **Inferior Wall Myocardial Infarction** or inferior wall muscle necrosis. The ST elevation implies current tissue injury. The slight ST depression noted in leads I and aVL is simply the reciprocal changes that appear in leads oriented toward the opposite uninjured myocardial surfaces.

Anatomically, the inferior wall of the left ventricle borders the diaphragm. Thus, the patient with an inferior wall myocardial infarction may be troubled with persistent hiccoughs as well as nausea, and/or vomiting.

Typically, the Right Coronary Artery supplies the inferior wall of the left ventricle. In most individuals, the Right Coronary Artery feeds both the SA node and the AV node (refer back to page 282). Compromise of the RCA can precipate an array of dysrhythmias. As a matter of fact, that is no doubt why this patient has a first degree heart block! And you know what else—this patient later developed Wenckebach! Remember Wenckebach? If not, review page 150.

What do you think? Is looking for EKG evidence of infarcts tough business? ☺

Let's try another one! The precordial (V) leads appear on the next page.   *These are EKG calibrations!

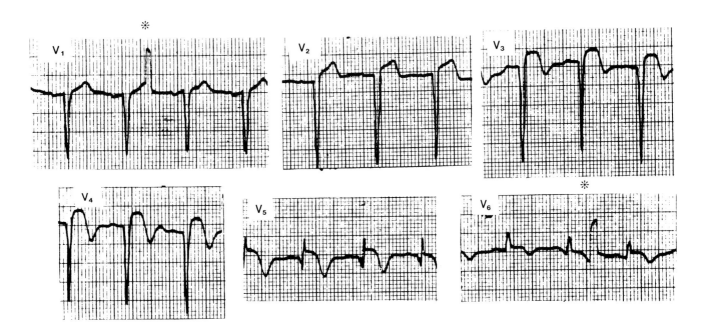

*To make certain that the EKG machine is properly calibrated, a standardized 1 millivolt pulse (10 vertical boxes) is periodically introduced into the tracing.

Remember, look at each lead!

Lead I looks rather "squatty" (low voltage) and the T waves are inverted. There is probably an initial Q wave, but it's difficult to tell for certain. There may also be slight ST elevation.

Leads II, III, and aVF appear normal, though there is slight ST sagging in leads *III* and *aVF*.

Lead aVL demonstrates very pronounced Q waves and inverted T waves. Further, there is slight ST elevation.

Leads V_1–V_4 show no R waves, only large negative QS deflections. In addition, there is pronounced ST elevation in leads V_2, V_3 and V_4.

Lead V_5 shows abnormal Q waves, ST elevation, and deeply inverted T waves. Also the R waves are greatly diminished in size.

Lead V_6 shows diminished R waves, a slightly elevated ST segment and inverted T waves.

This one is tough! Look back to the chart (page 300) if you need assistance! Sometimes, if there are multiple pathologies, I begin in reverse order. For instance, *leads II, III, and aVF* are fairly normal, so I presume that the inferior wall of the left ventricle is uninvolved.

You will remember that *leads I and aVL* represent the high lateral wall of the left ventricle. Pathologic Q waves in both of these leads suggest high lateral wall myocardial infarction. Because there is accompanying slight ST elevation, I am assuming there is current injury. The inverted T waves tell me there is ischemia of the lateral wall as well. So, the Q waves in leads I and aVL probably represent a high lateral wall infarction. Does that make sense? Hope so!

Injury and infarction (STEMI) in upright leads typically presents as follows:

Moving on, leads V_1–V_4 show ST elevation and diminished or nonexistent R waves. Looking back at the chart on page 000, I see that leads V_1–V_4 reflect the electrical activity of the anteroseptal wall of the left ventricle. From the above changes in leads V_1–V_4, the patient's history of crushing chest pain and the elevated serum markers, I can assume the patient also has an anteroseptal infarction. That means there is probably occlusion of the Left Anterior Descending coronary artery (refer back to page 282).

Continuing on with analysis . . .

Lead V_5 demonstrates abnormal Q waves; leads V_5 and V_6 show ST elevation and inverted T waves. So, the Q waves represent necrosis, the ST elevation represents injury, and the inverted T waves represent ischemia. The following day, a prominent Q wave was evident in V_6, as well. Since leads V_5 and V_6 represent the low lateral or apical area of the left ventricle, it would appear that the patient suffered damage of the high and low lateral and anteroseptal walls of the left ventricle!

Ugh! Also, one should bear in mind that the more "lethal" types of dysrhythmias . . . Mobitz II and complete heart block . . . are associated with anterior wall myocardial infarction.

Identifying injury and Q-wave infarct patterns is a matter of looking at each lead *very carefully* to determine subtle or pronounced deviations from normal.

It should be emphasized that many factors distort and complicate EKG patterns, such as dysrhythmias, electrolyte imbalances, drug effects, and so forth. If only a portion of the heart muscle wall is involved, or an occlusion is intermittent, the EKG changes will be subtle. Thus, the diagnosis of myocardial infarction is *never* solely based on the EKG findings!

The patient suspected of having an acute myocardial infarction (A.M.I.) or the patient actually having an A.M.I. must be monitored closely and continuously. The cells in the injured area of the heart muscle are **electrically unstable.** You will recall from Section 4, ischemic tissue is thought to release a *substance* which is capable of increasing the automaticity of the Purkinje fibers, resulting in electrical instability. This electrical instability may predispose the patient to *lethal* ventricular dysrhythmias. When ventricular irritability is present, amiodarone is the antiarrhythmic drug therapy of choice.

The above patient has a confirmed acute inferior wall myocardial infarction. Notice the extreme ST elevation and the prominent Q waves in lead II. This same pattern was evident in leads III and aVF, as well. P.V.C.s are falling on the downstroke of the vulnerable T waves and are occurring in couplets. This patient is at high risk for ventricular tachycardia or ventricular fibrillation. Amiodarone therapy is the usual treatment of choice.

The rhythm strip on the bottom of page 304 was recorded following hospital admission for an acute inferior wall myocardial infarction. Note the extreme ST elevation and the pathologic Q waves. Near the end of the strip, a P.V.C. falls near the vulnerable T wave, warning of increasing ventricular irritability.

It is important to remember that decreased cardiac contractility occurs secondary to myocardial muscle injury. **Observe the acute myocardial infarct patient closely for signs of heart failure and shock-like symptoms.**

The treatment objectives and options for transient ischemia or persistent ischemia leading to acute myocardial infarction will be discussed in Section 12. **Principally, it is the degree of left ventricular muscle mass involvement, and secondarily, the occurrence of lethal dysrhythmias, that determine patient prognosis post infarct.**

At the outset of acute myocardial infarction, anti-platelet or thrombolytic drug therapy ("clot busters") may be used in an attempt to restore the patency of the blocked coronary artery. Please see the discussion on platelet inhibitor and thrombolytic drug therapy, Section 14, page 382.

Before moving on to the practice exercise, a few points regarding QT intervals are in order. (If you need a refresher on QT intervals, refer back to pages 126 and 264). Studies of QT intervals have reported a direct relationship between the duration of QT intervals and myocardial ischemia and injury. The duration of the QT interval and the QTd measurement appear to be markers of both the extension and severity of myocardial damage.

Ischemia and non-Q wave infarcts have shorter QT and QTd intervals; Q wave infarcts and sustained ischemia typically demonstrate QTd prolongation.

You will recall, the QTd interval (QT dispersion) is a measure of myocardial refractoriness. In this metric, the QT interval is measured on the same beat in all 12 EKG leads. The shortest QT interval measurement is then subtracted from the longest QT interval measurement. The resulting difference represents the degree of variation in refractoriness. (You may also remember, the greater the dispersion, the greater the presumed risk for ventricular tachycardia or ventricular fibrillation associated with proarrhythmic drug effects!)

Now, on to the Practice Range!

 Practice Exercise 2

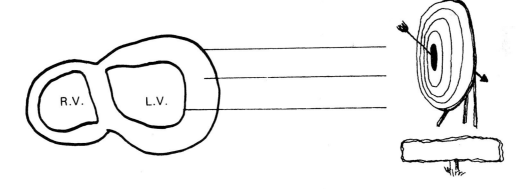

A. Above is a cross section view of the heart. Label the three muscle layers.

B. The diagnosis of large scale (Q-wave) myocardial infarction is based upon three criteria. List them!

1. _____

2. _____

3. _____

C. Draw a complex demonstrating a current injury pattern.

(Circle the correct word.)

D. Reciprocal ST (elevation / depression) will occur in the leads oriented toward the uninjured myocardial surfaces.

E. The hallmark of extensive myocardial infarction or necrosis is the _____

wave in positive leads and the _____ in negatively deflected leads.

F. To be pathologic, the abnormal Q waves must meet two criteria:

   1. The Q waves must measure at least _____ seconds in width or duration.

   2. The Q waves must be deeper than _____ the R wave amplitude.

G. Okay . . . here we go!

This patient was admitted to the hospital with crushing chest pain radiating to his left elbow. Leads I, II, III, and aVL were essentially normal. Here are the precordial leads from his admission EKG. Study them closely, describe what you see, and make an interpretation using the chart on page 300.

V₁   V₂   V₃   V₄   V₅   V₆

_____

_____

_____

_____

_____

_____

_____

_____

_____

_____

H. The following patient presented with indigestion-type pain, nausea, vomiting, and elevated serum markers. Study the leads carefully, describe what you see, and make an interpretation using the chart on page 300.

_____

_____

_____

_____

_____

_____

_____

_____

_____

_____

_____

I. Below are five examples of various EKG lead patterns. On the following page are five descriptions of EKG patterns. Study the EKG patterns closely! Then, write the number of the example EKG pattern next to the phrase that correctly identifies the strip. (See phrases on page 309).

(number)

_____ Prominent Q waves in leads II, III, and aVF. Inverted T waves in leads II, III, and aVF. Probable old inferior wall infarction with ischemia of the inferior wall.

_____ Marked ST depression and T wave inversion in leads I and aVL. Prominent Q waves and ST elevation in leads II, III, and aVF. Probable acute inferior wall myocardial infarction with reciprocal ST-T wave changes in the lateral leads.

_____ Pathologic Q waves in leads I and aVL. Inverted T waves in lead aVL. Probable old lateral wall infarction. The inverted T waves denote ischemia.

_____ Leads V_1–V_6 appear within normal limits. No pathology evident.

_____ Leads V_1–V_4 show abnormal QS deflections with marked ST elevation. There is marked ST elevation in leads V_5 and V_6. Probable acute anteroseptal wall infarction with injury extending to the low lateral wall of the left ventricle.

J. Evaluate this rhythm strip. Describe the rhythm and your impressions.

_____

_____

_____

_____

_____

_____

K. This next strip is a "Thinking Only" exercise. If perplexed, refer to Feedback 2.

✔ For **Feedback 2,** refer to page 315.

Input Section 11.3: Posterior Wall Myocardial Infarction

Seemingly, Section 11 has continued forever!

So, this final discussion on **posterior wall myocardial infarction** will be brief!

You will recall, there are no leads directly viewing the posterior wall of the left ventricle. That presents some-what of a problem! When using a 12 lead EKG, injury and infarction of the posterior surface is evidenced by changes in leads opposite the posterior surface.

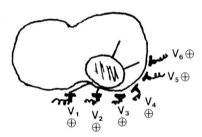

Leads V_1 and V_2 represent the anterior surface of the left ventricle and are directly opposite to the posterior left ventricular surface.

In other words, leads V_1 and V_2 lie opposite to the posterior surface of the heart.

So when observing for a posterior wall infarction, one needs to view leads V_1 and V_2!

Electrocardiographic findings associated with posterior wall infarctions appear in leads V_1 and V_2 and present as *the opposite* of electrocardiographic findings associated with anterior wall infarctions. So, one must remember patterns associated with an anterior wall infarct!

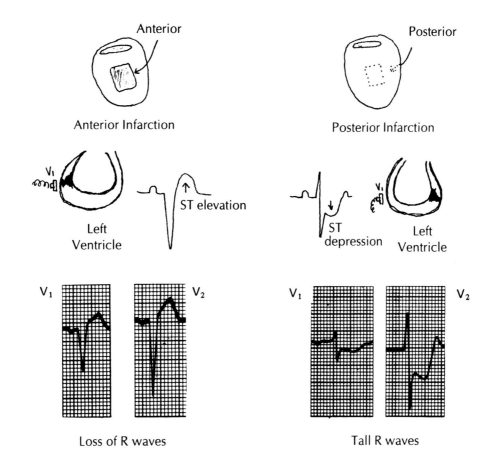

Anterior Infarction

Posterior Infarction

Loss of R waves

Tall R waves

Important: With an acute posterior wall myocardial infarction, one will see *tall R waves in leads V_1 and V_2* (instead of loss of R waves), *slight ST depression in leads V_1 and V_2* (rather than ST elevation), and tall, upright, symmetrical T waves. (Additional electrode positions V_7–V_9 can be utilized for a more direct visualization of the posterior surface).

The other factor to consider is that a posterior wall infarct is usually due to occlusion of the Right Coronary Artery, or one of its branches. It is not uncommon, then, for concurrent injury to occur in both the inferior and posterior walls of the left ventricle.

P.S. Watch out for dysrhythmias!

As you might suspect, the posterior wall infarct patient may present with back pain, and sometimes this pain is mistaken for "renal" or other pathology.

> **... Beware of the patient that presents with back pain ...**
> **(A warning from the management.)**

Since this exercise is **brief,** let's try some practice!

Practice Exercise 3

A. Leads _____ and _____ lie opposite the posterior surface of the left ventricle.

B. When looking at leads V_1 and V_2, the three EKG criteria arousing suspicion of a posterior wall infarction are:

1. _____

2. _____

3. _____

C. The following patient was admitted to the hospital with crushing chest pain radiating into his back. He was diaphoretic and nauseated. Look at each lead closely and describe what you see. Refer back to the chart on page 300 to help you with your interpretation.

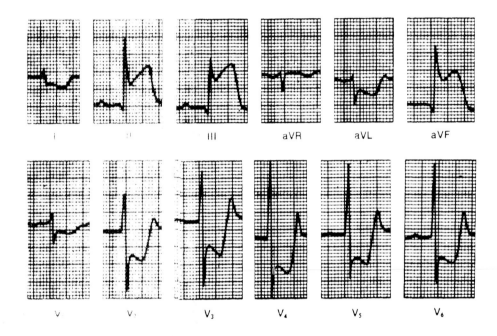

_____

_____

_____

_____

_____

_____

_____

_____

✔ For **Feedback 3**, refer to page 317.

Input Section 11.4: Serum Markers

Important Notes about Serum Markers

As noted earlier in this Section, the *textbook* identification of acute myocardial infarction is based upon (1) a positive patient history; (2) the presence of serum markers; and (3) specific EKG changes. Unfortunately, not all patients resemble textbook cases! Progressive clinical research has demonstrated that a substantial percentage of patients with an acute myocardial infarction may not exhibit ST elevation (injury pattern) or a pathologic Q wave. In those cases, the diagnosis is based on patient presentation and serum marker elevations.

It is worth emphasizing that earlier cardiac enzyme measures (CPK, LDH, SGOT) have been abandoned for serum markers (proteins) that demonstrate more site specificity and time sensitivity. Serum markers CK-MB, myoglobin and cardiac troponin (I and T), represent the current studies utilized to identify acute myocardial infarct. Biochemical researchers continue to search for even more precise markers to expedite the diagnosis and treatment of acute coronary syndromes. Specifically, research is ongoing to determine if future generations of assays for cardiac troponin may detect release of protein that occurs during reversible injury (ischemia without infarction).

Ck-Mb (Creatine Kinase-Myocardial Band)

CK-MB is dominantly a cardiac specific isoenzyme found in the serum of all acute myocardial infarct patients. (However, small concentrations (1–3%) are also found in skeletal muscles. Thus, severe trauma may cause a rise in CK-MB levels.) CK-MB begins to rise within 3–9 hours post infarct and is present for 48 hours. CK-MB is measured in ng/ml and reported as a % relative index. Levels of less than two percent are consideredinsignificant; levels of two to four percent are considered borderline; and, levels greater than four percent are considered positive. However, depending upon laboratory methods and instrumentation, percentage limits for both normal and abnormal values may vary slightly. Just for the record, occasionally CK-MB is referenced as CPK-MB.

Myoglobin

Myoglobin is a large molecule protein released secondary to muscle injury. This protein is non-specific to cardiac muscle and therefore, may be elevated with trauma and other muscle injury. Myoglobin normal values are less than 85 ng/ml. When associated with muscle damage, the myoglobin level begins to rise within the first one to two hours post injury and remains elevated during the first 24 hours. Though non-specific to cardiac muscle, myoglobin is considered an *early marker* and raises diagnostic suspicions when associated with classic cardiac physical symptoms.

Cardiac Troponins (T and I)

Cardiac troponins are the most specific markers for the definitive diagnosis of necrosis associated with cardiac muscle injury. The cardiac troponins begin to rise within four to nine hours following an ischemic event. Cardiac troponin I remains elevated for a longer period (10 to 14 days) than cardiac troponin I (7–10 days). Clinical research has demonstrated that elevated cardiac troponin I values associated with *non-Q wave* infarcts are associated with higher mortality rates. The accepted normal troponin I value is ≤ 0.4 ng/ml.

Of the three markers discussed above, myoglobin is considered an *early riser*; while CK-MB and the troponins are *late risers*. For the quick diagnosis of myocardial ischemic disorders, an early and late riser analysis are combined, often through serial blood draws.

The following graphic illustration demonstrates the timing of serum marker elevation.

SERUM MARKER EVALUATION

Hours

Myoglobin CPK-MB Troponin

Based on the previous discussion, it is clear that a single sampling of an isoenzyme or serum marker is inconclusive for the identification of an acute coronary syndrome.

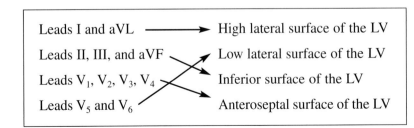

✔ **Feedback 1**

How did you do? If all your answers are correct, you may advance to the head of the class!

A. The 12 lead EKG allows one to look at the electrical activity of the heart from various <u>angles or from various points of reference</u>.

B. The most important chamber of the heart is the left ventricle because it functions as "The Pump" or the driving force for systemic circulation.

C.

Leads I and aVL	High lateral surface of the LV
Leads II, III, and aVF	Low lateral surface of the LV
Leads V_1, V_2, V_3, V_4	Inferior surface of the LV
Leads V_5 and V_6	Anteroseptal surface of the LV

For review, reference page 285.

D. By definition, *ischemia* is the myocardial change that results from a <u>temporary, insufficient</u> blood supply.

E. Myocardial ischemia presents on the EKG as <u>ST and T wave</u> changes in the leads looking at the ischemic surfaces.

F. Lead I shows a depressed and flat ST segment and a flattened T wave.

Leads II and III show slight ST depression and inverted T waves.

In lead aVL the ST segment is depressed.

In lead aVF the T wave is inverted.

Leads V_2, V_3, V_4, V_5, and V_6 show ST depression and T wave inversion (generalized ischemic changes).

G. An STEMI presents on the EKG as ST elevation measuring 1 mm or greater in 2 or more contiguous leads. A LBBB pattern may be evident as well. In a NSTEMI, no ST elevation is present. Instead, ST depression measuring 0.5 mm or less is evident in 2 or more contiguous leads. There may also be marked symmetrical T wave inversion in multiple precordial leads.

✔ Feedback 2

Whew! How did you do with this practice section? Sometimes, learning this material is a S-L-O-W process. It may help to read it through several times!

A.

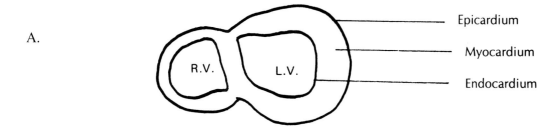

B. The diagnosis of myocardial infarction is based upon three criteria.

1. <u>Positive patient history.</u>
2. <u>Elevated serum markers.</u>
3. <u>Specific EKG changes.</u>

C. The first complex demonstrates a current injury pattern (ST elevation) in an upright lead. The second complex depicts a current injury pattern in a negatively deflected lead.

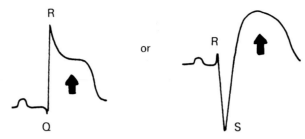

D. Reciprocal ST (elevation / depression) will occur in leads oriented toward the uninjured myocardial surfaces.

E. The hallmark of extensive myocardial infarction or necrosis is the **abnormal Q** wave in positive leads and the **loss of R wave** (QS pattern) in negatively deflected leads.

F. To be pathologic, the abnormal Q waves must meet two criteria:

1. The Q waves must measure at least 0.04 seconds in width or duration.

2. The Q waves must be deeper than ¼ the R wave amplitude.

G. **Interpretation:**

There are abnormal QS patterns and marked ST elevation in leads V_1–V_4. Leads V_5, and V_6 demonstrate Q waves and ST elevation. These changes represent probable acute anteroseptal wall myocardial infarction, including infarction of the apical surface of the left ventricle.

H. **Interpretation:**

Lead I shows depression of the ST segment.

Lead aVL shows ST depression and inverted T waves.

Leads II, III, and aVF demonstrate prominent Q waves and pronounced ST elevation.

Leads V_1–V_6 appear normal.

This EKG represents probable acute inferior wall myocardial infarction with reciprocal ST-T wave changes in the lateral leads.

I. **1** Prominent Q waves in leads II, III, and aVF. Inverted T waves in leads II, III, and aVF. Probable old inferior wall infarction with ischemia of the inferior wall.

3 Marked ST depression and T wave inversion in leads I and aVL. Prominent Q waves and ST elevation in leads II, III, and aVF. Probable acute inferior wall myocardial infarction with reciprocal ST-T wave changes in the lateral leads.

5 Pathologic Q waves in leads I and aVL. Inverted T waves in aVL. Probable old lateral wall infarction. The inverted T waves denote ischemia.

4 Leads V_1–V_6 appear within normal limits. No pathology evident.

2 Leads V_1–V_4 show abnormal QS deflections with marked ST elevation. There is marked ST elevation in leads V_5 and V_6. Probable acute anteroseptal wall infarction with injury extending to the low lateral wall of the left ventricle.

J. **Interpretation:**

Hope this rhythm strip did not fool you! This is a sinus rhythm (rate 94) with a left bundle branch block. (If you need a review of LBBB, turn back to page 166.) REMEMBER: IN LBBB, ST SEGMENT DISTORTION OCCURS SECONDARY TO THE ABNORMAL ACTIVATION OF

THE LEFT VENTRICLE. It is the delayed activation of the LV that causes abnormal ventricular repolarization (recovery). Thus, a current injury pattern cannot be determined in the presence of left bundle branch block!

K. Someone inadvertently labeled (II) this strip upside down! To correct, turn the book upside down and again view the strip. When a rhythm strip makes no sense whatsoever, consider human error!

✔ Feedback 3

If you answered all three questions correctly, you are entitled to the "official" EKG merit badge. (Please cut along the dotted lines.)

A. Leads V_1 and V_2 lie opposite the posterior surface of the left ventricle.

B. When looking at leads V_1 and V_2, the three EKG criteria arousing suspicion of a posterior wall infarction are:

1. Tall R wave

2. Slight ST depression

3. Tall, upright symmetrical T waves

P.S. Remember, the diagnosis of acute myocardial infarction is never solely based on the EKG findings.

C. **Interpretation:**

Leads I and aVL show significant ST depression.

Leads II, III, and aVF show prominent Q waves and marked ST elevation.

Lead V_1 demonstrates a small R wave and ST depression.

Lead V_2 shows a tall R wave, ST depression, and a tall, upright T wave.

Leads V_3–V_6 show a fairly normal progression of R waves and severely depressed ST segments. The T waves remain upright.

The pathologic Q waves and ST elevation in leads II, III, and aVF suggest an acute inferior wall myocardial infarction. The ST depression noted in leads I and aVL is simply the reciprocal change occurring in leads oriented toward the uninjured myocardial surface.

Though by itself, V_1 is only suspicious of a posterior wall myocardial infarction, V_2 confirms any doubts. The ST depression noted in V_3–V_6 is no doubt reciprocal in nature.

. . . So, there appears to be acute injury and necrosis of both the inferior and posterior surfaces of the left ventricle! **Ugh!**

A *Summary of Coronary Artery Compromise* is included on page 318 for future reference!

SUMMARY OF CORONARY ARTERY COMPROMISE

Stages of Compromise	Patient Symptoms	Cellular	Electrical	Mechanical	Wave Forms	Serum Markers
Transient ischemia (< 20 minutes)	Intermittant chest pain; diaphoresis; nausea and vomiting	Intermittant disruption of O^2 and CO^2 exchange	Ectopic activity associated with irritability may be present	No disruption	Inverted T waves; flattened T waves; modest ST depression	No serum marker release
Persistent ischemia (> 20 minutes)	Persistent chest pain; pain may radiate to arms, neck or jaw: diaphoresis: nausea and vomiting	O^2 and CO^2 exchange disrupted; cells rupture, leaking enzymes into the blood stream	Ectopic activity associated with irritability may be present	Disruption related to any significant ectopic activity	ST segment depression pronounced (NON-STEMI)	No serum marker release
Current injury (30–40 minutes)	Persistent chest pain; may be crushing in nature and/or may radiate; diaphoresis; nausea and vomiting	O^2 and CO^2 exchange severely compromised; cells rupture expelling total contents into the blood stream	Ventricular irritability (P.V.C.s) often present	May be compromised depending upon the extent of injury	ST elevation in leads overlying the injury; reciprocal ST segment depression (STEMI)	No serum marker release
Tissue necrosis and death (begins 1–2 hours post occlusion)	Crushing chest pain, pain may radiate; diaphoresis; nausea and vomiting; shock-like symptoms often present (hypotension, altered mental status, pulmonary edema)	O^2 and CO^2 exchange disrupted. Cells necrose and die	Ventricular irritability usually observed; depending on the affected vessel(s), various forms of heart block may be observed.	Compromised secondary to loss of muscle contractility associated with cellular death {ventricular failure}; may be further compromised secondary to dysrhythmias	When associated with extensive damage, pathologic Q waves (or loss or R waves) develop in leads overlying the areas of damage	Early markers begin to rise 1–2 hours post occlusion
4–9 hours post occlusion						Definitive diagnosis based on rise of cardiac specific serum markers

Notes

Notes

The Diagnosis and Treatment of Acute Coronary Syndromes

Objectives

When you have completed Section 12, you will be able to describe or identify

1. the general diagnostic approaches for coronary artery disease (CAD)

2. the general treatment options for coronary artery disease

3. differences in treatment options for non-emergent vs. acute coronary syndromes

Text by
Stephanie L. Woods, Ph.D., R.N.

The diagnosis and treatment of coronary artery disease (CAD) is made under a variety of conditions, both emergent (acute) and non-emergent. In the acute scenario, a patient often arrives in the emergency department with chest pain, palpitations and/or shortness of breath. In that setting, national guidelines and, the American Heart Association standards of Advanced Cardiac Life Support (ACLS) are used to determine treatment (AHA, 2003).

To simplify your learning of this complex material, two algorithms are provided (See pages 325, 329). An algorithm is like a recipe. It provides sequenced guidance . . . *Do this, then do that.* Best of all, an algorithm provides one with just the critical facts. Having access to, or memorizing algorithms, allows one to diagnose and treat in a methodological way and according to accepted guidelines.

The most important thing to understand regarding the diagnosis and treatment of coronary artery disease is that **time is of the utmost importance**. Both the Non-Emergent Algorithm for Diagnosis and Treatment of Coronary Artery Disease and the Diagnosis and Treatment of Acute Coronary Syndrome algorithms begin with assessment of the patient. Based upon assessment findings (acute symptoms vs. no distress), diagnosis and treatment may occur immediately, or can be scheduled electively. Treatment options are based upon the information gained in the assessment and the results of the diagnostic tests.

Input Section 12.1: Coronary Artery Disease and Progression to Acute Coronary Syndrome

Diet, sedentary lifestyles and genetics predispose individuals to atherosclerosis. Atherosclerosis is the process whereby lipids (fats) are deposited within the walls of arteries. This process results in decreased blood flow to vital organs including the heart, brain and kidneys. For the purposes of this discussion, atherosclerosis will be related to the coronary arteries and the resulting decreased blood flow to the heart.

Coronary artery disease (CAD) begins with early plaque formation in the coronary arteries. Plaques are made up of lipids (fats) that are deposited along the wall of the artery. As this lipid-laden plaque builds up in the vessel wall, blood flow turbulence and inflammatory changes predispose the plaque to rupture. When the plaque ruptures, the fatty contents of the plaque protrude toward the center of the artery. As blood flows past the ruptured plaque, platelets are snagged and begin to stick to one another (agglutination) and clump (aggregation). A thrombus (blood clot) begins to form when clotting factors such as fibrinogen and thrombin are generated. Micro-emboli (small blood clots) can also break off of the original thrombus, sending small clots to occlude the smaller branches of the coronary arteries.

The thrombus may partially occlude, intermittently occlude or completely occlude arteries, blocking blood flow to the heart.

☆ Partial occlusions can produce symptoms associated with ischemia (decreased blood flow): angina (chest pain), shortness of breath (SOB), diaphoresis (sweating) and fatigue

☆ Intermittent occlusion may cause the symptoms associated with ischemia and progression to myocardial necrosis (death of heart muscle) without a resulting Q wave (a non-Q wave myocardial infarction, NSTEMI)

☆ Occlusion for a prolonged time usually produces a Q wave on the 12-lead EKG.

Input Section 12.2: Non-Emergent Diagnosis and Treatment of Coronary Artery Disease

The algorithm on page 325 summarizes how the diagnosis of coronary artery disease (CAD) proceeds in the non-emergent setting.

It is definitely preferable to diagnose and treat coronary artery disease in the non-emergent setting. Most typically, CAD is initially considered as patients seek routine medical advice and as their caregivers identify a high risk profile. Depending upon the presence of suspicious symptoms or high risk factors, diagnosis will occur using minimally invasive versus invasive diagnostic tests. Based upon diagnostic test results, treatment options are chosen.

Minimally Invasive Diagnostic Tests

Minimally invasive means that nothing more invasive than a small needle is used (phlebotomy, injection of a radioisotope). *Invasive* diagnostic tests require percutaneous approaches (through the skin) using large bore needles, threading of catheters, infusion of radiopaque dyes, infusion of drugs, and use of electrical energy (pacemaking, ablation).

The minimally invasive diagnostic tests cluster under three major headings: electrocardiography, medical imaging, and laboratory.

➤ **Electrocardiography**—You know the importance of obtaining a 12-lead EKG in the diagnosis of ischemia, injury, and infarction (Section 11). And, throughout this study of dysrhythmias, you have seen the value of rhythm strips. However, both the 12 lead EKG and rhythm strips are transient, representing a snapshot in time. The Holter monitor is a device capable of recording a 24 hour rhythm. There are also more sophisticated monitors which can record and store information for up to 30 days. If, while wearing the device, a patient feels he is experiencing a dysrhythmia, most of these have telephonic capability, allowing the patient's rhythm to be transmitted over the phone to a diagnostic center.

➤ **Medical Imaging**—The echocardiogram is a sonogram of the heart, produced by the soundwaves generated with systole. Echocardiograms allow one to estimate chamber size and cardiac output, evaluate valve function and look for presence of blood clots in the atria (often associated with atrial fibrillation).

Stress tests are used to diagnose ischemia while the heart responds to exercise ($\uparrow$ HR, $\uparrow$ contractility). Scanning is accomplished with an imaging camera while radioisotopes are injected into the patient's vein. As the patient exercises, the radioisotope flows through the coronary arteries "lighting up" the well-perfused areas of the heart. Under-perfused areas show up as "cold spots" (ischemic areas). **MRI and Single Photon Emission Computed Tomography (SPECT)** are sophisticated non-invasive scans that allow for imaging of the heart. Again radioisotopes are injected and the patient is scanned to evaluate both the coronary arteries and myocardial perfusion.

➤ **Laboratory**—Cardiac serum markers are drawn to determine if actual damage is occurring to the myocardium (see page 313).

Invasive Diagnostic Tests

➤ **Coronary Angiography** is often referred to as cardiac catheterization or in clinical lingo a "cardiac cath." **A cardiac cath is considered the "gold standard" for evaluating the coronary arteries and is undertaken before surgery or other interventions are considered.** A patient is taken to the catheterization laboratory and placed on an xray table. A surgical cutdown is performed on both an artery and a vein (usually femoral). An arterial catheter is advanced antegrade (against the flow), up through the abdominal aorta, up to the aortic arch and then through the coronary sinus to the coronary arteries. Radiopaque dye is injected to "light up" the coronary arteries. Stenotic (narrowed) areas as well as areas of blockage will show up. A venous catheter is advanced with venous flow through the vena cava up to the superior vena cava into the right atrium and ultimately, the right ventricle. Again, radiopaque dye can be used to evaluate chamber size and blood flow across the valves. Pressures in the right atrium, ventricle and pulmonary artery can also be directly measured (to be discussed in Section 13!) A precise measure can also be made of cardiac output.

➤ **Chemical Stress Tests**—For patients who are physically unable to tolerate a standard treadmill test, a chemical stress test is done. The patient is given a drug that increases heart rate and contractility (mimicing the effects of exercise) and a scan is done to identify the "cold spots" as discussed earlier.

➤ **Electrophysiology studies** (EPS) were briefly discussed in Section 2. These studies, accomplished in specialized catheterization labs, are used to both diagnose and treat patients with various dysrhythmias, particularly tachydysrhythmias. Special catheters are used to identify the areas from which the dysrhythmias originate. Then, treatment options are pursued that best resolve the dysrhythmia. Primarily radiofrequency ablation (RFA), specialized implantable pacemakers and defibrillators, and various drug therapies are used as treatments.

Elective Treatment Options

Elective treatment options are medical management, interventional procedures, and surgical procedures.

➤ **Medical Management Options** include the use of drugs to control or diminish the patient's symptoms. Most patients with CAD require some form of medical treatment. It is noteworthy that there is a large population of patients who are *poor risks* for interventional or surgical options. Therefore, those patients have only a medical management option. **Vasodilators** increase the diameter of the coronary arteries allowing better blood flow to the myocardium. **Anti-Platelet (platelet inhibitors) and Lipid-Lowering Drugs** change the properties of the blood itself. Lipid-lowering drugs decrease the amount of circulating lipids (fat, cholesterol) in the blood stream. Therefore, less lipids can be deposited as fatty plaque (atheromas) in the walls of the coronary arteries. Additionally, when circulating lipids are reduced, the viscosity (thickness) of the blood is decreased, allowing better blood flow through narrowed arteries. Anti-platelet drugs make the blood less likely to form clots in the narrowed coronary arteries (refer to Section 14, page 383).

➤ **Interventional Options** actually increase the diameter of diseased coronary arteries. This is accomplished through the use of balloons, roto-rooters, or springs!! These percutaneous coronary interventions (PCI) are done in concert with a cardiac catherization and are performed in the cardiac catheterization lab by an interventional cardiologist. **Percutaneous transluminal coronary angioplasty (PTCA)** uses an inflatable *balloon tipped catheter,* threaded across the narrowed area (stenosis) in the coronary artery. The balloon is inflated to compress and fracture the fatty plaque. When the balloon is deflated, the anticipated result is a larger diameter vessel, with less fatty plaque blocking blood flow. **Athrectomy** is accomplished using a catheter with a very small whirling blade or diamond tipped drill. Athrectomy works *roto-rooter style* to pulverize fatty plaque in the coronary artery. The resulting fragments are so small they are of little danger in the circulation. **Stents** are *slinky-like* springs that are loaded onto a catheter that is threaded across the narrowed area in the coronary artery (stenosis). Once the catheter is positioned at the stenosis, a balloon is inflated, expanding the spring. The spring actually holds open the coronary artery by compressing the fatty plaque against the vessel wall.

➤ **Surgical Options** are used when interventional options are not possible. **Coronary Artery Bypass Grafting (CABG)** uses vein grafts (the patient's own or those of a cadaver) that are sewn into the patient's aorta and distal to (below) the area of stenosis. This creates a "bypass" around the stenotic area, thus creating a source of oxygenated blood. **Valve replacement** is done when either valvular stenosis (narrowing of the opening) or valvular regurgitation (backward flow of blood) is leading to a decrease in cardiac output. Valvular stenosis in either the tricuspid or mitral valves decreases ventricular filling, therefore compromising stroke volume. Pulmonic and aortic stenosis obstructs ejection of blood from the ventricles. When blood flow is obstructed across the valve, the ventricles must work harder to pump out

ALGORITHM FOR THE DIAGNOSIS AND TREATMENT OF NON-EMERGENT CORONARY ARTERY DISEASE

Patient has no acute distress

| **Patient seeks medical advice** | **\<OR\>** | **M.D. or R.N. identifies *high risk indicators* of coronary artery disease (CAD)** |

➤ Usual doctor office visit
➤ Visit to doctor secondary to new symptoms
  • Chest pain
  • Palpitations (skipped beats)
  • Fatigue
  • Dizziness or fainting

➤ Age
➤ Associated conditions
  • Chronic Obstructive Pulmonary Disease (COPD)
  • Diabetes
  • Hypertension
➤ Cardiac murmur or click
➤ Dysrhythmias

➤ Metabolic Syndrome:
  • Central Obesity
  • Dyslipidemia (↑triglycerides, ↓HDL)
  • Raised B/P (130/85 or higher
  • Insulin resistance or glucose intolerance
➤ Prothrombotic state (high fibrinogen or plasminogen activator)
➤ Proinflammatory state (↑high-sensitivity C-reactive protein)

Depending on the level of suspicion (suspicion index) that the patient has CAD, diagnosis is made by:

| **Minimally invasive diagnostic tests** | **More invasive diagnostic tests** |

➤ 12 lead EKG
➤ Cardiac serum markers
➤ Holter monitor
➤ Echocardiogram
➤ Stress test (treadmill)
  • Thallium
  • Technetium
➤ MRI
➤ Single photon emission computed tomography (SPECT)

➤ Coronary angiography (cardiac catheterization)
➤ Chemical stress tests
  • Dobutamine
  • Dipyramidole
➤ Electrophysiology study (EPS)

| **Elective Treatment Options** |

➤ Medical (drugs)
  • Vasodilators
  • Anti-platelet
  • Lipid-lowering
  • Anti-dysrhythmics
  • Anti-hypertensives
  • Hypoglycemics

➤ Interventional
  • Percutaneous transluminal coronary angioplast (PTCA)
  • Arthrectomy
  • Stent
  • Pacemaker/AICD

➤ Surgical
  • Coronary artery bypass graft (CABG)
  • Valve replacement

blood. This chronic overwork leads to ventricular hypertrophy (enlargement) and ultimately, to failure. A hypertrophied ventricle requires a greater blood supply. In the patient with CAD, this increased demand cannot be met and ischemia results. Valvular regurgitation in the mitral and tricuspid valves allows for backward flow of blood into the atria during ventricular systole. Since part of the blood does not leave the heart as cardiac output, blood flow to the lungs and/or the body is compromised. Replacement valves are either mechanical or porcine (pig).

Input Section 12.3: Diagnosis and Treatment of Acute Coronary Syndrome (ACS)

> Diagnosis and Treatment are based upon the following:
> *Time Since Symptoms Started + Elevated Serum Markers + EKG Evidence*

The algorithm on page 329 summarizes the diagnosis and treatment of acute coronary syndrome. **Acute coronary syndrome** (ACS) describes a cluster of signs and symptoms in patients presenting with ischemic chest pain and one of the following diagnoses:

➤ unstable angina

➤ ST elevation myocardial infarction (STEMI), or

➤ Non-ST elevation myocardial infarction (NSTEMI)

These three diagnoses are related, in that all are a part of a progressive continuum of coronary artery disease. An assessment of symptoms, cardiac serum markers studies, and 12-lead electrocardiograms **over time**, determine where a patient is on this continuum.

Ask-Assess-Treat

One of the greatest challenges in caring for the patient with acute coronary syndrome is that one must be able to ask questions, assess, and treat all at the same time! When a patient enters the emergency department with chest pain, you must focus your "asking and assessing" while treating the chest pain as ischemia. This is challenging for the inexperienced practitioner, but after some experience, quite doable. The goal is to classify the type of acute coronary syndrome the patient is experiencing within **10** minutes of arrival!

ASK Targeted Questions: You are most interested in knowing **"when did the symptoms start?"** Every minute of ischemia counts when it comes to saving heart muscle. A patient with chest pain should be triaged quickly and evaluated within ten minutes of arrival. **Twelve hours or less** since symptom development is the cut-off time for use of fibrinolysis (clot-busting) drugs. Since thrombolytic drugs break down blood clots, it is imperative to ask **"have you had a recent stroke?"** Clot-busting drugs are contraindicated for patients with a recent stroke history. Additionally, you want to know **"are you taking any blood thinners or herbal medicines?"** Many herbal medications can cause bleeding when combined with traditional medications. Finally, you want to ask, **"do you have a family or personal history of cardiovascular or pulmonary disease, or diabetes?"** since these all relate to coronary artery disease (CAD).

Conduct a Targeted ASSESSMENT: Vital signs may or may not be definitive; however, look for **signs of shock (low blood pressure, cool and clammy skin, scant urinary output)**. Then, of course, listen to breath sounds and carefully assess for **rales** (a sign of cardiogenic shock) and evaluate the **pulse oximetry reading**. The 12-lead EKG must be observed for **waveforms indicating ischemia, injury, or infarct** (discussed in Section 11) as well as for dysrhythmias. Now as you are doing this, make certain that a chest x-ray is taken and that **serum markers**, coagulation and electrolyte studies are being drawn!

INTERVENE AS IF THIS IS ISCHEMIC PAIN: During the history and assessment phase (and while firing off orders for the various tests), start a large bore IV and oxygen at 4L/min with your free hand! Oh, and don't forget to give the patient 160–325 mg of aspirin and possibly a nitroglycerine tab under his tongue. (Are YOU having chest pain yet??)

Classifying Patients According To 12-Lead EKG Evidence

ST Elevation MI (STEMI)

➤ ST elevation > or equal to 1mm in 2 or more contiguous leads
  ☆ Anterior leads
  ☆ Inferior leads
  ☆ Lateral leads
  ☆ Antero-lateral leads
  ☆ Posterior leads
➤ New (or presumably new) LBBB

Non-ST-Elevation MI (NSTEMI) (Includes High-Risk or Unstable Angina)

➤ ST depression < or equal to 0.5 mm in two or more contiguous leads
➤ Marked symmetrical T-wave inversion in multiple precordial leads
➤ ST-T wave changes with chest pain

Indeterminate/Low Risk Unstable Angina (Includes Normal or Non-Diagnostic Changes in ST Segment or T Waves)

➤ ST depression < 0.5 mm
➤ T wave inversion or flattening in leads with dominant R waves
➤ Normal EKG

Treatment Plans

Once the patient is classified according to 12-lead EKG evidence, serum marker results have been received and time since symptom onset is established, a treatment plan begins.

☆ Adjunctive treatments are supportive in nature and have been proven to improve outcomes. In ACS, STEMIs and non-STEMIs receive adjunctive treatments. Additionally, patients without significant EKG changes who are unstable, are new onset of angina, or who are troponin positive will receive these treatments.

☆ Time since onset of symptoms and resources available also affect the treatment plan. As has been stated, the critical time frame for myocardial tissue is 12 hours. Access to a catheterization laboratory, cardiologists capable of performing percutaneous coronary interventions (and who have done high volumes of such procedures), and ability to do cardiac surgery, if necessary, all impact choices of treatment.

If fibrinolysis is a treatment option, the goal is to infuse these drugs within thirty minutes of the patient's arrival in the emergency department (door to drug).

If percutaneous coronary interventions (PCI) are an option, the goal is to have the patient in the catheterization lab and begin intervention within 90 minutes, plus or minus 30 minutes, from the time of patient's arrival in the emergency department (door to balloon).

In summary, early identification of high risk patients is the goal. This is best done non-emergently. However, when patients present, **time is critical**. By following research-based guidelines, care can be standardized and outcomes improved.

Practice Exercise

Critical Thinking Questions

1. When considering the following treatment options, match them to a commonly understood plumbing concept!

    _____ Thrombolysis   A. *Roto-Rooter-like* clearing out of a sewer line

    _____ Athrectomy   B. Dissolution of a clog in a drain

                               C. Using a plunger to unstop a sink drain

2. A stent is a spring or mesh-like device placed in a coronary artery to hold open the narrowed vessel. Given this device is a foreign object, what sort of complications might compromise the stent and/or the patency (flow through) the artery?

    _____

    _____

    _____

    _____

3. Which of the following is *not* a characteristic of metabolic syndrome?

    a. Dyslipidemia

    b. Glucose intolerance

    c. B/P > 140/90

    d. Central obesity

    e. Elevated troponin

THE DIAGNOSIS AND TREATMENT OF ACUTE CORONARY SYNDROME (ACS)

PATIENT INFORMANTION

ASK ⟶ WHILE

➤ When did the symptoms begin?
  • less than 12 hours ago
  • more than 12 hours ago
➤ Is there a medical history?
  • Cardiac disease
  • Vascular disease
➤ Have you had a recent stroke?
➤ Do you have diabetes?
➤ Do you have pulmonary disease?
➤ Is there any related family history?
➤ Are you taking anti-coagulants or herbal preparations?

PHYSICAL DATA

ASSESSING ⟶ WHILE

➤ Vital signs
➤ STAT 12-lead EKG with a rhythm strip
➤ O_2 saturation
➤ Cardiac serum markers
➤ Coagulation studies
➤ Electrolytes
➤ Portable chest x-ray requested and reviewed within 30 minutes

INTERVENTION

TREATING AS ISCHEMIA

➤ Start IV
➤ O_2 @ 4L/min.
➤ Aspirin 160–325 mg
➤ Nitroglyccrin sublingual or spray
➤ Morphine sulfate IV if pain unrelieved by nitroglycerin

CLASSIFY TYPE OF ACS, DETERMINE TREATMENT OPTIONS BY EKG EVIDENCE, ELEVATED SERUM MARKERS AND TIME SINCE ONSET OF SYMPTOMS

ST ELEVATION MI (STEMI)

NON-STEMI

NORMAL OR NON-DIAGNOSTIC CHANGES IN ST-SEGMENT OR T-WAVE

START ADJUNCTIVE THERAPIES
➤ Beta-adrenoceptor blockers IV
➤ Nitroglycerin IV
➤ Heparin IV
➤ Ace-inhibitors (after 6 hrs or when stable)

START ADJUNCTIVE THERAPIES
➤ Beta-adrenergic blockers IV
➤ Nitroglycerin IV
➤ Heparin
➤ Aspirin 160–325 mg daily
➤ Glycoprotein IIb/IIIa receptor inhibitors

Yes ⟵

Is patient unstable *or* is this new onset of angina *or* troponin +?

No

HOW LONG HAS PATIENT HAD SYMPTOMS? WHAT RESOURCES ARE AVAILABLE?

IF < I2 HRS:
➤ Fibrinolytics (<30 min. Door to Drug)
➤ Cardiac catheterization
➤ Choose Reperfusion strategy:
  • Percutaneous coronary intervention (PCI) (Door to Balloon 90 ± 30 min.)
  • CABG

IF > I2 HRS: ⟵ Yes
➤ Cardial catheterization
➤ Re-vascularize if possible?
  • PCI
  • CABG

IS PT. HIGH RISK?
➤ Persistent s/s
  • Chest pain, SOB, N/V
  • L-Sided CHF
  • EKG changes in multiple leads
  • Prior history of MI, CABG, PCI

No ⟶ **ADMIT & MONITOR:**
➤ Serum markers
➤ Serial EKGs
➤ Consider cardiac imaging

Based in part on the ischemic chest pain Algorithm & the acute coronary syndrome algorithm, ACLS guidelines, American Heart Association, 2003.

4. You are asked to speculate on the cost-effectiveness of:

PCI vs. CABG

Provide a brief answer with your rationale.

_____

_____

_____

_____

_____

5. Describe the differences between minimally invasive and invasive testing.

_____

_____

_____

_____

_____

✔ Feedback

Critical Thinking Questions

1. When considering the following treatment options, match them to a commonly understood plumbing concept!

   (B) Thrombolysis   A. *Roto-Rooter-like* clearing out of a sewer line

   (A) Athrectomy   B. Dissolution of a clog in a drain

   C. Using a plunger to unstop a sink drain

2. A stent is a spring or mesh-like device placed in a coronary artery to hold open the narrowed vessel. Given this device is a foreign object, what sort of complications might compromise the stent and/or the patency (flow through) the artery?
   Coating and closing off of the stent due to platelet adhesion and aggregation. Closure of the vessel secondary to scar tissue.

3. Troponin is a cardiac marker and does not relate to metabolic syndrome.

4. You were asked to speculate on the cost-effectiveness of:

PCI vs. CABG

The average length of hospital stay for a patient who is having a PCI (stent, athrectomy or angioplasty) procedure is 2 days. However, the average length of stay for a patient having a CABG is 5 days. Therefore, PCI procedures are more cost-effective.

5. The difference between minimally invasive and invasive testing is that with minimally invasive testing, nothing more than a small needle is used. Invasive testing may require percutaneous approaches, use of large bore needles and threading of catheters, injection of dyes and isotopes, and/or the use of electrical energy.

Notes

Notes

The Fundamentals of Hemodynamic Monitoring

Objectives

When you have completed Section 13, you will be able to describe or identify

1. blood flow through the heart identifying chambers, valves, and major vessels

2. normal right atrial, right ventricular, pulmonary artery, and pulmonary capillary wedge pressures

3. typical pressure waveforms associated with right heart chambers and the pulmonary artery

4. relationships among pulmonary artery diastolic pressure, pulmonary capillary wedge pressure, and left ventricular end-diastolic pressure

5. causes for abnormal pressures

6. this section as a future reference!!

Text by
Stephanie L. Woods, Ph.D., R.N.

Input Section 13.1: Hemodynamic Monitoring and Cardiac Output

Hemodynamics is defined as the *flow of blood*. Hemodynamic monitoring is the study of blood flow to, and oxygenation status of, the body tissues. Blood flow is accomplished via the heart and vasculature, and oxygenation occurs in the lungs. Specific hemodynamic measures and techniques allow a practitioner to monitor the ability of the heart, lungs and vasculature to deliver oxygen to the body tissues. While the EKG allows the practitioner to assess the electrical functioning of the heart, hemodynamic monitoring allows the assessment of the heart's mechanical action (pumping).

Hemodynamic parameters can be monitored both non-invasively and invasively. *Non-invasive* monitoring does not require puncturing the skin or the insertion of catheters. Topical applications of technology allow for the monitoring of blood pressure, pulse rate, respiration rate and oxygen saturation. *Invasive* hemodynamic monitoring, requiring both the puncture of the skin and insertion of catheters, is reserved for critically ill and unstable patients. Invasive hemodynamic monitoring requires the insertion of a pulmonary artery catheter (PAC), also known as the Swan-Ganz catheter. A PAC can be inserted at the bedside. Appropriate patient populations include, but are not limited to, myocardial infarction, congestive heart failure, pulmonary hypertension, and septic shock.

Invasive monitoring provides specific clinical data to guide precise therapeutic intervention. Invasive hemodynamic monitoring allows differentiation between cardiac and pulmonary disease, and provides data regarding the extent of pathology. Hemodynamic monitoring can be done continuously or intermittently. For example, a patient with congestive heart failure (CHF), may have a PAC inserted, pressures obtained, and the catheter removed. The obtained pressures, guide treatment.

Blood Flow through the Heart

It is important to remember that the primary functions of the cardiovascular system are to deliver oxygen and nutrients to the cells and to remove wastes.

In order to perform this nutrient/waste exchange, the left heart circulates oxygenated blood from the pulmonary vasculature throughout the system to the cells via arteries. The oxygen/waste exchange occurs at the cellular level. Deoxygenated blood and waste is then returned via the veins to the right heart.

As can be seen in the following diagram, deoxygenated blood enters the right atrium (RA) via the inferior and superior vena cava. From the right atrium (RA), the blood crosses the tricuspid valve into the right ventricle (RV). The right ventricle (RV) pumps deoxygenated blood across the pulmonic valve into the pulmonary artery (PA). The blood then flows through the pulmonary vascular beds, a passive activity owing to the absence of contracting vessels and valves. Carbon dioxide (CO_2) is exchanged for oxygen (O_2) as the blood flows through the pulmonary vasculature.

The oxygenated blood then returns to the left atrium (LA) via the pulmonary veins. After passing across the mitral valve, the blood begins to fill the left ventricle (LV). The left ventricle has both the largest and strongest muscle mass of any of the four heart chambers. This muscle mass allows the left ventricle (LV) to generate a pressure of sufficient magnitude to eject the blood past the aortic valve into the aorta, and out to the vascular beds (systemic circulation).

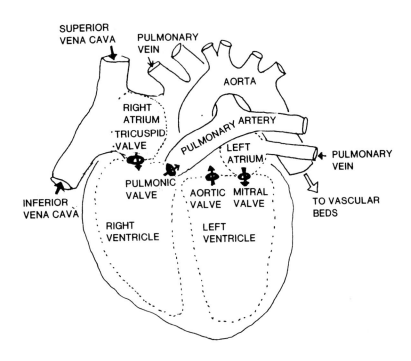

The blood flow cycle can be broken down into two major phases: (1) *systole*, or the contraction/ejection phase; and (2) *diastole*, the relaxation/filling phase. During each phase, the pressure and blood volume in each chamber differs. It is this pressure difference that permits the cardiac valves to open and close appropriately. The valves (tricuspid, pulmonic, mitral, and aortic) perform gatekeeper functions, keeping the blood flowing in a forward direction.

Filling of the chambers occurs during diastole. As blood flows into the right and left atria, atrial chamber pressures increase. These increasing pressures force the tricuspid and mitral valves open, allowing the right and left ventricles to fill. The increased pressure in the atrial chambers and electrical activation (depolarization) stimulates the atria to contract. The P wave seen on the EKG monitor corresponds with ventricular diastole or filling. You will remember that the P wave represents atrial depolarization.

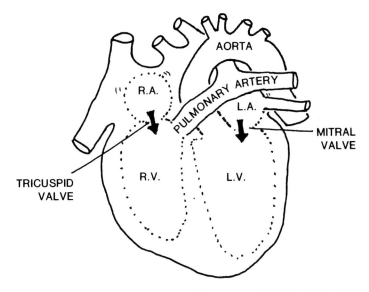

Ventricular filling. Increasing atrial pressures force open the Tricuspid and Mitral valves.

Ejection of blood occurs during systole. Ventricular systole occurs when the pressure and volume in the right and left ventricles exceed atrial pressures. The rising ventricular pressures force the mitral and tricuspid valves closed. The aortic and pulmonic valves are then forced open, allowing blood to flow out of the ventricles. Blood is ejected from the right ventricle into the pulmonary artery where it is taken to the right and left lungs for oxygenation.

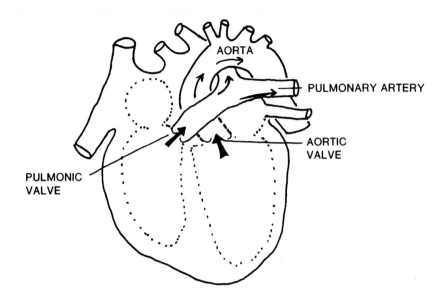

Blood returns to the left atrium via the pulmonary veins. This oxygenated blood will be ejected against the high resistance in the arterial system. The more muscular wall of the left ventricle contracts (systole) with great force, opening the aortic valve and allowing flow to the system.

Ventricular muscle contraction immediately follows electrical activation (depolarization) of the ventricles. Electrical depolarization produces the QRS seen on the EKG monitor!

This systole and diastole business is sometimes confusing! It may be helpful to remember . . .

> **Diastole = relaxation and filling**
> **Systole = contraction and ejection**

The diagram on the next page depicts the relationships between the EKG waveforms, diastole and systole, pressure changes and valve openings and closures.

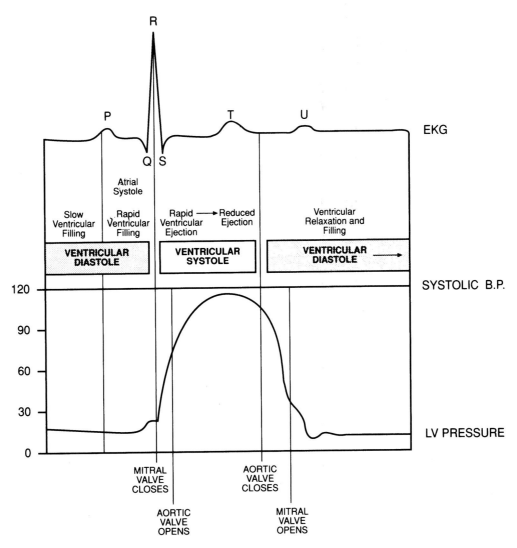

Cardiac cycle demonstrating EKG relationship to ventricular diastole, systole and valve function.

The Effects of Pressure, Vessel Characteristics, Viscosity, Resistance and Volume

Hemodynamies, or blood flow, is affected by pressure, vessel characteristics, viscosity, resistance, and volume.

Pressure:

☆ Blood tends to flow from areas of **high pressure to low pressure (pressure gradient).** The greater the pressure difference between flow into and out of a blood vessel, the greater the pressure gradient. If there is *no* pressure difference, then there is no flow. For instance, the pressure in the left ventricle must be higher than the pressure in the aorta, for blood to be ejected during systole.

Vessel Characteristics:

➤ The longer the **length of a vessel**, the lesser the flow. A practical example of this can be observed in the backyard. If a gardener desires to water flowers far out by the back fence, he may need to attach multiple water hoses. The more water hose extensions he attaches, creating a longer hose, the less water flow will occur at hose end! Likewise in the body, the further the distance blood must travel, the lesser the flow at the end point.

➤ The larger the **diameter of a vessel,** the greater the flow (*vasodilation*). The smaller the diameter the vessel, the lesser the flow (*vasoconstriction*). When a person is under stress, the stress hormone norepinephrine causes vasoconstriction. As a result, flow is compromised to the periphery of the body. When under stress, the feet and hands often become cold. This is a sign of reduced blood flow, due to reduced diameter (vasoconstriction) of the blood vessels in the feet and hands. The disease process of atherosclerosis also affects the diameter of arterial vessels. As fatty deposits called atheromas build up within the vessel wall, flow is diminished.

➤ The greater the **viscosity of blood,** the lesser the flow. Viscosity is the thickness of blood. In states of dehydration or increased cell counts, blood becomes thicker. Thicker blood flows less well than thinner blood. Simply speaking, iced tea pours (flows) more rapidly into a glass than does a milkshake.

➤ **Resistance** is that factor that impedes blood flow. When blood vessels are constricted, resistance is increased. When vessels are dilated, resistance is decreased.

➤ **Volume** is related to pressure. When volume is increased within a vessel, pressure is increased. When pressure within vessels increases, the diameter of the vessel also increases. In response to the increased diameter, resistance decreases. This ability to respond to changes in pressure is called *distensibility*. Veins are much more distensible than arteries. A very personal example of distensibility *may* be found in your closet. There are two vintage pairs of favorite jeans:

- One pair of jeans has a fixed waist band and button closure, thus limiting distensibility. Despite some acquired distensibility from hundreds of washings, a few extra pounds (increased volume) may create extreme pressure when buttoning those jeans!

- The second pair of jeans has an elastic waist band and possibly a Velcro closure! The elastic in the waist band allows greater distensibility following a big meal, thus reducing the pressure felt!

As long as the jeans are distensible, volume can increase within reason, without greatly increasing pressure. In the human body, as long as the vessels are distensible, volume can increase within reason, without greatly increasing pressure.

Understanding Cardiac Output

Cardiac output is affected by all the previously discussed concepts: pressure, vessel characteristics, viscosity, resistance, and volume. **Cardiac output (CO) is defined as the amount of blood ejected from the left ventricle in one minute**. The normal cardiac output is **4–8 L/minute**. This normal however, is a gross measure. To determine if a cardiac output is adequate for an individual, the cardiac output should be indexed to the individual's height and weight. This is calculated by dividing the cardiac output by the body surface area (derived from a height and weight nomogram.)

The equation for calculating CO is **heart rate times stroke volume**. From a practical standpoint, stroke volume cannot be calculated at the bedside. Therefore more practical measures of cardiac output are needed.

The Four Components of Cardiac Output

There are four components of cardiac output: **preload, contractility, heart rate and afterload.**

☆ **Preload** – Maximum muscle contractility is achieved when the myocardial muscle fiber is stretched from 2.0–2.2 microns. The sarcomeres (bundles of muscle fibers) of the ventricles are stretched with blood volume received from the atria. The optimal stretch of a sarcomere requires a normal to slightly higher blood volume. This volume is called **preload**.

Preload is the blood volume from the veins that returns to the right side of the heart. Theoretically, whatever returns to the right side of the heart also returns to the left side. Since the left heart is the major pump of the heart, we are most interested in the left ventricular volume at the end of diastole. This volume generates a pressure known as the left *ventricular end diastolic pressure*, or (**LVEDP**). LVEDP or preload is measured as a *pulmonary capillary wedge pressure* (**PCWP**).

$$\boxed{\text{PRELOAD} = \text{PCWP} = \text{LVEDP}}$$

When blood volume is increased, preload is increased. When blood volume is decreased, preload is decreased. One must have a normal or slightly higher volume to achieve a maximum cardiac output. In a volume overload situation (preload), the sarcomeres are overstretched and produce a lesser cardiac output.

The relationship between optimal volume (preload) and optimal sarcomere stretch is explained as Starling's Law.

Starling's Law (Scientifically Speaking)

The force of contraction is proportional to the muscle fiber length up to a critical length. When the critical length is exceeded, myocardial contractile force decreases.

Starling's Law (Simply Speaking)

When the normal, or slightly above normal amount of blood volume flows from the atria into ventricles, the ventricular muscle fibers are stretched to an optimal length. Optimal stretch leads to a strong contraction that moves blood forward to the lungs and body leaving very little blood left in the ventricles.

Starling's Law is often compared to a rubber band stretching. The rubber band length can be compared to myocardial fiber length. If the rubber band (muscle fiber) is stretched (diastole) a SHORT distance, contraction (systole) is *weak*. If, however, the rubber band is **fully** stretched (diastole) to its optional length, contraction (systole) is *forceful* and *efficient*! If a rubber band is repeatedly **overstretched** (diastole), it becomes *weakened* and its contractile force (systole) is *diminished.* And so goes the Starling Theory of rubber bands!

☆ **Contractility** – As discussed above, contractility and preload are intimately related. In addition to the effect of preload, contractility is affected by the integrity of muscle fibers, sympathetic nervous system effects, and calcium.

Myofibrils are the muscle fibers in the heart which allow for contractility. Made up of actin (thin) and myosin (thick) filaments, these filaments interweave to form bands. When these filaments interact, contraction occurs. The adequate pumping of blood requires intact, functional myofibrils. Conditions that impair integrity of the myofibrils include ischemia, injury, infarction, and inflammation. Sarcomeres are groups of myofibrils. They encompass fluid and mitochondria which supply energy to the heart.

The *sympathetic nervous system* (SNS) affects the heart via beta adrenergic affects. *Beta-1* effects are increased heart rate (*chronotropy*), increased speed of impulse conduction (*dromotropy*) and increased strength of contractility (*inotropy*).

Calcium interacts with "active" sites on the actin filament leading to contraction. Influx of calcium into the cardiac cell also affects the *cardiac action potential* (impulse formation).

> CALCIUM = CONTRACTILITY

☆ **Heart rate** is also an important dimension of cardiac output.

Within a given target range, as heart rate increases, so does cardiac output. It often becomes necessary to control heart rate in order to maximize cardiac output.

☆ **Afterload.** Finally to further optimize cardiac output, the vasculature must be able to accept blood ejected from the left ventricle. With vascular vasoconstriction, there is greater resistance; with vascular vasodilation, there is lesser resistance. This resistance is called *afterload*. There are specific mathematical equations for calculating afterload. Afterload for the right ventricle is referred to as *pulmonary vascular resistance* (PVR). Afterload for the left ventricle is referred to as *systemic vascular resistance* (SVR). Afterload is measured in resistance units known as dynes/second. Changes in afterload affects cardiac output. When afterload is high, cardiac output falls. When afterload is low, cardiac output is high.

> AFTERLOAD for the Left Heart = SVR

Systemic Vascular Resistance (SVR) = Resistance the left ventricle must overcome to eject blood into the systemic circulation. It is calculated:

$$SVR = \frac{\text{Mean Arterial Pressure } - \text{ Right Atrial Pressure}}{\text{Cardiac Output}} \times 80$$

(Normal SVR = 900–1400 dynes/sec)

> AFTERLOAD for the Right Heart = PVR

Pulmonary Vascular Resistance (PVR) = Resistance the right ventricle must overcome to eject blood into the pulmonary vascular beds. It is calculated:

$$PVR = \frac{\textit{(Mean Pulmonary Artery Pressure} - PCWP)}{Cardiac\ Output} \times 80$$

(Normal PVR = 150–250 dynes/sec)

In summary, the four components of cardiac output are **contractility, preload, heart rate and afterload**.

How Does A Pulmonary Artery Catheter Work?

The development of the pulmonary artery (PA) catheter, also known as the Swan-Ganz catheter, permitted indirect invasive measurement of cardiac output. Though the pulmonary artery catheter is placed in the right side of the heart, this right-sided catheter allows the practitioner to monitor the left-sided pressures of the heart.

The PA catheter is usually inserted via the subclavian vein through the superior vena cava, into the right atrium. A small balloon on the tip of the PA catheter is inflated to assist the catheter flow across the tricuspid valve into the right ventricle (RV). From the RV, it floats across the pulmonic valve out into the pulmonary artery (PA). It then wedges into one of the small diameter pulmonary capillaries.

There are no valves in the pulmonary vessels. When the mitral valve is open during diastole, left ventricular pressure can be measured. If one thinks of the cardiac circulatory system being laid "end to end," it is easier to understand how a right heart catheter can measure pressures in the left ventricle. (It is much like being able view the back room of a *shotgun house* if all the interior room doors are open!)

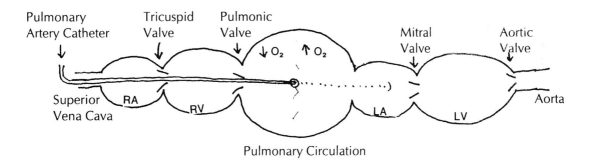

How a right-sided catheter is used to measure left-sided pressures

Practice Exercise 1

A. Invasive hemodynamic monitoring is accomplished via a _____ catheter.

B. The size (mass) and strength of the left ventricle allows oxygenated blood to be ejected past the

_____ valve into the _____, and out to systemic circulation.

C. Correctly label the four cardiac valves

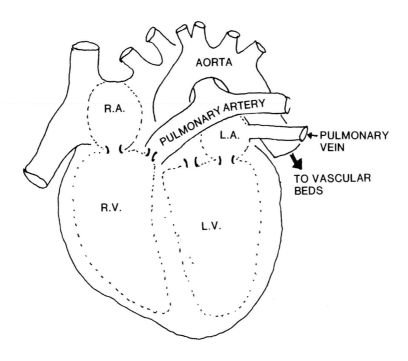

D. The contraction/ejection phase of the blood flow cycle is termed _____;

the relaxation/filling phase of the blood flow cycle is known as _____.

E. If a muscle fiber is stretched (diastole) a short distance, contraction (systole) is _____.

If a muscle fiber is fully stretched to its critical length, contraction is _____. If a

muscle fiber is repeatedly overstretched, contractile force is _____.

F. Starling was a

☐ bird

☐ plane

☐ law man

(sense of humor poll conducted by the management)

G. List the four components of cardiac output.

1. _____

2. _____

3. _____

4. _____

✔ For **Feedback 1**, refer to page 360.

Input Section 13.2: The Pulmonary Artery Catheter (Swan-Ganz)

The pulmonary artery catheter (PA) is a hollow latex tube with three internal lumen (channels). In addition, a thermistor runs through the length of the catheter. A thermistor measures blood temperature. If one were to cut the catheter in half, it would look like the following diagram.

Cross Section: Pulmonary Artery Catheter

Proximal Lumen—This lumen opens into the right atrium. Right atrial pressure (**RAP**) is measured via this lumen. RAP is also called the central venous pressure (**CVP**). This lumen can be used for fluid administration as well as for monitoring pressure.

Distal Lumen—This lumen runs the entire length of the catheter and opens into the pulmonary artery.

Infusion Port—Some PA catheters have an extra lumen used for fluid and medication infusion.

Thermistor—This lumen is used to measure the patient's core temperature and to measure cardiac output (when connected to a cardiac output computer).

Balloon Port—This port allows inflation of a small balloon located near the end of the catheter. The balloon is inflated during catheter insertion and for obtaining the pulmonary capillary wedge pressure.

Cardiac Output (CO) can be measured in a number of ways. The PA catheter measures cardiac output using the thermodilution method. A known volume of fluid (10cc) at a known temperature (room temperature) is injected into the right heart via the proximal lumen of the pulmonary artery catheter. As the fluid mixes with the blood and passes by the thermistor, an attached external computer calculates the cardiac output. **Normal cardiac output ranges between 4–8 liters/minute.**

 Practice Exercise 2

Go for it ☆ *?!!*

A. The pulmonary artery catheter (Swan-Ganz catheter) has three internal lumens, and a

_____ which is used to measure core temperature.

B. Which pulmonary artery catheter port is utilized for fluid administration _____

_____

C. _____ atrial pressure is monitored at the proximal lumen opening.

D. An inflated pulmonary artery catheter balloon causes the catheter to _____ into a small pulmonary vessel.

E. Normal cardiac output (CO) ranges between _____ and _____ liters per minute.

✔ For **Feedback 2**, refer to page 361.

Input Section 13.3 Pressures and Waveforms

Hemodynamic monitoring requires an understanding of normal pressures and waveforms originating from the cardiac structures. Beyond the placement of a pulmonary artery catheter (PAC), hemodynamic monitoring requires both a bedside monitor and, transducer to measure pressures and display waveforms.

A *transducer* system is utilized to convert the mechanical pumping action into an electrical waveform displayed on a monitor. A transducer is much like a bathroom scale! When weight or pressure is applied to a bathroom scale, the gauge on the scale moves.

When pressure is applied to a transducer, the resulting waveform rises on the monitor and then falls as pressure is removed. Easy so far, right? As you progress through this section, you will learn that each cardiac chamber presents unique pressures and waveform characteristics!

You will recall from Section I, page 24, that monitor paper has both a time and amplitude dimension. Moving across monitor paper measures time.

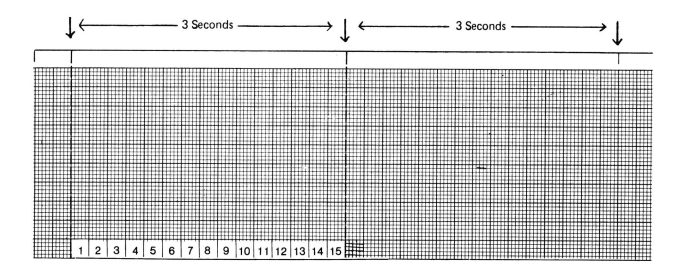

Moving vertically measures amplitude. Each small square represents 1mm amplitude, and each large square represents 5mm amplitude. As we move forward in the section, waveforms and the pressure they represent will be measured in amplitude dimension. Waveforms with great pressure differences are read as sytole over diastole. Lower pressure waveforms are read as mean or average measures.

Right Atrium

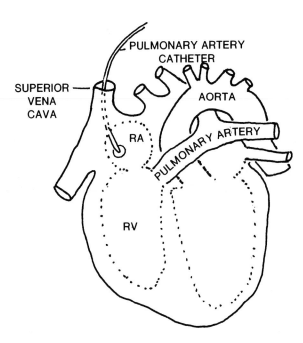

The pulmonary artery catheter is situated in the right atrium.

The above diagram demonstrates the placement of pulmonary artery catheter in the right atrium. You will recall that blood enters the right atrium (RA) passively. Intrathoracic pressure changes occurring secondary to respiration assist blood return to the right heart. Owing to its small muscle mass, the normal right atrial pressure is low. The low pressure produces a low amplitude, oscillating waveform demonstrated in the following diagrams. Because there is only a minimal difference between right atrial systolic and diastolic pressures, a mean or averaged RA pressure is utilized.

Right Atrial (RA) Pressure Waveform

"a" = Atrial Contraction

"c" = Closure of Tricuspid Valve

"x" = Atrial Diastole

"v" = Atrial Filling

"y" = Atrial Empting

Mean (averaged) RA Pressure
2-5 mm. Hg.

Right Atrial (RA) Pressure

Note the low amplitude, oscillating waveform

Normal mean (averaged) right atrial pressure = 2–5mm Hg.

Low RA pressure may indicate hypovolemia or vasodilation. Elevated pressures may indicate fluid overload, RV failure, tricuspid insufficiency, chronic left heart failure or pulmonary disease.

Right Ventricle

Before you move forward, a bit of review is in order! Earlier in this section, the cardiac valves and their gate-keeper function were discussed. The cardiac valves serve to keep blood flowing in a forward direction. The tricuspid valve (see page 335) is located between the right atrium and the right ventricle. When the tricuspid valve opens, the blood volume in the right atrium (RA) flows into the right ventricle (RV). You will recall from page 336 that filling pressure is the same as diastolic pressure. So, the right ventricular diastolic pressure is equal to the mean right atrial filling pressure of 2–5mm Hg.

Right ventricular (RV) diastolic pressure = 2–5mm Hg.

As ventricular systole begins, pressure increases. The systolic or emptying pressure of the right ventricle ranges between 20–30mm Hg. This pressure is low in comparison to the systolic pressure of the left ventricle. This is due to the marked difference between the small muscle mass of the right ventricle and the large muscle mass of the left ventricle. Under normal conditions, pulmonary vascular resistance is low. Therefore, it only requires a small muscle mass to pump blood to the lungs.

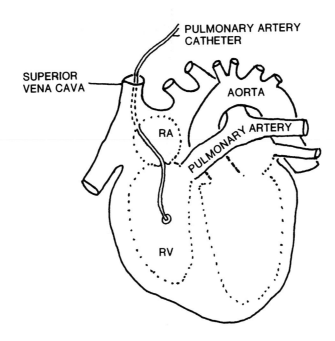

The above diagram demonstrates the placement of a pulmonary artery catheter in the right ventricle.

$$\text{Normal right ventricular (RV) pressure} = \frac{\text{20–30mm Hg. (systolic)}}{\text{2–5mm Hg. (diastolic)}}$$

The following diagrams demonstrate normal right ventricular (RV) waveforms.

Right Ventricular (RV) Pressure Waveform

$$\text{RV PRESSURE} = \frac{\text{20–30 mm. Hg. (SYSTOLIC)}}{\text{2–5 mm. Hg. (DIASTOLIC)}}$$

Note: The RV waveform and pressure can *only* be recorded during catheter insertion. There is no catheter opening into the right ventricular chamber. As the catheter is inserted, pressure in the right ventricle is noted, and then the catheter is floated out into the pulmonary artery.

Right Ventricular (RV) Pressure

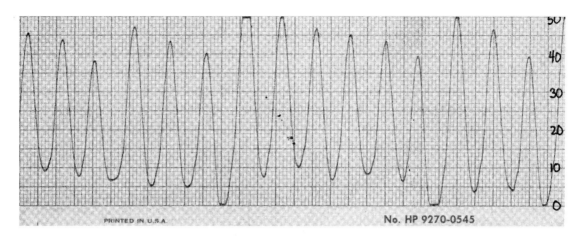

RV pressure is affected by the volume of blood in the ventricle (preload), the pumping ability of the muscle (contractility), and the resistance to ejection found in the pulmonary artery and the lungs (after load). When preload, contractility or afterload changes, so does RV pressure.

Changes in preload (volume)

Hypervolemia ————————————➤ RV pressure ↑

Hypovolemia ————————————➤ RV Pressure ↓

Changes in contractility

Right ventricular infarction ——————➤ ↓ RV contractility ——————➤ Decreased volume of blood is pumped out ——————➤

Volume accumulates ————————➤ RV pressure ↑

Changes in afterload (resistance)

Pulmonary hypertension (↑ resistance in pulmonary artery) ➤ ↓ blood is pumped out ——————➤

Volume accumulates ————————➤ RV pressure ↑

*Chronic obstructive lung disease (COPD) is a common cause of pulmonary hypertension that increases RV pressure. Over time, the right ventricle fails as a pump and right-sided CHF results.

How are you doing thus far! At best, the hemodynamic monitoring concepts should create a stretch in your thinking!

(STARLING STRETCH CONCEPTS, INC.)

Pulmonary Artery

When the pulmonic valve opens secondary to increasing right ventricular pressure, blood and the pulmonary artery catheter moves out of the right ventricle into the pulmonary artery (PA). Though the pulmonary artery has no contractile properties, both systolic and diastolic pressures can be measured.

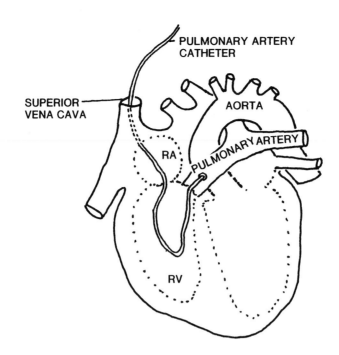

The above diagram demonstrates the pulmonary artery catheter placed in the pulmonary artery. Pulmonary artery filling occurs with right ventricular contraction and emptying. The pressure generated (systolic pressure) by the right ventricle is the same as the pulmonary artery (PA) systolic pressure!

> **RV Systolic Pressure = PA Systolic Pressure**
> 20–30mm Hg.   20–30mm Hg.

Let's backtrack a minute. You will remember that right atrial (RA) pressure measures 2–5mm Hg. Right atrial (RA) pressure drives the filling of the right ventricle (RV). As the RV fills, the right ventricular muscle stretches, forcing the pulmonic valve open. This stretch stimulates the RV muscle to contract. As the muscle contracts, it generates a higher pressure, thus allowing complete emptying of the RV chamber. In the healthy heart, emptying pressure measures 20–30mm Hg. When the pulmonic valve opens, the RV volume is ejected into the pulmonary artery. So the highest or systolic pressure in the pulmonary artery is also 20–30mm Hg.!

Pressure Points Summary

	Right Atrium (RA)	Right Ventricle (RV)	Pulmonary Artery (PA)
Systolic		20–30mm Hg.	20–30mm Hg.
Mean	2–5mm Hg.		
Diastolic		2–5mm Hg.	

Makes sense, right!

Following pulmonary artery filling, the pulmonic valve closes to prevent blood from flowing backwards. Valve closure creates a "back slosh" of blood against the valve, producing a distinctive notching in the waveform. This notching is referred to as the *dicrotic notch*. Please see the following diagram.

Pulmonary Artery (PA) Pressure Waveform

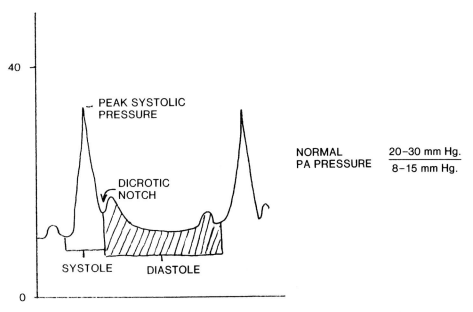

The dicrotic notch is produced by closure of the pulmonic valve.

Low systolic pulmonary artery (PA) pressures would signify hypovolemia or vasodilation. Elevated pressures may be associated with a number of causes including pulmonary emboli, mitral insufficiency, left ventricular failure, cardiac tamponade, mechanical ventilation or COPD.

From the pulmonary artery, blood then flows passively through the pulmonary vasculature. Remember, there are no valves or "other blood flow controlling devices" in the pulmonary beds. Oxygenation occurs as the blood flows through the pulmonary system. As the blood disperses across the pulmonary vascular beds, the pressure drops to a resting or diastolic level. The pulmonary artery (PA) diastolic pressure ranges between 8–15mm Hg.

In summary, a normal pulmonary artery pressure (PAP) will reflect the following norms:

$$\frac{\text{Pulmonary Artery}}{\text{Pressure (PAP)}} = \frac{\text{20–30mm Hg. (systolic)}}{\text{8–15mm Hg. (diastolic)}}$$

Left Atrium

Earlier discussion indicated that there are no valves present in the pulmonary vascular system. Thus, blood flows passively from the pulmonary artery under low pressure to left atrium (LA). Since the PA catheter stops in the PA, there is no waveform or direct pressure reading from the LA. Indirectly, the PA diastolic correlates with the LA pressure.

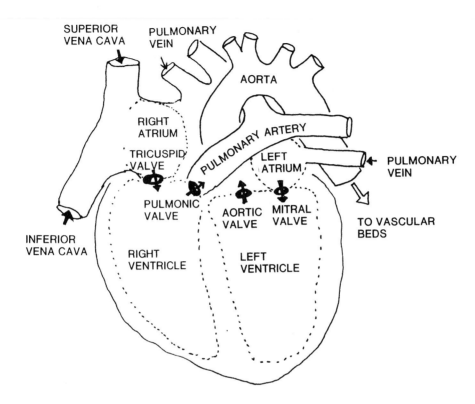

The following table maps pressure relationships from the right atrium to the left atrium.

	Right Atrium (RA) Pressure	Right Ventricle (RV) Pressure	Pulmonary Artery (PA) Pressure	Left Atrial (LA) Pressure
Pressure Points (continued)				
Systolic		20–30-mm Hg.	20–30-mm Hg.	
Mean	2–5-mm Hg.			8–15mm Hg.
Diastolic		2–5-mm Hg.	8–15mm Hg.	

Clear as a foggy day, right! Bear in mind that no one masters hemodynamic concepts on the first pass. Mastery is gained through repetition and practice.

Important Detail:

Before going further, it is important to point out that the pulmonary artery catheter cannot be passed beyond the pulmonary artery! Therefore, left atrial and left ventricular pressure measurements cannot be made directly using the pulmonary artery catheter. Read on for clarification . . .

Pulmonary Capillary Wedge Pressure (PCWP) vs. Left Atrial Pressure

The notion that a catheter inserted into the right heart can measure left heart functioning is confusing. The secret is the 1.5cc latex balloon at the tip of the pulmonary artery catheter. When inflated with a syringe, the balloon occludes or wedges into a small branch of the pulmonary artery and blocks any information coming *from the right heart*. At the tip of the catheter, distal to the balloon, there is a pressure reading device. When the balloon is inflated, the device reads pressure in the left atrium at the end of diastole. Remember, this is filling pressure or preload!

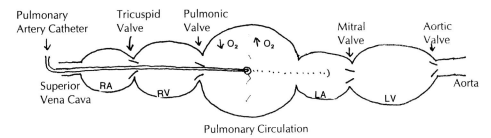

A right-sided catheter used to measure left side pressures.

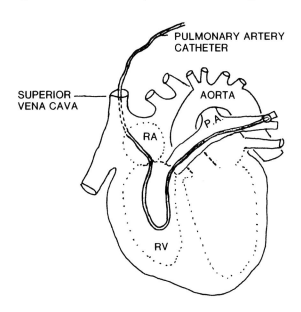

The inflated balloon on the pulmonary catheter is wedged into a small branch of the pulmonary artery.

Both the pulmonary capillary wedge pressure (PCWP) and the left atrial pressure (LA), should be 8–15mm.Hg. (mean values) under normal circumstances.

	Right Atrial (RA) Pressure	Right Ventricle (RV) Pressure	Pulmonary Artery (PA) Pressure	Pulmonary Capillary Wedge Pressure (PCWP)	Left Atrial (LA) Pressure
Pressure Points (continued)					
Systolic		20–30mm Hg.	20–30mm Hg.	8–15mm Hg.	8–15mm Hg.
Mean	2–5mm Hg.				
Diastolic		2–5mm Hg.	8–15mm Hg.		

The pulmonary capillary wedge pressure (PCWP) waveformation is presented in the next two diagrams.

Pulmonary Capillary Wedge Pressure (PCWP)

"a" wave   = atrial contraction

"x" descent = atrial diastole

"v" wave   = passive ventricular filling

"y" descent = passive atrial emptying

Mean PCWP = 8-15 mm. Hg.

The PA waveform "flattens out" as the pulmonary artery catheter balloon is inflated and subsequently wedges in the pulmonary artery. The resulting waveform has little systolic-diastolic pressure change. Thus, as with the RAP, the PCWP is reported as a mean pressure.

The following diagram demonstrates a pulmonary artery catheter moving from the right ventricle into the pulmonary artery. Note that both the RV and PA pressures are elevated.

Pulmonary Capillary Wedge Pressure (PCWP)

Note the elevated pulmonary capillary wedge pressure (PCWP).

Pulmonary Capillary Wedge Pressure (PCWP) vs. Left Ventricular End Diastolic Pressure (LVEDP)

Finally, the last topic in the hemodynamic monitoring process is to relate previously discussed pressures to left ventricular (LV) function. The left ventricle is the major pump of the heart! The left ventricle (LV) has the greatest muscle mass of the four cardiac chambers.

Earlier we presented the concept that the right ventricular (RV) diastolic or filling pressure is equivalent to the mean right atrial (RA) pressure. These pressures are equivalent owing to the *passive* flow of blood from the right atrium to the right ventricle. **Voila!** The same phenomenon occurs in the left side of the heart!

The left ventricular filling or diastolic pressure should equal the left atrial mean pressure because blood flows passively from the left atrium into the left ventricle. Makes sense, right? Thus, at the conclusion of the left ventricular filling phase, the *left ventricular end diastolic pressure* (LVEDP) equals the mean left atrial pressure. Whew!

Now, have a look at the entirety of pressure relationships.

Pressure Points

	(RA) Pressure	(RV) Pressure	(PA) Pressure	(PCWP)	(LA) Pressure	(LV) LVEDP
Systolic		20–30mm Hg.	20–30mm Hg.			
Mean*	2–5mm Hg.			8–15mm Hg.	8–15mm Hg.	
Diastolic		2–5mm Hg.	8–15mm Hg.			8–15mm Hg.

*means pressures are reported for the right and left atria and PCWP because minimal differences exist between systolic and diastolic pressures in those chambers/vessels.

Key:
RA = Right Atrium   PCWP = Pulmonary Capillary Wedge Pressure
RV = Right Ventricle   LA = Left Atrium
PA = Pulmonary Artery   LVEDP = Left Ventricular End Diastolic Pressure

So, in reviewing the pressure points, the PA diastolic, PCWP, LA, and LVEDP should be equal pressures. Thus, a catheter placed in the right heart *can* assess left heart function!!

The left ventricular end diastolic pressure (LVEDP) is a critical measure of left ventricular function. If the LVEDP rises, it is an indication that left ventricular emptying is incomplete. Incomplete left ventricular emptying may occur secondary to pump failure (left ventricular failure) caused by acute myocardial infarction (muscle injury and necrosis). Incomplete LV emptying may also result from *aortic stenosis.* In aortic stenosis, the aortic valve fails to open completely, thus restricting the free flow of blood out of the left ventricular chamber.

Hint: Aortic stenosis reminds me of a Sunday morning church service finale, where 200 people attempt to exit a single door obstructed by a bastion of hand shakers! The hand shakers create congestion and crowd backup. This "obstructed emptying" causes tension (pressure) to rise!

A decrease in the pulmonary capillary wedge pressure (PCWP)/left ventricular end diastolic pressure (LVEDP) results from a reduced preload. A reduced preload is often due to hypovolemia, dehydration, or extreme vasodilation of the venous system.

Cardiac Output Can Be Assessed Without Invasive Hemodynamic Monitoring

There are times when invasive hemodynamic monitoring may not be indicated. However, the measurement of cardiac output is still important. One can assess *some* information regarding cardiac output indirectly. While the information is not specific, it may guide treatment decisions.

➤ Increases and decreases in **preload** may be reflected, in part, by changes in

- Volume status – Intake and output, daily weights

- Edema

- Changes in serum sodium or hematocrit (due to dilution or concentration)

➤ Increases and decreases in **contractility** may be reflected, in part, by changes in

- Skin temperature

- Pulse strength

- Neurological status

- Urine output

➤ Fast, slow or irregular **heart rates** can affect cardiac output.

➤ Increases and decreases in **afterload** may be reflected, in part, by changes in

- Skin temperature. Warm, flushed skin reflects vasodilation and therefore, decreased afterload.

- Skin temperature. Cold skin reflects vasoconstriction and therefore, increased afterload.

Practice Exercise 3

Note: Difficulty Ahead . . . Be Prepared to Stop for Review

A. Owing to its (circle one) small/large muscle mass, the normal right atrial pressure is low/high.

B. Minimal differences between systolic and diastolic pressures are reported as _____ pressures.

C. Mean right atrial pressure normally ranges between _____ and _____ mm Hg.

D. Correctly match right atrial pressure abnormalities with probable pathologies by placing the letter L or H in the spaces provided.

L = Low right atrial pressure   _____   Right ventricular failure

H = High right atrial pressure   _____   Fluid overload

                                   _____   Vasodilation

                                   _____   Tricuspid valve insufficiency

                                   _____   Chronic left heart failure

                                   _____   Hypovolemia

E. Explain why the right ventricular diastolic pressure equals the mean right atrial pressure (to cheat, turn to page 347).

_____

_____

_____

_____

F. Normal right ventricular (RV) pressure is (circle one).

2–5mm Hg.   20–30mm Hg.   20–30mm Hg.
                                                2–5mm Hg.

G. The dicrotic notch in the pulmonary artery waveform is produced by

_____

_____

_____

• Check (X) if you are alive and well . . .

• Check (X) if you are uncertain!

H. Correctly match systolic pulmonary artery pressure abnormalities with suspect pathologies by placing the letter L or H in the spaces provided.

L = Low systolic PA pressures   _____ Pulmonary emboli

H = High systolic PA pressures   _____ Hypovolemia

_____ Mechanical ventilation

_____ Left ventricular failure

_____ Vasodilation

I. Normal pulmonary artery pressure (PAP) is _____mm Hg.

8–15mm Hg.

J. The pulmonary artery (PA) resting or diastolic pressure equals the mean left atrial (LA) pressure because there are no _____ in the pulmonary vascular system or left atrial junction. The absence of _____ allows the pressures to equalize.

K. If the diastolic PA pressure is 10mm.Hg., the mean LA pressure will be _____ mm Hg.

L. The pulmonary artery catheter cannot be passed beyond the _____!

Break Time . . .
Please return in 15mm Hg. ☞
· · · · · · · · · · ·

☐ I returned on time

☐ I was tardy

M. Left ventricular filling or end diastolic pressure equals the left atrial mean pressure because _____

_____

_____

N. Correctly match left ventricular end diastolic pressure (LVEDP) abnormalities with associated pathologies by placing the letter H (high) or L (low) in the spaces provided.

H = elevated LVEDP (> 15mm Hg.)   _____ Hypovolemia

L = low LVEDP (< 8mm Hg.)   _____ Aortic stenosis

_____ Incomplete LV emptying

_____ Left Ventricular failure

_____ Dehydration

O. In the spaces provided, write the words represented by the following abbreviations. *Then*, note normal pressures for the various hemodynamic measures!

Pressures

RA = _____

RV = _____

PA = _____

PCWP = _____

LA = _____

LVEDP = _____

P.

> **There are four components of cardiac output: Preload, Heart Rate, Contractility and Afterload**
>
> Please review the following list of drugs, factors, and interventions. Evaluate how each of these would increase or decrease the patient's preload, heart rate, contractility and/or afterload. Some of the drugs, factors, and interventions will impact one of the four components, others may impact two or more of the components. Use an arrow up for increase and an arrow down for decrease. See Digoxin as an example.

Drugs, Factors and Interventions	Preload	Heart Rate	Contractility	Afterload
Digoxin		↓	↑	
Anxiety				
Lasix				
Nitroglycerin				
Blood Transfusion				
Fever				
Bolus of IV fluids				
Atropine				
Caffeine				
Hypoxia				
Thyroid Hormone				
Calcium				
Hemodialysis				
Elevate Head of Bed				
Cooling Blanket				
Pacemaker Insertion				
Nicotine				

Bravo

✔ For Feedback 3, refer to page 361.

✔ **Feedback 1**

Great Job!

A. Invasive hemodynamic monitoring is accomplished via a <u>pulmonary artery</u> catheter.

B. The size (mass) and strength of the left ventricle allows oxygenated blood to be ejected past the <u>aortic</u> valve into the <u>aorta</u> and out to systemic circulation.

C.

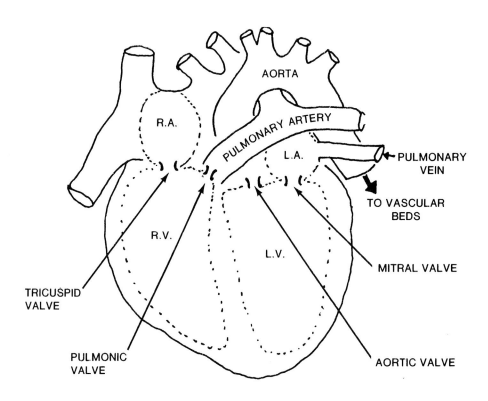

D. The contraction/ejection phase of the blood flow cycle is termed <u>systole</u>; the relaxation/filling phase of the blood flow cycle is known as <u>diastole</u>.

E. If a muscle fiber is stretched (diastole) a short distance, contraction (systole) is <u>weak</u>. If a muscle fiber is fully stretched to its critical length, contraction is forceful. If a muscle fiber is repeatedly overstretched, contractile force is <u>diminished</u>.

F. Starling was a   ☐ Bird

☐ Plane

☒ Law man

G. Cardiac output (CO) is a measure of <u>myocardial contractile force</u>.

✔ Feedback 2

A. The pulmonary artery catheter (Swan-Ganz catheter) has three internal lumens, and a <u>thermistor</u> which is used to measure core temperature.

B. The <u>proximal</u> pulmonary artery catheter port is utilized for fluid administration.

C. <u>Right</u> atrial pressure is monitored at the proximal lumen opening.

D. An inflated pulmonary artery catheter balloon causes the catheter to <u>"wedge"</u> into a small pulmonary vessel.

E. Normal cardiac output (CO) ranges between <u>4</u> and <u>8</u> liters per minute.

✔ Feedback 3

A. Owing to its small muscle mass, the normal right atrial pressure is low.

B. Minimal differences between systolic and diastolic pressures are reported as averaged or mean pressures.

C. Mean right atrial pressure normally ranges between <u>2</u> and <u>5</u>mm Hg.

D. L = Low right atrial pressure   <u>H</u> Right ventricular failure

   H = High right atrial pressure   <u>H</u> Fluid overload

                                              <u>L</u> Vasodilation

                                              <u>H</u> Tricuspid valve insufficiency

                                              <u>H</u> Chronic left heart failure

                                              <u>L</u> Hypovolemia

E. When the tricuspid valve opens, the blood volume in the RA flows passively into the RV. It is the mean right atrial pressure that forces the valve open. That pressure is maintained in the action stage of right atrial ejection and the relaxation stage of RV filling via the open tricuspid valve. Whew!

F. Normal right ventricular (RV) pressure is   <u>20–30mm Hg.</u>

                                               2–5mm Hg.

G. The dicrotic notch in the pulmonary artery waveform is produced by <u>the back slosh of blood against the pulmonic valve. The pulmonic valve closes following pulmonary artery filling</u>.

H. L = Low systolic PA pressures   <u>H</u> Pulmonary emboli

   H = High systolic PA pressures   <u>L</u> Hypovolemia

                                              <u>H</u> Mechanical ventilation

                                              <u>H</u> Left ventricular failure

                                              <u>L</u> Vasodilation

I. Normal pulmonary artery pressure (PAP) is   <u>20–30mm Hg.</u>

                                                 8–15mm Hg.

J. The pulmonary artery (PA) resting or diastolic pressure equals the mean left atrial (LA) pressure because there are no <u>valves</u> in the pulmonary vascular system or left atrial junction. The absence of <u>valves</u> allows the pressures to equalize.

K. If the diastolic PA pressure is 10mm Hg., the mean LA pressure will be <u>10</u>mm Hg.

L. The pulmonary artery catheter cannot be passed beyond the <u>pulmonary artery</u>!

M. Left ventricular filling or end diastolic pressure equals the left atrial mean pressure because <u>the blood flows passively from the left atrium into the left ventricle via the open mitral valve</u>.

N. Correctly match left ventricular end diastolic pressure (LVEDP) abnormalities with associated pathologies by placing the letter H (high) or L (low) in the spaces provided.

H = elevated LVEDP (> 15mm Hg.)   <u>L</u>   Hypovolemia

L = low LVEDP (< 8mm Hg.)   <u>H</u>   Aortic stenosis

                                   <u>H</u>   Incomplete LV emptying

                                   <u>H</u>   Left ventricular failure

                                   <u>H</u>   Dehydration

O. In the spaces provided, write the words represented by the following abbreviations. <u>Then</u> note NORMAL pressures for the various hemodynamic measures!

	Pressures
RA = right atrium	2–5mm Hg.
RV = right ventricle	<u>20–30mm Hg.</u>
	2–5mm Hg.
PA = pulmonary artery	<u>20–30mm Hg.</u>
	8–15mm Hg.
PCWP = pulmonary capillary wedge pressure	8–15mm Hg.
LA = left atrium	8–15mm Hg.
LVEDP = left ventricular end diastolic pressure	8–15mm Hg.

P. Answers to question P on next page.

Answer Key

There are four components of cardiac output: Preload, Heart Rate, Contractility and Afterload

Please review the following list of drugs, factors, and interventions. Evaluate how each of these would increase or decrease the patient's preload, heart rate, contractility and/or afterload. Some of the drugs, factors, and interventions will impact one of the four components, others may impact two or more of the components. Use arrow up for increase and an arrow down for decrease. See Digoxin as an example.

Drugs, Factors and Interventions	Preload	Heart Rate	Contractility	Afterload
Digoxin		↓	↑	
Anxiety	↑	↑	↑	↑
Lasix	↓			↓
Nitroglycerin	↓			↓
Blood Transfusion	↑			
Fever		↑	↑	↓
Bolus of IV fluids	↑			
Atropine		↓		
Caffeine	↓	↑	↑	↑
Hypoxia		↑	↑	
Thyroid Hormone		↑	↑	
Calcium			↑	
Hemodialysis	↓			
Elevate Head of Bed	↓			
Cooling Blanket	↑			↑
Pacemaker Insertion		↑		
Nicotine		↑	↑	↑

☆ *Stellar performance!*

Notes

Antiarrhythmic, Thrombolytic and Platelet Inhibitor Agents

Objectives

When you have completed Section 14, you will be able to describe or identify

1. the body's handling of drugs

2. the autonomic nervous system control of heart rate

3. drug actions at receptor sites

4. the four classifications of antiarrhythmic drugs

5. general therapeutic and toxic effects of the four antiarrhythmic drug classifications

6. treatment for specific rhythm disorders

7. thrombolytic and platelet inhibitor drug therapy for acute coronary syndromes

8. the use of drug-eluting stents

Text by
Mike Lucey, Pharm. D.

Antiarrhythmic Drugs, An Introduction

Arrhythmias are often "fun" to analyze, but once identified, one needs to consider "what next!" Should the dysrhythmia be treated? If so, how?

These are really "loaded" questions! The introduction of new technologies and drugs, combined with surprising results from clinical trials, continue to result in a whirlwind of change.

The preferred treatment for an arrhythmia is likely to change rapidly as research continues.

Since we usually think that arrhythmias are "bad" or represent "disease," one may make the assumption that making the arrhythmia go away is a good thing. Certainly, in life-threatening disorders (ventricular fibrillation or sustained ventricular tachycardia, for example), treatment is required immediately since perfusion to vital organs is diminished or absent.

The long-term treatment of "non-emergent" arrhythmias like recurrent P.V.C.s or atrial fibrillation is less clear. Some clinical trials have found that a drug treatment may effectively treat an arrhythmia, but ironically the treated patients may have a higher mortality than the untreated group! Many of the more recent clinical trials are examining the effects of drug treatment on mortality more closely than before.

All antiarrhythmic drugs have been associated with a ***proarrhythmic effect***. This means that sometimes an arrhythmia will worsen or a new arrhythmia will appear after the initiation of antiarrhythmic drug therapy. Of special concern are drugs which prolong the QT interval (or the QTc interval—the QT interval corrected for heart rate). The arrhythmia described *as torsades de pointes* is a type of proarrhythmic effect by drugs causing prolongation of the QT interval. Many other medications used for a variety of conditions, also cause a prolongation of the QT interval. The FDA recommends extra caution for use of such medications in patients with conditions that predispose to torsades de pointes. Those predisposing conditions include (though not limited to) bradycardia, electrolyte imbalances, concurrent use with other drugs that prolong the QT interval, or the presence of congenital QT prolongation.

Accurate diagnosis and careful patient selection is fundamental to arrhythmic drug administration since harmful, even fatal, effects can occur from drug use. Some types of arrhythmias respond well to proper drug treatment, while other rhythm disorders are completely resistant to drug effects.

The presence of physical symptoms, underlying cardiac disease (CHF or a recent MI), resultant undesirable changes (hypotension, reduced cardiac output, changes in heart rate), or high-risk status for a serious event (atrial embolization) will influence the decision to use an antiarrhythmic drug.

If an arrhythmia is caused by a correctable condition (electrolyte imbalance, hypoxia, drug or chemical toxicities, ischemia), treatment should be aimed at correcting the underlying condition. An antiarrhythmic drug may be needed only temporarily until the condition has been resolved.

Finally, each drug is assigned a generic name, unique for its chemical substance. Drug manufacturers attach a *brand* or *trade* name to a drug which is *usually* easier to remember than the generic name. There can be several brands of the same generic drug, which may be confusing. Throughout this Section, generic drug names are mentioned first; brand names, if significant, follow in parentheses. Generally, drug manufacturers include packaging information specifying both drug indications and contraindications. ***Indications*** are those conditions, diseases or symptoms a particular drug has been proven useful in relieving or preventing. ***Contraindications*** *(or precautions)* are patient characteristics (age, gender, race, etc.) or conditions (CHF, impaired kidney function, drug allergies, etc.) for which the administration of a particular drug should be avoided owing to an increased risk of harm to the patient. For example, calcium channel blockers, adenosine, beta blockers, and digoxin are contraindicated in patients having second- or third-degree heart block unless artificial pacing is employed.

Input Section 14.1: Pharmacologic Processes and Therapeutic Ranges

The Body's Four Processes for Drug Handling

In order for a drug to be effective, it must travel to its site of action (a receptor) in sufficient quantities to produce the desired effect. If an insufficient quantity of drug is present at the receptor, the treatment will be ineffective. Conversely, if an excessive amount of drug is present, toxicity is likely to occur.

Questions regarding drug route, dosage and dosage frequency have more to do with the way the body handles a drug than on how the drug affects the body! There are four basic **pharmacologic processes** governing the body's handling of drugs. Those processes are:

➤ Absorption

➤ Distribution

➤ Metabolism

➤ Excretion

Read on for the details!

➤ Absorption

Absorption is the process whereby a drug enters the bloodstream from the site of drug administration. The speed of the absorption process and how much of the drug is absorbed depends on the route of administration.

The intravenous route of drug administration places 100% of the administered drug directly into the bloodstream; this bypasses a "true" absorption step, and therefore produces more immediate effects. Therefore, the intravenous route is ideal for emergencies.

Drugs given intramuscularly are injected into the tissue of skeletal muscle. From there, the drug diffuses into the capillaries of the muscle which lead to veins leading back to the heart. This process takes time. Giving a drug intramuscularly results in a slower onset (or beginning) of action than the intravenous route.

Drugs administered orally are usually absorbed from the small intestine, rather than the stomach. This means that absorption does not occur until the drug dissolves and the stomach empties its contents into the small intestine (called gastric emptying). Depending on stomach contents and gastric motility, gastric emptying and subsequent absorption across the intestinal membrane can take a long time, even hours sometimes. Thus, the oral route of administration is not suitable for the emergency treatment of an arrhythmia.

Some drugs are poorly absorbed from the intestine, making the oral route of administration unusable. In these cases, the intravenous or intramuscular route of administration may be necessary to get the drug to the site of action.

In a pinch, when an intravenous route is unavailable during cardiac arrest, some antiarrhythmics (**lidocaine, atropine**) can be given through an endotracheal tube. The endotraceal tube will put the drug directly into the lungs, where absorption takes place across the capillary membrane in the lung tissue. However, this absorption is limited by the poor blood flow through the lungs during cardiac arrest. A recent study concluded that the intratracheal route of administration was associated with poorer patient outcomes than drugs administered via an intravenous route.

➤ Distribution

Once the drug is in the bloodstream (following absorption), it is distributed by blood flow throughout the system. Most drugs are distributed widely throughout the body, regardless of the intended site of action. (The body has no way of knowing that the circulating drug is intended to act at a specific site!) A drug may concentrate in certain tissues depending on its chemical characteristics.

Highly perfused organs, such as the brain, heart, lungs, kidneys, and liver, are exposed to administered drugs more quickly and in greater amounts initially than are organs with less perfusion—i.e., bone, muscle, skin, and adipose tissue. Eventually, less perfused tissues will take up the drug from the circulation.

Drug distribution during cardiac arrest (asystole or ventricular fibrillation) is impaired since there is no effective blood flow to move the drug from the site of administration to the heart, the intended site of action. During cardiac arrest, blood flow is dependent on the provision of effective CPR.

Peripheral blood flow is minimal during cardiac arrest, thus inhibiting drug distribution to the intended site of action. **During cardiac arrest, a "significant delay" should be anticipated following intravenous drug administration via *peripheral veins* before the drug reaches the heart, even if effective CPR is being provided.**

When possible, the **central venous route**, including the jugular and subclavian veins, is the preferred route for drug administration in order to minimize this time delay. Peak drug concentrations reaching the heart are lower when drugs are administered via a peripheral vein. Therefore, saphenous (leg) veins and veins in the hands and wrists are less desirable than more proximal veins.

➤ Metabolism

Metabolism of a drug is the process whereby the **drug is changed chemically**. Most drug metabolism is performed by proteins called enzymes located in various parts of the body. The liver is the most important location for these drug-metabolizing enzymes. In drug metabolism, the drug molecules are modified by the addition of a chemical part, the subtraction of a chemical part, or some combination of the two processes.

The chemical alteration of a drug yields a **metabolite** which has different actions and toxicities than its **parent drug**. Most metabolites are **inactive**, meaning they do not possess the antiarrhythmic actions of the parent drug.

The metabolism of some drugs, however, such as procainamide, disopyramide, lidocaine, and encainide, results in production of **active metabolites** which share the antiarrhythmic activity of the parent drug. Most active metabolites have less activity than the parent drug, but for some drugs the metabolite is responsible for most of the drug's action! How is your mental metabolism?

➤ Excretion

Excretion is the process whereby **drugs and drug metabolites are eliminated from the body**. The two major routes for excretion are the urinary tract and the biliary tract.

A common measure for describing the rate of drug elimination from the body is called **half-life**. Half-life is the time required to reduce (by metabolism and/or excretion) the amount of drug in the body by one half. The following table reveals a wide range of half-lives for various antiarrhythmic drugs.

Half Life of Various Antiarrhythmic Drugs	
Drug	**Half-life**
amiodarone (Cordarone)	25 days
digoxin (Lanoxin)	1.5 days
sotalol (Betapace)	12 Hours
esmolol (Bevibloc)	8 minutes
adenosine (Adenocard)	5 seconds

Note the wide *differences* among the above half-life values! Some half-life values are measured in seconds, others in days, and some, in nearly a month. These wide differences in elimination rates require that specific drugs be administered on dosage schedules tailored to elimination rates.

The processes of absorption and distribution determine the time to the onset, or beginning, of drug action. A drug must be given by an administration route that results in good absorption at an acceptable rate. What is "acceptable" is determined by the patient's clinical condition.

Metabolism and excretion determine the duration of drug action, since these processes remove the drug from the site of action. Metabolism and excretion also determine the necessary frequency of drug administration and dosage. Therefore, a drug with a rapid rate of metabolism, like **lidocaine**, must be administered frequently to maintain an effective or therapeutic drug level. In clinical practice, lidocaine is administered via continuous infusion to assure the desired therapeutic effects.

Serum Drug Concentrations and the "Therapeutic Range"

The Therapeutic "Range"
(Pharm Art, Inc.)

Some antiarrhythmic drugs are more effective when the serum (blood) drug concentration exceeds a certain minimum value. Likewise, toxicity is more frequent when the serum drug concentration becomes excessive. For some antiarrhythmic drugs, a desirable range of serum concentrations has been established which effectively controls most arrhythmias, and avoids excessive toxicity. This desired range of drug concentrations is called the **therapeutic range**. Drug concentrations below the range are likely to be ineffective. The therapeutic range is intended to be a guideline which can assist in determining the optimal dosage for a particular patient and in determining the presence of drug toxicity.

The following table provides a sampling of drug therapeutic ranges for commonly administered antiarrhythmic drugs.

Table of Therapeutic Ranges

Drug	Therapeutic Range
digoxin	0.5–2 ng/ml
amiodarone	1–2.5mcg/ml
lidocaine	1–5 mcg/ml
propafenone	0.5–2.0 mcg/ml

Keying = nanograms
    Mcg = micrograms

Practice Exercise 1

"Pharmacist-Wanna-Be" Practice

A. Cardiac cells may interact with or respond to different types of drugs because _____

_____

_____.

B. Antiarrhythmic drugs work by affecting one or more of the following cardiac tissue properties:

   1. _____.

   2. _____.

   3. _____.

C. Drug absorption depends on the _____.

D. The intravenous route of drug administration produces "near-immediate" effects because one of the following processes is bypassed. Check the omitted process.

❏ Absorption

❏ Distribution

❏ Metabolism

❏ Excretion

E. During a code arrest situation, a central venous route of drug administration is recommended because

_____

_____

_____.

F. The _____ is the primary location for drug metabolism.

G. Drug "half-life" refers to _____

_____

_____

✔ For **Feedback 1**, refer to page 386.

Input Section 14.2: Control of Heart Rate by Autonomic Nerves

The SA node is the heart's normal pacemaker since it has the most rapid rate of spontaneous depolarization. However, the heart must be able to vary its rate to accommodate changing perfusion demands (stress, varying temperature, activity, and so forth). How can the rate of SA node firing be varied under these conditions?

The SA node (and other key cardiac tissues) has nerve connections from the autonomic nervous system. These nerves communicate with the heart by releasing chemicals from the nerve endings called neurotransmitters. Norepinephrine and acetylcholine are the main neurotransmitters used for this purpose. The body has a number of other neurotransmitters with interesting names as well.

Neurotransmitters bind to special proteins called *receptors* that sit on the surface of SA nodal cells and cells in other cardiac tissues, too. A neurotransmitter will bind to *only* one type of receptor.

The receptor for norepinephrine is different than the receptor for acetylcholine. Both are proteins, yet they are different. These receptor types have funny names, as well.

When a rapid heart rate is required under conditions such as exercise, danger, or stress, the sympathetic nerve connections to the heart are stimulated. This stimulated nerve releases norepinephrine near the SA node, which binds to the **beta-adrenergic receptors** on the SA cells. This binding of norepinephrine increases the frequency of SA node depolarization, which increases the heart rate.

Likewise, if a decrease in heart rate is required, the parasympathetic nerve connections to the heart are stimulated to release acetylcholine near the SA node. The acetylcholine binds to **muscarinic receptors** on the surface of the SA node cells. This binding causes a decrease in both the automaticity and frequency of SA node depolarization, and a subsequent decrease in heart rate.

This sequence of *nerve stimulation* ⟶ *neurotransmitter release* ⟶ *receptor binding* ⟶ *cardiac action* is helpful in understanding drug actions.

Some antiarrhythmic drugs work by acting at these same "beta-adrenergic" and "muscarinic" receptors. For example, the class II antiarrhythmics, the "beta-blockers," block the effect of norepinephrine at the beta-adrenergic receptor. Another example is the drug atropine, which blocks the action of acetylcholine on the muscarinic receptor.

Practice Exercise 2

A. The SA node is the heart's normal pacemaker since it has the most rapid rate of spontaneous _____

_____.

B. A "proarrhythmic effect" means _____

_____.

✔ For **Feedback 2**, refer to page 386.

Input Section 14.3: Antiarrhythmic Drugs: Actions at Receptor Sites

Cardiac cells have a number of other proteins on their surfaces which are needed to make the cells work properly. Many antiarrhythmic drugs produce their actions by attaching ("binding") to these proteins, causing changes in cell functions. For example, certain proteins control the movement of sodium into the cell (called "sodium channels"). Other proteins control the movement of calcium into the cell ("calcium channels"), too. Some antiarrhythmic drugs act on these sodium and calcium channels to produce their effects. The proteins that *receive* the antiarrhythmic drugs are also referred to as drug *receptors*.

A specific receptor will usually bind only to one drug or type of drug. However, a cardiac cell may have many different receptor types on its surface, and may therefore interact with many different types of drugs. Receptors for various drugs can be found in the SA node, the AV node, cardiac muscle cells, and the His-Purkinje system. Once a drug binds to the receptor, chemical changes take place producing an effect or action.

The following table demonstrates receptor sites for various antiarrhythmic drugs.

Drug or Drug Class	Receptor
Class I Antiarrhythmics	Sodium Channels
Class II Antiarrhythmics ("beta-blockers")	Beta-adrenergic receptors
Class III Antiarrhythmics (act at differing receptors)	
Amiodarone	Sodium, calcium, and potassium channels. Adrenergic mechanisms.
Sotalol	Beta receptors, potassium channels
Class IV Antiarrhythmics ("calcium channel blockers")	Calcium channels

Mechanisms of Action

Once an antiarrhythmic drug is delivered to its site of action (the receptor), it usually works by affecting one or more of the following cardiac tissue properties. The particular way in which an antiarrhythmic drug works is called its *mechanism of action*.

➤ **Automaticity**: Some antiarrhythmic drugs exert their effects by decreasing the rate of ectopic pacemakers discharge. For instance, intravenous lidocaine is often employed to reduce ventricular ectopy.

➤ **Rate of impulse conduction**: Other drugs act by slowing the movement of depolarization through cardiac tissues, including the myocardium, AV node, and the Purkinje system. The class IC drugs are especially potent in this regard.

➤ **Duration of the refractory period** (or, the time needed for repolarization): Drugs acting in this way hold up the whole process of impulse conduction by prolonging the refractory period. Prolonging cellular repolarization or recovery results in a slowing of tissue receptiveness to the next stimulus. Prolongation of the refractory period is the specialty of the class III antiarrhythmics.

You will be happy to know there is no practice exercise associated with Input Section 14.3!

Input Section 14.4: The Classification of Antiarrhythmic Drugs

Antiarrhythmic drugs can be classified (or grouped) according to their mechanism of action or EKG effects. By grouping drugs in this manner, one does not need to memorize each drug's effects separately! Rather, one should focus on remembering the drug effects produced by different drug groups. The most common classification system used is the *Harrison modification of the Vaughn Williams system*.

In this system, there are four distinct drug classes: Class I, Class II, Class III, and Class IV. Though not everyone is satisfied with this classification scheme, it remains the "accepted" method.

It is important to note, however, the classification system has not been useful in reliably predicting whether a drug will be effective in the treatment of a particular arrhythmia. Treatment of arrhythmias should use an **evidence-based** approach. Evidence-based means that controlled research has shown that a treatment actually improves patient outcomes in a statistically measurable way, such as prolonging survival, or decreasing hospitalization, or alleviating a target symptom. *It is not enough to merely demonstrate that a treatment eliminates the arrhythmia.* Sometimes, the elimination of an arrhythmia with a treatment actually negatively affects patient outcomes.

There is another antiarrhythmic drug classification system designed to address the limitations of the Vaughn-Williams system. Called the *Sicilian Gambit*, this system acknowledges that antiarrhythmics often act on more than one receptor, and may have more than one mechanism of action. This system describes how drugs affect a number of factors, including ion channels, adrenergic and adenosine receptors, cellular "pumps" like the Na/K ATPase pump, clinical actions such as cardiac output and sinus rate, and EKG effects."

Class I Drugs

Earlier, you learned that cardiac cell depolarization occurs when sodium cations come "whooshing" into the cell. These sodium ions come through tiny alleys called *sodium channels*. All class I drugs work by binding to the sodium channel (their receptor), slowing the passage of sodium through to the cell. This slowing of sodium passage serves to decrease the rate of depolarization which may be important in treating rapid ectopic rhythms. That's it! . . .

. . . however, there is one *minor* glitch. Not all sodium channel blockers (i.e., class I drugs) produce the same electrocardiographic effects. So, to make matters complicated, class I drugs were subdivided into classes IA, IB,

	Class I Drugs and Actions	
Class	**Actions**	**Drugs: Generic name (Trade name)**
IA	➤ Moderate slowing of conduction (widened QRS) ➤ Repolarization prolonged (prolonged QT interval) ➤ Increased P-R interval)	quinidine procainamide (Pronestyl, Procan SR) disopyramide (Norpace)
IB	➤ Little effect on conduction ➤ Repolarization shortened (QT interval may shorten)	lidocaine (Xylocaine) mexiletine (Mexetil) phenytoin (Dilantin) tocainide (Tonocard)
IC	➤ Conduction slows significantly ➤ Repolarization: little effect ➤ Marked increase in P-R and QRS duration	flecainide (Tambocor) propafenone (Rhythmol)

and IC. *All the class I drugs decrease automaticity, but the subgroups (IA, IB, IC) have different effects on conduction and repolarization!* Whew! Those differences are shown in the table at the bottom of page 373.

The Class IA antiarrhythmics are referenced as **broad spectrum drugs** because they have been used for a *variety* of *supraventricular* and *ventricular* arrhythmias, including paroxysmal supraventricular tachycardia, atrial flutter and fibrillation, PVCs, and ventricular tachycardia.

Though many of the Class I drugs successfully control dysrhythmias, they have been found to be associated with a higher than expected patient mortality. In other words, an improved EKG pattern has not been a predictor of patient outcome! In particular, Class IA and Class IC drugs have been suspected as causative of sudden death when administered to patients with significant structural disease. Patient survival benefits are questionable given the proarrhythmic effect of these drugs. A *proarrhythmic effect* is a drug induced worsening of an existing dysrhythmia.

As a result of these findings, the use of the Class I drugs has decreased markedly. Current Class I drug therapy includes Lidocaine, (Class IB) for control of ventricular dysrhythmias, in the acute care setting, and Class IC drugs for carefully selected patients with atrial dysrhythmias. Drug therapies continue to evolve in response to current clinical trials and longitudinal studies.

Class II Drugs: Beta-Blockers

Class II drugs are beta-adrenergic antagonists (usually called beta-blockers). These agents block (reverse or prevent) the cardiac actions of epinephrine or norepinephrine at the beta-adrenergic receptor.

Class II Drugs and Actions *Beta-Blockers*

Class II Drugs and Actions		
Class	**Actions**	**Drugs: Generic name (Trade name)**
II	➤ Blocks beta-receptors	propranolol (Inderal)
	➤ Decreases SA node automaticity	atenolol (Tenormin)
	➤ Decreases heart rate	acebutolol (Sectral)
	➤ Decreases ectopy secondary	metoprolol (Lopressor)
	to sympathetic overstimulation	esmolol (Brevibloc)
	➤ Increases duration of AV node	nadolol (Corgard)
	refractory period	carvedilol (Coreg)

The beta-blockers are frequently administered to control supraventricular tachyarrhythmias such as atrial fibrillation, atrial flutter, or paroxysmal supraventricular tachycardia. Though a beta-blocker will not usually eliminate the supraventricular dysrhythmia, it will decrease the rate of ventricular response by antagonizing sympathetic nerves going to the AV node. This antagonism increases the AV node refractory period, which limits the number of impulses conducted through to the ventricles.

For example, a rapid atrial fibrillation (ventricular rate 130 per minute) might be reduced to a controlled rate atrial fibrillation (ventricular rate less than 100 per minute); or, a 2:1 atrial flutter might be reduced to a 3:1 atrial flutter. If you need review, see page 73.

Beta-blockers are also used to treat ventricular dysrhythmias caused by either extreme sympathetic nervous system overactivity or excessive amounts of circulating epinephrine (pheochromocytoma) or hyperthyroidism.

Clinical trials have demonstrated that the long-term administration of **beta-blockers following acute myocardial infarction consistently reduces mortality**. The mortality reduction averages around 20 percent compared to control groups.

Beta-blockers are also used to treat hypertension and angina pectoris. Propranolol (Inderal) has also been used to prevent migraine headaches.

Beta-blockers can cause bronchospasm in patients with existing respiratory disease (asthma and COPD). They can also precipitate CHF in susceptible individuals. Beta-blockers **should never be suddenly discontinued** in patients with a history of severe coronary artery disease or angina pectoris—precipitation of **anginal attacks, arrhythmias, or myocardial infarction may result**. Fatigue, depression, and sleep disturbances may be associated with the use of beta-blockers.

It should also be noted that Betapace (sotalol) and amiodarone, though class III drugs, have beta blocking effects as well.

Class III Drugs

The Class III drugs are a "mixed bag" of chemical agents which bear little resemblance to one another except for their *prolongation of ventricular repolarization.*

Class III Drugs and Actions		
Class	**Actions**	**Drugs: Generic name (Trade name)**
III	➤ Prolongs repolarization	amiodarone (Cordarone)
	➤ Increases refractory period	sotalol (Betapace)
		ibutilide (Corvert)
		dofetilide (Tikosyn)

Amiodarone and sotalol are drugs reserved for *life-threatening* ventricular arrhythmias (ventricular tachycardia or ventricular fibrillation). Sometimes, amiodarone is used to treat stubborn supraventricular arrhythmias. Amiodarone can be a toxic antiarrhythmic agent. A certain percentage of patients may not tolerate this drug due to one or more of the following effects: corneal microdeposits, liver toxicity, lung fibrosis, hyper- and hypothyroidism, skin discoloration, photosensitivity, and worsening of arrhythmias. Amiodarone rivals lidocaine as the first line of drug intervention for ventricular tachycardia.

Ibutilide (Corvert) is given by the intravenous route for conversion of atrial fibrillation or atrial flutter to sinus rhythm. Ibutilide, released to market in 1996, causes polymorphic ventricular tachycardia, also known as torsades de pointes, as an adverse proarrhythmic effect in 1.7% of patients treated.

Dofetilide is indicated for the conversion of atrial fibrillation or atrial flutter to sinus rhythm, or for the maintenance of sinus rhythm in highly symptomatic atrial fibrillation or flutter patients. Dofetilide may also cause torsades de pointes.

Class IV Drugs *Calcium Channel Blockers*

Class IV drugs are called calcium channel blockers. There are many calcium channel blockers on the market currently, but the majority are used to treat hypertension or angina pectoris. The only two of interest in terms of arrhythmia treatment are verapamil and diltiazen.

These two drugs inhibit the flow of calcium into cardiac cells, thereby decreasing conduction through the AV node, slowing the ventricular response to rapid supraventricular rhythms. So, really, the calcium channel blockers do not usually normalize the arrhythmia at all, but limit the effect of these supraventricular rhythms on the ventricular rate. Sometimes they are used in combination with digoxin or a beta-blocker to further slow conduction through the AV node.

Class IV Drugs and Actions

Class	Actions	Drugs: Generic name (Trade name)
IV	➤ Blocks calcium channels ➤ Decreases AV node conduction ➤ Increases P-R interval ➤ Decreases ventricular rate in atrial fibrillation	verapamil (Calan, Isoptin, Verelan) diltiazem (Cardizem, Dilacor XR)

Both diltiazem and verapamil are available in injection and oral dosage forms.

Intravenous **verapamil** can cause hypotension, AV block, bradycardia, and decreased cardiac output. It is contraindicated in patients with Wolff-Parkinson-White syndrome, sick sinus syndrome, AV block, hypotension, and severe heart failure.

Diltiazem may be the calcium channel blocker of choice for use in paroxysmal supraventricular tachycardia (PSVT) and atrial fibrillation since it causes less depression of cardiac "contractility" (cardiac muscle strength) than verapamil.

Important Antiarrhythmics without "Class"

Certain drugs, important in the treatment of dysrhythmias, are not included in the Vaughn-Williams classification scheme:

Atropine blocks acetylcholine from binding onto the muscarinic receptors on the SA and AV nodes. **Atropine increases the heart rate and improves AV conduction**. These effects are useful for the treatment of first degree AV block, Mobitz type I AV block, in some patients with bradyasystolic cardiac arrest, and in sinus bradycardia with associated symptoms of hypotension, confusion, or junctional escape rhythms.

Caution must be used when atropine is administered to patients with acute myocardial infarction or severe angina pectoris. This is because an increase in heart rate may increase the oxygen requirements of cardiac muscle, and ischemia or an extended area of infarction may result.

Adenosine (Adenocard) is administered by injection to terminate **paroxysmal supraventricular tachycardia** (PSVT), including PSVT caused by the Wolff-Parkinson-White syndrome. It has a shockingly short half-life of only **5 seconds**! It induces a profound block at the AV node, and a period of asystole is common when adenosine is used. Shortness of breath, flushing, chest pain, and transient arrhythmias may also occur.

Digoxin is a drug commonly used for treating congestive heart failure. Digoxin increases the force of cardiac muscle contraction and works by inhibiting the "pump" on cardiac cells that keeps potassium in and sodium out.

Further, digoxin slows conduction in the AV node, thereby decreasing the ventricular rate, an action which makes it a useful therapy for rapid supraventricular dysrhythmias. Lowering the ventricular rate provides the ventricles more filling time, thus improving pump efficiency. (Remember the flushing toilet example on page 61)

Therapeutic serum concentrations of digoxin produce characteristic EKG changes: prolonged P-R intervals, flattened T waves, S-T segment depression, and a shortened Q-T interval. The hallmark of digoxin effect is ST segment changes.

Digoxin produces a gradual downward sloping of the ST segment. This downward sloping of the ST segment may resemble a check mark as seen above or, may slope more gradually with a symmetrical appearance (scooped) . . . more or less like the hull of a boat, as evidenced below.

That's precisely why EKG interpretation is so difficult! Your *best bet* is to describe the appearance of the ST segment. It is much easier to determine ST segment appearance when viewing a lead that has no demonstrable S wave!

Digoxin induced ST depression is most usually seen in leads that have the *tallest* R waves . . . and this effect is characteristic of therapeutic digoxin usage. When characteristic ST segment changes are observed in *most* leads (including leads without tall R waves), digitalis toxicity should be suspected. Digoxin is eliminated slowly; and the margin between an effective dosage and a toxic dosage is narrow.

Following are *some* of the conditions that **predispose** the patient to *digitalis toxicity.*

➤ advanced age

➤ renal (kidney) impairment

➤ elevated serum Ca^{++}

➤ liver impairment

➤ acute hypoxia

➤ cor pulmonale

➤ hypothyroidism

➤ low serum K^+ (*adequate potassium serves to buffer the irritating effects of digitalis*)

➤ recent myocardial infarction

It takes approximately twice as much digoxin to produce toxicity when the serum K^+ is 5.0 mEq./L. compared to 3.0 mEq./L.!!

There are several non-EKG manifestations of digoxin toxicity, such as *anorexia, nausea, vomiting, diarrhea, lethargy, confusion, tinnitus* (ringing in the ears) and *distortion in yellow-green color perception* . . . though a patient may exhibit none of these symptoms.

It is rumored that Vincent Van Gogh (the painter) had a heart condition. As was typical for the times (late 1800's), he took digitalis leaf for that condition. It is thought that he became digitalis toxic, which might explain his erratic behavior, his use of yellow-greens in his paintings, and why he cut off his ear! Anyway . . . that's the story!

Digoxin in excessive amounts retards AV conduction and can produce the various forms of heart block—sinus block, first degree AV block, second degree AV block, blocked P.A.C.s, paroxysmal atrial tachycardia with block . . . etc. Ironically, a variety of ectopic rhythms result from digoxin toxicity, as well.

The *most common* dysrhythmias seen as a result of digitalis toxicity include

> P.C.V.s
> Multifocal P.C.V.s
> Bigeminy P.C.V.s
> Ventricular tachycardia
>
> (WARNING)

Unfortunately, digoxin-induced ventricular dysrhythmias are rarely responsive to antiarrhythmic drugs. Typical therapy involves correcting electrolyte imbalances and supporting the patient. Magnesium, in particular, may counter ventricular dysrhythmias. In severe cases of toxicity, Digiband or dilantin may be administered. (Dilantin, a Class IB drug, depresses ectopic activity in the atria, AV junction and ventricles and shortens ventricular repolarization time. Digibind is an antidote made from sheep antibodies.)

Magnesium. Though not classified as an antiarrhythmic drug, magnesium has antiarrhythmic effects, exhibiting calcium channel blocking properties. Magnesium slows cardiac conduction and increases cardiac refractoriness. It is used for the treatment of torsades de pointes (refer to page 126) and for resistant ventricular tachycardia and ventricular fibrillation associated with hypomagnesmic states. Magnesium is also utilized as an antiarrhythmic agent for severe ventricular dysrhythmias associated with digoxin toxicity. Current studies are investigating the efficacy of magnesium in controlling rapid ventricular rates precipitated by atrial and supraventricular tachyarrhythmias.

A low magnesium level (hypomagnesemia) causes an increase in the QTc interval (see page 264 for a quick review). A prolonged QTc interval predisposes the patient to ventricular dysrhythmias. Often times, hypomagnesemia is found in association with hypokalemia.

Practice Exercise 4 *Class Act Practice* ☆

A. Antiarrhythmic drugs are classified in accord with their _____

and _____.

B. Class I antiarrhythmic drugs are infrequently prescribed owing to their
_____ effect.

C. Class II antiarrhythmics are called _____ blockers. Class II drugs are frequently
administered to control _____.

D. Calcium channel blockers, Class IV drugs, inhibit the flow of calcium into the cardiac cells and
function by _____

_____

_____

_____.

E. Digoxin works by _____

_____

_____

_____

F. Draw a cardiac cycle (PQRST) demonstrating digitalis effect.

G. Though not an antiarrhythmic drug, magnesium has antiarrhythmic properties. Magnesium acts by
_____ cardiac conduction and _____ cardiac refractoriness.

✔ For **Feedback 4**, refer to page 387.

Input Section 14.5: Treatment of Specific Rhythm Disorders

Atrial Fibrillation and Atrial Flutter

Atrial fibrillation is one of the most frequently encountered dysrhythmias; its occurrence increases with patient age. Atrial fibrillation can decrease cardiac output through loss of the "atrial kick" which assists in left ventricular filling. Long term atrial fibrillation can lead to formation of blood clots in the atrium because blood flow through it is "turbulent" (i.e. not smooth). These clots can embolize and result in strokes. Conversion of longstanding atrial fibrillation to normal sinus rhythm (by cardioversion or drugs) can result in ejection of emboli from the atrium into the circulation, also leading to strokes. Therefore, any attempted conversion of long term atrial fibrillation to normal sinus rhythm should be preceded by anticoagulation for 3 weeks. If atrial fibrillation has been present for 48 hours or less, anticoagulation may not be needed.

The treatment of atrial fibrillation is designed to either

1. Attempt conversion to normal sinus rhythm, or
2. Control the elevated ventricular rate associated with atrial fibrillation.

Conversion to normal sinus rhythm is more likely to be successful if the atrial fibrillation is less than 12 month's duration and there is no enlargement of the left atrium. DC cardioversion is the method of choice to attempt conversion of atrial fibrillation to normal sinus rhythm. If cardioversion is undesireable, drugs used for conversion to normal sinus rhythm include amiodarone, procainamide, ibutilide, and others. Importantly, the AFFIRM substudy (J. American College of Cardiology, 2003:42) concluded that amiodarone is more effective at maintaining sinus rhythm and preventing the recurrance of atrial fibrillation when compared to sotalol or class I antiarrhythmic drugs.

If conversion is not likely or not successful, ventricular rate control is the goal of drug treatment. Medications which reduce conduction of impulses at the AV node are selected, such as a calcium channel blocker (diltiazem or verapamil), a beta blocker (such as metoprolol or atenolol), or digoxin.

Rate controlled atrial fibrillation.

Ventricular Ectopy: PVCs

Clinical trials continue to challenge ideas regarding drug therapy for PVCs. The most visible study was the Cardiac Arrhythmia Suppression Trial (abbreviated CAST). The CAST studied patients who had arrhythmias (ventricular ectopy) following acute myocardial infarction. Some patients received drug therapy (encainide, flecainide, or moricizine), while others received a placebo.

The study found that the mortality, or death rate, was higher in the patient groups receiving drug therapy than in the placebo group! The findings were surprising since drug treatment did suppress ventricular ectopy. However, successful arrythmia treatment did not improve mortality. It was felt that deaths were attributable to drug-induced worsening of the arrhythmias, called a **proarrhythmic effect**.

Beta blockers, however, have been shown to reduce mortality when administered following an acute myocardial infarction, even if P.V.C.s are not a significant problem. Therefore, many patients are given beta-blockers immediately following a myocardial infarction for periods of months or even years. Some patients have conditions which contraindicate the use of beta-blockers, however. Respiratory disease or congestive heart failure are common contraindications to beta-blocker administration.

More recently, class III drugs (amiodarone and sotalol) have been administered to control ventricular ectopy. PVCs occurring *during* acute myocardial infarction are preferentially treated with amiodarone (though lidocaine and procainamide remain acceptable alternatives) to prevent lethal ventricular dysrhythmias.

Sustained Ventricular Tachycardia

The treatment for sustained unifocal or monomorphic ventricular tachycardia is dependent upon the degree of hemodynamic compromise. When associated with hypotension, congestive heart failure, unconsciousness or pulselessness, ventricular tachycardia is considered *unstable*. Unstable VT may quickly degenerate into ventricular fibrillation. Thus, DC cardioversion is immediately indicated. Pulselessness requires CPR support.

A patient's tolerance of the dysrhythmia is referred to as *stable* ventricular tachycardia. Tolerance implies that neither cardiac output nor blood pressure are significantly impaired. In this situation, treatment options will be considered in light of underlying pathology or abnormalities. Consideration will be given to any or all of the following factors: (1) the baseline QTc interval, a measure of the total time for ventricular depolarization and repolarization, corrected for heart rate (refer to page 264); the presence of acute injury; compromised cardiac output (ejection fraction < 40%); the presence of CHF; the presence of pulmonary pathology and so forth.

Sotalol or procainamide are the preferred drugs for treating a stable ventricular tachycardia when cardiac function is unimpaired. In the presence of compromised cardiac functioning, amiodarone or lidocaine are the recommended drug treatment options, though amiodarone is contraindicated for patients with baseline QTc prolongation.

Polymorphic ventricular tachycardias are treated with beta-blockers, lidocaine, amiodarone, procainamide or sotalol. In the presence of a prolonged baseline QT interval or torsades de pointes, the correction of electrolyte imbalances (particularly hypokalemia and hypomagnesemia) is often the first order of treatment (refer to page 126 for a quick review). As noted earlier, magnesium exhibits calcium channel blocking properties, slowing cardiac conduction and increasing cardiac refractoriness. Other drug interventions may include lidocaine, isoproterenol or phenytoin. When unresponsive to drug therapy, certain patients may require overdrive pacing to correct the dysrhythmia.

IMPORTANT NOTE: It is a patient's clinical presentation that determines the sequence of therapeutic interventions; it is the patient's clinical history that drives drug selection. On the monitor, a ventricular tachycardia is a ventricular tachycardia. The patient's response to that dysrhythmia determines whether the dysrhythmia is termed stable or unstable ventricular tachycardia!

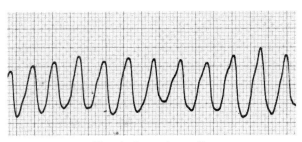

Ventricular tachycardia

Ventricular Fibrillation and Pulseless Ventricular Tachycardia

Immediate CPR and *prompt* defibrillation are the first order interventions for ventricular fibrillation and pulseless ventricular tachycardia. (Many treatment protocols specify similar treatments for ventricular fibrillation.) Drug therapy plays a secondary role, being much less important than the proper administration of CPR and electrical defibrillation. The time necessary to prepare and administer drugs with questionable efficacy delays the proven lifesaving treatments of CPR and defibrillation.

If initial defibrillation attempts are unsuccessful, epinephrine or vasopressin is commonly administered to stimulate ventricular activity that may respond to further electrical defibrillation attempts. If successive defibrillation attempts are then unsuccessful, antiarrhythmics such as amiodarone, lidocaine or procainamide may be administered. When hypomagnesemia is suspected, magnesium will be administered.

NOTE: The preferred treatments for severe dysrhythmias requiring emergency treatment (sustained ventricular tachycardia, ventricular fibrillation, PSVT, symptomatic bradycardia, etc.) are outlined in the current *Standards and Guidelines for Cardiopulmonary Resuscitation and Emergency Cardiac Care* published by the American Heart Association. These guidelines are presented in algorithm fashion to guide therapeutic decision making and patient management.

Practice Exercise 5

A. The primary objective for treating atrial fibrillation is to _____

_____.

B. P.V.Cs occurring during acute myocardial infarction are preferentially treated with _____, a class _____ drug, to prevent lethal ventricular dysrhythmias.

C. _____ have been shown to decrease mortality in the post-myocardial infarction period.

✔ For **Feedback 5**, refer to page 387.

Input Section 14.6: Platelet Inhibitor and Thrombolytic Drug Treatment for Acute Myocardial Infarction

Developments continue in the treatment of acute myocardial infarction (AMI). The introduction of GPIIb/IIIa inhibitors offered treatment options beyond the arsenol of thrombolitic agents.

To understand the role of these agents, the pathophysiology of an acute myocardial infarction must be understood. The genesis of acute myocardial infarction (AMI) is usually atherosclerotic disease in the coronary arteries. In atherosclerosis, plaques of fatty-like material adhere to the inside walls of coronary arteries. Accumulation of plaque limits the amount of blood that can flow through the artery. Reduction in blood flow can result in angina pectoris, heart failure, and arrhythmias.

When plaques tear or damage the smooth inner lining of a coronary artery, proteins are exposed which activate the blood clotting sequence at the site of the injury. Blood clotting involves a series of clotting factors, which are enzymes, acting together to make a fibrin plug. Fibrin is a protein which is made of smaller building blocks called fibrinogen. Thrombin, a clotting enzyme, takes the fibrinogen pieces and assembles them into fibrin.

Usually, fibrin's *job* is to *plug up* sites of bleeding in the circulatory system. However, a fibrin plug in a coronary artery can obstruct or severely minimize vital blood flow. Changes in platelet function contribute to this occlusive process. Damage to the inner lining of the coronary artery exposes platelets to proteins which bind to receptors causing a clumping of platelets at the injury site. So a coronary thrombus is made up of a fibrin mesh, thrombin and platelets. The resulting lack of blood supply to the cardiac muscle results in ischemia, damage, and, if prolonged, death (necrosis) of cardiac muscle. Because necrosis occurs progressively, damaged cardiac muscle can be *saved* if blood flow can soon be restored in a timely manner.

Mechanism of Action–Thrombolytic Agents

The body has a naturally occurring enzyme, plasmin, which digests fibrin. Plasmin comes from the activation of plasminogen. Thrombolytic drugs act by converting plasminogen to plasmin. The plasmin subsequently *digests* fibrin in the clot occluding the coronary artery.

When the clot is dissolved soon enough, the subsequent restoration of blood flow limits further heart muscle damage. The opening of a previously clotted artery is called **reperfusion**.

The timely reperfusion of an occluded coronary artery results in improved cardiac function and survival. Signs that reperfusion has occured include relief of chest pain, reduction of ST segment elevation, and the onset of arrhythmias called *reperfusion arrhythmias*. Though these arrhythmias may require treatment, they signal restored perfusion. ("Good" arrhythmias!)

Thrombolytic Agents	
Generic Name	**Trade Name**
streptokinase	Kabikinase, Streptase
alteplase (TPA)	Activase
anistreplase	Eminase
retaplase	rpa
tenecteplase	TNKase

Thrombolytic agents should be administered as soon as possible following the identification of acute myocardial infarction (clinical symptoms and ST elevation) in order to save the greatest amount of heart muscle. Little benefit is anticipated if treatment is initiated 12 or more hours following the onset of pain.

Thrombolytic drugs not only dissolve "bad" clots in coronary arteries, but also dissolve "good" clots plugging areas of bleeding anywhere in the body. Thus, the major side effect associated with thrombolytic agent administration is bleeding from any site of injury. There is also a paradoxical effect in that thrombolytics activate platelet aggregation or clumping.

Bleeding can range from a minor problem (a little oozing from cuts or IV sites) to serious, life-threatening intracranial bleeding. Therefore, patients must be *carefully* screened for conditions that predispose the patient to bleeding. Thrombolytic drugs *should be avoided* in patients with a history of recent surgery, childbirth, or trauma. Pregnancy, uncontrolled severe hypertension, recent stroke, and coagulation abnormalities are also contraindications for the use of thrombolytic drugs.

Patency, secondary to thrombolytic drug administration is restored in approximately 60–80 percent of the time, though full myocardial perfusion occurs slightly more than 50 percent of the time. Heparin (an anticoagulant) is commonly administered for several days following successful thrombolytic treatment to prevent *reocclusion*, or a repeat thrombus formation in the same artery. Recent combinations of thrombolytic agents with GPIIb/IIIa inhibitors accelerate reperfusion time and decrease the risk of reocclusion.

Thrombolytic drugs differ from one another in terms of source of drug, allergenicity, dosage, administration, duration of thrombolytic effect, cost . . . and here's the controversial part . . . efficacy and toxicity. TPA is a human protein and is therefore *less likely* to produce allergic reactions than streptokinase or anistreplase, which are produced by streptococcal bacteria. The "GUSTO" trials found TPA to be more effective than streptokinase in reperfusing coronary arteries in acute myocardial infarction.

Thrombolytic agents are usually administered intravenously, though they can be administered directly into the coronary artery during a cardiac catheterization procedure.

Mechanism of Action–GPIIb/IIIa Inhibitors

Platelet Inhibitors are a special class of drugs that interfere with platelet aggregation. Common aspirin (ASA) is a weak platelet inhibitor. A subset classification of platelet inhibitors is **GPIIb/IIIa Inhibitors**. Currently used GPIIb/IIIa agents are tabled below.

Platelet Inhibitor Agents

Generic Name	Trade Name
• aspirin	Bayer
• clopidrogel	Plavix

GPIIb/IIIa Inhibitor Agents

Generic Name	Trade Name
• abciximab	Reopro
• tirofiban	Aggrastat
• eptifibitide	Integrilin

As introduced previously, damage to the inner lining of a coronary artery (plaque rupture) exposes platelets to proteins which activate the glyoprotein (GP) IIb/IIIa receptors causing platelet aggregation or *clumping* (known as "white clots"). This clumping can further occlude a compromised vessel. More specifically, platelets are activated by several agonists which result in the activation of fibrinogen receptors on the platelet surface known as GPIIb/IIIa *receptors*.

These GPIIb/IIIa *receptors* then bind to fibrinogen, VonWillebrand factor and maybe other proteins, forming a web that includes other platelets. This process produces a clot which can further occlude a compromised vessel.

A group of antiplatelet drugs, GPIIb/IIIa receptor *inhibitors* (noted above), were developed to bind with the GPIIb/IIIa receptors, thus preventing their binding with fibrinogen. In other words, the GPIIb/IIIa inhibitors prevent clot formation or clot extension. **They do not dissolve existing clots as do the thrombolytic drugs.**

There are currently three GPIIb/IIIa inhibitor agents in use.

- Reopro (abciximab), an antibody of human and mouse origin

- Aggrastat (tirofiban), a drug modeled after an anticoagulant substance found in the venom of the African saw-scaled viper

- Eptifibitide (Integrilin), a drug modeled after a snake venom from the Pygmy rattlesnake.

The GPIIb/IIIa inhibitor drugs are primarily indicated for the treatment of acute coronary syndromes (ACS), in those patients treated medically or those patients for whom percutaneous coronary intervention (PCI) is planned. They are especially used with PCIs because the stretching and trauma of the coronary artery wall and the placement of a foreign body (metal stent) makes for a very ***thrombogenic*** (clot forming) situation. Thus, the GPIIb/IIIa inhibitor drugs are used to decrease the incidence of clot formation associated with acute myocardial infarction and to reduce mortality associated with PCI procedures.

All three of the GPIIb/IIIa drugs are administered intravenously by ***loading dose*** or bolus, followed by a continuous intravenous infusion. The loading dose is designed to achieve an effective blood concentration for immediate effect. The continuous infusion maintains the effective blood concentration by replacing the drug that is eliminated through metabolism and excretion processes.

Following the conclusion of continuous intravenous therapy, the duration of IIb/IIIa inhibitor drug action varies. The approximate times for platelet function to return to normal are listed below.

Abciximab: 24–48 hours
Eptifibitide: 4–6 hours
Tirofiban: 4–8 hours

The following notes are included for information purposes.

Notes

1. If a PCI procedure fails and emergency surgery is warranted, the patient having received the IIb/IIIa inhibitor abciximab will probably present a higher risk for bleeding problems because of its longer duration of action.

2. There may be differences in efficacy among the three drugs in this class. It has yet to be determined whether the differences are due to the intrinsic properties of the drugs or differing levels of knowledge regarding administration (dosing, timing in relation to a patient's condition, duration of action, etc.). Clinical studies are ongoing.

3. Earlier clinical trials (GUSTO-5 and ASSENT-3) supported the combined use (with certain risk and age advisories) of a GPIIb/IIIa inhibitor (such as Reopro) and a thrombolytic agent (such as Activase) to accelerate reperfusion time and diminish the risk of reocclusion.

4. GPIIb/IIIa inhibitor agents have contraindications similar to those of thrombolytic agents.

5. Because both thrombolytics and GPIIb/IIIa inhibitors have differing dosing and mixture requirements, it is important to consider the situation and location. For instance, a patient presenting in a more rural facility may be treated with a single dose, longer duration thrombolytic agent in anticipation of transfer to a cardiac center. Conversely, a symptomatic patient (ST elevation) presenting in a *high-tech* facility may be treated with a short acting GPIIb/IIIa inhibitor such as Reopro, then sent directly to a cardiac catheterization lab for study.

☆ ***Remember,*** the treatment for acute coronary syndromes is forever evolving.

How about some practice?!

Practice Exercise 6

A. Thrombolytic drugs are proteins that act by _____

_____

_____.

B. GPIIb/IIIa inhibitors work by _____

_____

_____.

C. A reperfusion arrhythmia is _____

_____

_____.

✔ For **Feedback 6**, refer to page 388.

Input Section 14.7: The Use of Drug-Eluting Stents in Percutaneous Coronary Interventions

Coronary artery disease, the cause of angina pectoris and myocardial infarctions, is characterized by the buildup of fatty plaques within the lumen of the artery. These plaques restrict blood flow to the myocardium and can rupture, setting off clot formation and total occlusion of the artery.

Many strategies have been developed to reverse, bypass, or reopen coronary arteries affected by this process. Coronary artery bypass surgery uses vessels harvested from elsewhere in the body (usually leg vessels) to route blood around the area of the blockage. Lipid-lowering medications are being researched for the possibility of reducing plaque formation.

Percutaneous Coronary Interventions (PCI's) are procedures involving the use of a catheter routed to the problem artery, usually threaded through the skin (that's where the "percutaneous" comes from ☺), through an artery in the groin or arm, and into the coronary vessel.

These interventions can take different forms. Balloon angioplasty is a technique in which an inflatable balloon is placed in the narrowed artery and inflated for a short period of time. This stretches the artery open, permitting improved blood flow. Another option is atherectomy, a procedure for removing plaque via a specialized catheter procedure.

Stent placement is an improvement on simple balloon angioplasty. A stent is a wire mesh tube which is routed to the narrowed area of the coronary artery, in collapsed form around a deflated angioplasty balloon. When in position, the balloon is inflated, expanding the stent to an open position, thus improving blood flow. The stent holds the artery open more successfully than the balloon angioplasty procedure alone. Over time, the lining of the coronary artery grows a coating of cells and other material over the stent, making the inside of the artery again *look normal* to the blood flowing through it.

The problem with both balloon angioplasty and stent placement is the risk of restenosis (re-closure) of the vessel after a period of time. This restenosis can happen quickly after the procedure as a result of clot formation, or can occur slowly over months of time as a result of **neointimal proliferation**. Neointimal proliferation is a result of cell growth, arterial smooth muscle proliferation and migration, and remodeling of extracellular material. Restenosis occurs about 35–45% of the time with balloon angioplasty, and about 25% of the time with stenting.

Researchers have incorporated different medications into various coatings applied to the metallic stents in an effort to stop neointimal proliferation. A variety of medications have been tried, but as of this publication, the most successful are sirolimus (CYPHER drug eluting stent made by Johnson & Johnson/Cordis) and paclitaxel (TAXUS Express2 Paclitaxel-Eluting Coronary Stent System, made by Boston Scientific). Both drugs slow the growth of vascular smooth muscle, reducing the restenosis problem by half or more. Expect more research and innovation in the development of improved drug-eluting stents!

There is no practice exercise associated with this section!

✔ Feedback 1
Great Work!
What is your retention half life?!

A. Cardiac cells may interact with or respond to different types of drugs because <u>cardiac cells have many different receptor types on the cell surfaces</u>.

B. Antiarrhythmic drugs work by affecting one or more of the following cardiac tissue properties:

1. <u>automaticity</u>.

2. <u>rate of impulse conduction</u>.

3. <u>duration of refractory period</u>.

C. Drug absorption depends on the <u>route of administration</u>.

D. The intravenous route of drug administration produces "near-immediate" effects because one of the following processes is bypassed. Check the omitted process.

☒ Absorption

E. A continuous infusion of lidocaine is necessary to maintain an effective blood concentration because <u>lower perfusion tissues remove lidocaine from circulation. The drug distribution steals lidocaine away from its intended site of action</u>.

F. The <u>liver</u> is the primary location for drug metabolism.

G. Drug "half-life" refers to <u>the time required to reduce (by metabolism or excretion) the amount of drug in the body by one half</u>.

✔ Feedback 2

A. The SA node is the heart's normal pacemaker since it has the most rapid rate of spontaneous <u>depolarization</u>.

B. A proarrhythmic effect means <u>that an arrhythmia may worsen or a new arrhythmia may appear secondary to antiarrhythmic drug therapy</u>.

✔ Feedback 4
"Best One in Your Row" Distinction!

A. Antiarrhythmic drugs are classified in accord with their <u>mechanism of action</u> and <u>EKG effects</u>.

B. Class I antiarrhythmic drugs are infrequently prescribed owing to their <u>proarrhythmic</u> effect.

C. Class II antiarrhythmics are called <u>beta</u>-blockers. Class II drugs are frequently administered to control <u>supraventricular tachyarrhythmias</u>.

D. Calcium channel blockers, Class IV drugs, inhibit the flow of calcium into the cardiac cells and function by <u>decreasing conduction through the AV node (thereby slowing supraventricular rhythms)</u>.

E. Digoxin works by <u>increasing the force of muscle contraction and by slowing conduction in the AV node</u>.

F.

Scooped ST segment demonstrating digitalis effect

G. Magnesium acts by <u>slowing</u> cardiac conduction and <u>increasing</u> cardiac refractoriness.

✔ Feedback 5

A. The primary objective for treating atrial fibrillation is to <u>reduce the rapid ventricular rate. (If you need a quick review of atrial fibrillation, turn to page 73)</u>.

B. P.V.C.s occurring during acute myocardial infarction are treated with <u>amiodarone</u>, a class <u>III</u> drug, to prevent <u>ventricular fibrillation</u>.

C. <u>Beta blockers</u> have been shown to decrease mortality in the post-myocardial infarction period.

✔ **Feedback 6**

A. Thrombolytic drugs are proteins that act by <u>converting plasminogen to plasmin, which subsequently digests the clot occluding the coronary artery</u>.

B. GPIIb/IIIa inhibitors work by <u>interfering with, or inhibiting the binding of fibrinogen to the platelet receptor. This prevents the platelets from clumping</u>.

C. A reperfusion arrhythmia is a <u>dysrhythmia that presents secondary to restored coronary artery perfusion. Though reperfusion arrhythmias may require treatment, they are GOOD NEWS!</u>

Phabulous
Pharmacology,
Phrankly!

Before moving ahead to Section 15, begin to . . . .

Notes

Notes

Kidstuff

Objectives

When you have completed Section 15, you will be able to describe or identify

1. cardiac variants in children
2. normal heart rate norms for children
3. normal duration of P, P-R, QRS, and QT intervals
4. recognition of the following cardiac dysrhythmias in kids:

> sinus arrhythmia
> sinus bradycardia
> sinus tachycardia
> sinus arrest/sinus block
> sick sinus syndrome
> atrial tachycardia
> P.A.C.s
> atrial flutter
> atrial fibrillation
> wandering atrial pacemaker
> junctional escape rhythms
> premature junctional beats
> junctional tachycardia

> P.S.V.T.
> P.V.C.s
> ventricular tachycardia
> ventricular flutter
> ventricular fibrillation
> P.E.A.
> long QT syndrome
> W.P.W. syndrome
> first degree heart block
> second degree heart block
> third degree heart block
> bundle branch blocks

5. drug and electrolyte manifestations

Contributions by:
Jane D. Werth, M.S., R.N.

391

Back in the days of Michelangelo, painters frequently painted children as little adults—same body shape, same body proportions, and the same skin tone. It didn't work then and it doesn't work now. . . .

. . . *children are not just adults in miniature.* They have different health care problems and different body function norms . . . so follows the reason for this section. It is important to understand both the similarities and differences between adult and pediatric electrocardiography.

Birth through 18 years of age covers a wide time span! However, for the sake of simplicity we will use the term *pediatrics* to cover this age span in most references. The term *newborn* applies to babies 0–1 month of age, and the term *infant* applies to infants 1 month–one year.

So bearing that in mind, let's start! . . . Just one more thing. . . .

. . . you may find it helpful to read the corresponding "adult" version as you ponder pediatric dysrhythmias

. . . that's why the rest of this book is attached!

The stable EKG pattern seen in the normal adult does not completely develop in the child until around the age of ten. Most changes that do occur in pediatric EKGs are due to a shift from right ventricular dominance (seen in the newborn) to left ventricular dominance (seen in the adult).

At birth, the right ventricle is thicker than the left side counterpart. During the first month of life, there is a dramatic decrease in right ventricular pressure and a subsequent decrease in right ventricular wall thickness. It is also probably important to note that the size of the infant heart is large in comparison to the size of the thoracic cavity.

In many instances, dysrhythmias in children differ in *cause* and *frequency* from adults. For instance, ventricular dysrhythmias are seen less frequently in children owing to the absence of atherosclerotic heart disease. More commonly seen in children are the EKG dysrhythmias and abnormalities which occur secondary to structural problems in the heart. Now, just take a minute and remember atrial septal defects . . . tetralogy of Fallot . . . and patent ductus arteriosus (you may have studied those in Anatomy 101). Basically, many congenital heart

defects, like those named above, create artificial openings in heart chambers that can greatly increase chamber pressure gradients. These pressure increases can cause chamber **hypertrophy.** Since congenital heart defects occur in approximately eight to ten of every 1,000 newborns, hypertrophy induced EKG changes are very common.

Let's look at *atrial hypertrophy* for a moment. As you will recall, the P wave represents atrial depolarization. The P wave then reflects depolarization of both the right and left atria. In reality, the P wave can be divided into two components.

Right Atrial Component ↘   P   ↙ Left Atrial Component

(Remember, leads II, III, and aVF display the most prominent P waves.) In the presence of atrial hypertrophy, one observes an increase in the *amplitude* or the *duration* of the P wave.

Looking at atrial depolarization in lead II, right atrial hypertrophy is reflected as a prominent (often pointed) P with increased amplitude (greater than 3 mm). Lead V_1 is included here for comparison purposes.

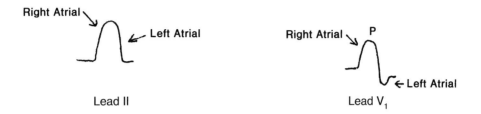

Left atrial hypertrophy may present either as a prolonged or a notched P wave.

When both right and left atrial hypertrophy are present, the P wave may reflect a combination of the above patterns.

Leading Statements

You will recall that leads view electrical activity from different perspectives or angles. Since ventricular dysrhythmias are less common in children, usually "kids" are monitored on leads which best reflect atrial activity. Commonly then, children will be monitored on leads II, III, and aVF. Generally speaking, the differences observed in normal or healthy adult and pediatric EKG tracings have to do with variations in the ventricular wall thickness and the position and orientation of the heart, itself.

Input Section 15.1: General Rules and Concepts

There are a few general rules and concepts that aide the understanding and identification of pediatric EKGs and rhythm anomalies. As one would suspect, the age of the infant is a critical factor in any rhythm analysis.

Heart rate norms vary in children from year to year (and sometimes month to month). Though the norms presented on page 394 are approximations, most authorities generally agree with these parameters.

Pediatric Heart Rate Norms		
Age	**Range**	**Average Rate**
0–1 month	90–200	160
2–3 months	90–200	150
4–12 months	100–180	140
1–3 yrs.	80–180	130
4–5 yrs.	70–150	100
6–8 yrs.	68–140	100
9–11 yrs.	60–120	88
12–16 yrs.	60–125	80
> 16 yrs.	60–90	75

As demonstrated above, there is a tremendous variation in the age-related norms. However, as a general rule . . .

Rule #1   As age ↑ heart rate ↓

In the absence of a rate guide, a *field* estimate of an age-specific heart rate is often determined by the following formula:

HEART RATE = 150 minus (5 × age in years)

In any case, *heart rate must be evaluated in relation to the age of the child and the underlying clinical condition.* Heart rate increases may be related to crying, agitation, fear, pain, fever, etc. In fact, the heart rate may increase eight to ten beats per minute for each Fahrenheit degree increase in temperature. (*Remember that?*) Decreases in heart rate may be related to sleep, increased vagal tone, abdominal distention, increased intracranial pressure, apnea, and a variety of *other* factors.

Another general rule that can be applied to pediatrics is . . .

Rule #2   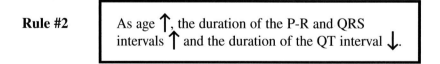 As age ↑, the duration of the P-R and QRS intervals ↑ and the duration of the QT interval ↓.

So . . . let's explore each of those intervals separately. In fact, let's explore all the wave forms!

The P Wave

You will recall that the P wave represents atrial excitation spreading from the SA node through the right and left atria. Normally the duration of the P wave is 0.06 ± 0.02 seconds in children.

Remember each small EKG paper square represents 0.04 seconds!

.06 ± .02

The maximum P wave duration is 0.10 seconds in children and 0.08 seconds in infants. A prolonged P wave may be due to atrial hypertrophy as was discussed on page 393.

The P-R Interval

You will remember that atrial activation and atrial repolarization are represented on the EKG as a P wave followed by a straight line, the P-R interval.

P-R interval

The P-R interval further represents the time for the impulse to pass from the SA node through the AV junction, through the ventricles to the Purkinje fibers. Like the duration of the P wave, the duration of the P-R interval tends to vary with age.

Pediatric P-R Intervals

Age	Duration of P-R Interval
0–4 months	0.08–0.12 seconds
4–12 months	0.08–0.13 seconds
1–3 years	0.09–0.14 seconds
4–5 years	0.10–0.16 seconds
6–8 years	0.10–0.17 seconds
9–16 years	0.10–0.18 seconds
> 16 years	0.12–0.20 seconds

A prolonged P-R interval represents increased conduction time and may be seen in conditions such as first degree heart block, myocarditis, excessive vagal stimulation or atrial septal defect. A shortened P-R interval may be seen in rhythms with accelerated conduction such as Wolff-Parkinson-White (W.P.W.) Syndrome.

QRS Duration

Remember, the duration of the QRS indicates the time elapsed during ventricular activation or depolarization. Normal pediatric QRS durations appear on the next page.

Kid's QRSs	
Age	**QRS Duration**
Premie	0.04 seconds
0–3 years	0.04–0.08 seconds
4–16 years	0.05–0.09 seconds
> 16 years	0.05–0.10 seconds

When the QRS is greater than the prescribed upper limit, i.e., ⌇⌄⋀⋁⌄⌇ a *ventricular conduction delay*

QRS

exists. This conduction delay may be caused by a number of factors including

➤ severe hyperkalemia

➤ quinidine toxicity

➤ procainamide toxicity

➤ bundle branch block

QT Interval

The QT interval represents the time for both ventricular depolarization and repolarization to occur. It is measured from the beginning of the Q wave to the end of the T wave. Just like the adult, the QT interval varies with heart rate and a variety of other factors. In the infant, however, the *QT interval principally varies with age!* In infants (less than 6 months), the maximum QT interval is 0.45 seconds. In children, the maximum QT interval is 0.44 seconds. As a comparison, the maximum QT interval for adults and adolescents is 0.425 seconds.

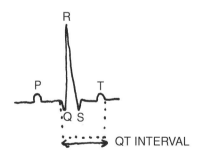

Though QT intervals may not be routinely measured, it is worthwhile noting that QT interval *prolongation* is associated with hypokalemia, hypocalcemia, myocarditis, and the administration of various antiarrhythmic drugs. The QT interval is also prolonged in long QT syndrome (LQTS), discussed on page 420. A *shortened* QT interval may be seen with hypercalemia and digitalis effect.

The ST Segment

The ST segment (straight line between the S and T wave) represents the early phase of ventricular repolarization. Similar to grown-ups, ST segment elevation may be associated with acute pericarditis (inflammation of enveloping membranes of heart) or acute myocardial infarct (a rarity). ST segment depression is principally associated with hypokalemia or digitalis effect.

As with adults, it is important to remember that EKGs are not diagnostic, only suggestive!

The T Wave

The T wave is the recovery phase (repolarization) following ventricular depolarization. Tall, peaked T waves may be seen in hyperkalemia and ventricular hypertrophy. Flat, low T waves may be seen in newborn infants as a normal phenomenon or associated with hypothyroidism, hypokalemia, pericarditis, myocarditis, or digitalis effect.

All these components come together for the *normal EKG lineup:*

➤ Rate—varies with age.

➤ Rhythm—regular.

➤ P waves—each QRS will be preceded by a P wave. All P waves will appear uniform.

➤ QRS—all QRS complexes will appear uniform in configuration.

➤ Conduction—each P will be followed by normal QRS.

➤ T wave—may be flipped (inverted) from birth to adolescence in the right precordial leads V_1, V_2.

➤ P-R interval and QRS duration normal for age

It is important to recognize that multiple subtle EKG pattern changes occur as an infant develops. Some of the major, early observed changes are now discussed.

Rule #3	Expect *subtle* EKG pattern changes.

Premie EKG (birth before 37 weeks gestation):

➤ Lower voltage QRS and T wave in limb leads (I, II, III).

➤ Shorter P-R, QRS, QT intervals.

Normal newborn EKG:

➤ Normal duration QRS in limb leads (this time you tell me . . . leads ____, ____, and ____).

➤ T wave in V_1 usually becomes flipped (inverted or negative) by third day and remains flipped until the age of five (this phenomenon occurs because of the changing nature of the developing heart)!

Before examining rhythm anomalies, let's review the steps you learned previously for analyzing EKGs—these steps are as appropriate for pediatric rhythms as they are for adult rhythms!

➤ Determine the heart rate using methods discussed on page 29

➤ Determine whether the rhythm is basically regular or irregular. Are there unexpected premature beats, pauses or dropped beats?

➤ Look at atrial activity (P waves). Is atrial depolarization occurring at an expected rate with a regular rhythm? Are the P waves so rapid that there are more atrial impulses than there are QRS complexes? Is it difficult to distinguish atrial activity?

➤ Observe ventricular activity. Are the QRSs of normal duration? Does a QRS following each P wave? Are the QRSs occurring regularly (consistent R-R interval)?

➤ Determine the relationship between atrial activity and ventricular activity. Is each P wave producing a QRS? Is the P-R constant?

Remember—*What's in a name?* A dysrhythmia by the *wrong* name may spell defeat! *It is more important to accurately describe what you observe than to apply a label.* (Unfortunately, people disagree over labels . . . actually, without labels, this is all very logical!)

Practice Exercise 1

A. The heart rate, the duration of P-R, QRS, and QT intervals all vary with _____.

Circle the correct answer in the following statements (B–E).

B. The heart rate increases/decreases with increasing age.

C. The P-R interval lengthens/shortens with increasing age.

D. The duration of the QRS is greater/lesser with increasing age.

E. The duration of the QT interval increases/decreases with increasing age.

F. Evaluate and describe this cardiac complex.

_____

_____

_____

✔ For **Feedback 1,** refer to page 433.

Input Section 15.2: Sinus Anomalies

Sinus rhythms are so called because they originate in the sinoatrial node. The SA node is the normal pacemaker of the heart because it has the fastest pacemaking capability or the *highest automaticity.* As with everything in pediatrics, the inherent rate of SA node discharge (thus the rate of conduction or heart rate in a normal heart) varies with age . . . so much for precision! Need a quick rate review? Please turn back to page 394.

Normal sinus rhythm in a normal newborn. The heart rate is 166 because the baby is crying!

Sinus Arrhythmia

The first dysrhythmia to be considered is *sinus arrhythmia*. Sinus arrhythmia is a slightly irregular rhythm that is initiated by the SA node. Usually the irregularity of the rhythm is related to respiration. The heart rate tends to increase with inspiration and decrease with expiration. Sinus arrhythmia is more pronounced in adolescence than in childhood.

A nonpathologic sinus arrhythmia. Note the irregular P-P interval.

Sinus arrhythmia is a variation of normal and can be differentiated from a truly abnormal arrhythmia by having the child hold his or her breath. In sinus arrhythmia, cessation of breathing will cause the heart rate to remain steady.

Let's look at sinus arrhythmia in detail.

➤ Rate—variable with age.

➤ Rhythm—irregular, but may be patterned when related to respiration

➤ P waves—
uniform in appearance
irregular P-P interval
precede each QRS complex

➤ P-R interval nonvarying.

➤ QRSs are all of normal configuration, but the R-R intervals are irregular.

Sinus arrhythmia is a common dysrhythmia that is usually a *variation of normal*. Though no treatment is required, one should be aware that it exists. Just for fun, measure the varying P-P and R-R intervals in this rhythm strip.

Normal newborn with sinus bradycardia and sinus arrhythmia secondary to maternal Inderal treatment for P.A.T.

Sinus Bradycardia

Bradycardia has a few drawbacks . . . remember bradycardia is a term used to describe a rate slower than the expected norm. Of course, the definition of bradycardia varies with age in pediatrics (and you're saying, "*What doesn't?*"). Generally speaking, *sinus bradycardia* is defined as a rate of less than 100 beats/minute in newborns and less than 70 beats/minute in children.

Getting back to the shortcomings of bradycardia . . . if sinus bradycardia develops gradually, compensatory cardiac changes (such as increased stroke volume and chamber dilation) may prevent a fall in cardiac output (*stable sinus bradycardia*). That's good! Unfortunately, if the bradycardia comes on more suddenly, the heart is less likely to compensate and cardiac output will be compromised (*unstable sinus bradycardia*).

So, keeping that in mind, let's look at *sinus bradycardia* in greater detail.

Sinus bradycardia with a heart rate of 62 per minute. This rhythm strip belongs to an eight year old girl.
Notice that the P-R interval approaches the upper limit of normal.

Criteria for *sinus bradycardia*

➤ Rate—less than 100 in newborns; less than 70 in children.

➤ Rhythm—regular.

➤ P waves precede each QRS; the P-R interval is constant; the P-P interval is regular.

➤ QRSs are all of normal configuration; the R-R interval is regular.

Some of the more common causes of sinus bradycardia include:

➤ hypoxia

➤ apnea in the healthy premature infant

➤ increased vagal tone (due to increased intracranial pressure, hypertension, abdominal distention, etc.)

➤ adolescent athletes (normal rhythm of *pint-size champions*)

➤ hypoglycemia

➤ following open heart surgery

Though rare, sinus bradycardia may be associated with sick-sinus syndrome, AV block or other congenital heart disease (primary disorder). In these instances, Atropine (0.02 mg/kg) may be the first line of treatment to augment the heart rate followed by the insertion of a pacemaker. Remember, atropine causes urinary retention!

Commonly, however, sinus bradycardia is a **secondary event** resulting from hypoxia. **Hypoxia suppresses the automaticity of the sinus node,** thus decreasing the rate of sinus impulse formation. If untreated, the hypoxia may result in hypotension and acidosis which, in turn, decreases cardiac contractility. A negative spiraling then ensues with the decrease in cardiac contractility causing further hypotension, hypoxia and bradycardia. Correcting the hypoxia and acidosis is critical. Epinephrine 0.01 mg/kg (1:10,000 solution) is the drug of choice for augmenting both the heart rate and myocardial contractility owing to its alpha- and beta-receptor stimulation.

Transcutaneous pacing may be used to treat symptomatic bradycardias unresponsive (refractory) to drug therapy.

In summary, *sinus bradycardia* is treated when there is evidence of decreased cardiac output (decreased responsiveness, lethargy, loss of consciousness, cyanosis). The underlying cause, however, should always be investigated and treated as necessary.

It is important to consider that an exaggerated slow heart rate may allow escape beats or escape rhythms to be initiated from a lower, more distal pacemaker. Commonly, one would see the escape beats originating from the AV junctional tissue. You will recall that escape beats are inscribed late, following the next anticipated normal beat. When escape beats originate in the AV junctional tissue, they are conducted normally through the ventricles. Thus, the QRS is within normal limits.

Notice that the heart rate gradually slows. An AV junctional pacemaker assumes
intermittent command following beat 4.

Sinus Tachycardia

Tachycardia is a term used to describe a heart rate of greater than 140 in children and greater than 160 in infants. *Sinus tachy* (as those of us who are close call it) is a regular sinus rhythm with an *increased* rate. Usually *sinus tachycardia* will not exceed a rate of 180 in children and 200 in infants. Whew!

Sinus tachycardia **has the following characteristics:**

➤ Rate—140–180 in children, 160–200 in infants.

➤ Rhythm-regular.

➤ P waves precede each QRS.

➤ P-P interval constant.

➤ P-R interval constant.

➤ A QRS follows each P wave; normal QRS configuration; R-R interval is regular.

➤ Usually has gradual onset; gradual slowing.

Look for yourself!

Sinus tachycardia in a three year old with an elevated temperature.

Some *culprits* that may be responsible for sinus tachycardia include agitation, fever, infection, anemia, hypovolemia, blood loss, CHF, sepsis, myocarditis, rheumatic fever, decongestants, etc. The treatment for sinus tachycardia consists of *discovering the underlying cause and treating it!* As with all rapid rhythms, ventricular fill time is reduced, thus diminishing cardiac output. When related to hypovolemia (hemorrhagic or non-hemorrhagic), the rhythm is considered unstable. Fluid replacement is the first line of treatment to restore hemodynamic equilibrium.

Sinus Arrest

Sinus arrest or *sinus pause* is the result of momentary failure of the SA node to initiate an impulse. Since there is no SA stimulus, no atrial or subsequent ventricular activity occurs. So there's no _____ and no _____. (If you said P wave and QRS, you may go to the head of the class!) The pause is usually of *short, but undetermined*, duration. Occasionally, an escape beat may interrupt the pause (a built-in safety device of the unit)! Let's take a look.

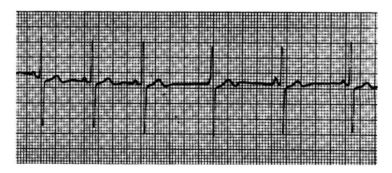

Notice the sinus pause following beat 3. A junctional escape beat interrupts the pause. The normal sinus pacemaker then resumes at a slower rate.

The specifics of *sinus arrest* are as follows.

➤ Rate usually within normal bounds.

➤ Rhythm irregular owing to pause(s).

➤ QRS follows every P wave; P-P interval regular and irregular.

➤ QRS of normal duration, R-R interval regular and irregular.

A close cousin of sinus arrest is *sinus block.* Although the sinus pacemaker fires on time, it is blocked somewhere within the sinus mechanism . . . in other words, *it never gets out of the gate!* Usually the pause in sinus block is the duration of two normal sinus impulses as seen in the diagram at the top of page 403.

duration of 2 sinus impulses

Sinus pause and sinus arrest are *most commonly caused* by increased vagal tone, hypoxia, and digitalis. Usually treatment is not required unless the pauses are pronounced or of frequent occurrence.

Sick Sinus Syndrome

Sick sinus syndrome was discussed back on page 77. It is seen when the good ol' SA node fails to function as the dominant pacemaker of the heart. Consequently, one sees a variety of dysrhythmias that are *together* labeled as *sick sinus syndrome*.These dysrhythmias include

➤ profound sinus bradycardia

➤ SA block

➤ sinus arrest with junctional escape beats

➤ P.A.T. (remember paroxysmal atrial tachycardia?)

➤ slow or fast ectopic atrial or junctional rhythms

Though rare, sick sinus syndrome may be found in children who have undergone extensive cardiac surgery. This is especially true when the surgery involves the atria and atrial septum.

Oftentimes these children develop frequent episodes of tachycardia requiring propranolol. Usually, the tachycardia episodes decrease as the child grows older. If bradycardia is pronounced, pacemaker therapy may be required.

The above strip demonstrates a sick sinus syndrome, though the heart rate is within normal limits.

Practice Exercise 2

A. The easiest way to determine rhythm irregularity is to measure the P-P interval or the
_____ interval.

B. Analyze the following rhythm strip. Bear in mind that the owner of this rhythm is six years old!

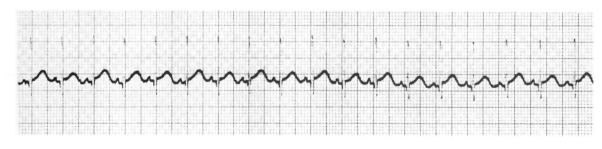

_____

_____

_____

_____

_____

C. Sinus bradycardia in a child is defined as a heart rate (circle the correct answer!)

    less than 90

    less than 70

    less than 80

    less than 60

✔ For **Feedback 2**, refer to page 434.

Input Section 15.3: Atrial Dysrhythmias

With no further ado, we are going to begin exploring atrial ectopic activity in children. You will remember that we are talking about pacemaker impulses that are generated in abnormal areas of the atria (outside the normal conduction system).

Atrial dysrhythmias are identified by *P waves or atrial deflections occurring prior to the QRSs*. The P waves may be premature or may vary in appearance from normal sinus P waves . . . or there may be multiple atrial deflections per QRS. Read on . . .

Premature Atrial Contractions (P.A.C.)

As the name implies, the P.A.C. is premature in its relationship to the sinus rhythm. You will recall that the premature P wave is different in configuration from the "normal" P wave.

Inspect this example!

Look closely! Every other beat is a P.A.C. (Bigeminy P.A.C.s). Notice that the P waves of
the P.A.C.s look distinctly different from the sinus P waves.

Get out the check list. . . . **Rhythms interrupted by P.A.C.s have the following features:**

➤ Rate—usually normal sinus rate . . . remember . . . the rate varies with age!

➤ Rhythm—irregular due to the interruption of the premature beats.

➤ P wave—of the P.A.C. is of different size and/or shape from normal P; P-R interval of normal beats is
   within normal limits; P-R of ectopic beats may vary from normal.

➤ QRS—normal duration; R-R interval irregular.

➤ Pause following the P.A.C. (allowing the sinus mechanism to reset the rhythm). An infant will have a
   complete compensatory pause (twice the R-R interval), while older children will demonstrate an
   incomplete compensatory pause (less than twice the R-R interval).

P.A.C.s are frequently observed in children with

➤ atrial enlargement

➤ electrolyte imbalances

➤ hypoxia

➤ hypoglycemia

➤ following atrial surgery

. . . and *surprise*, P.A.C.s are *common* in **healthy** children and newborns!!
The treatment of P.A.C.s depends on the underlying cause. If the cardiovascular system is healthy, no treatment is usually necessary. If the premature beats are frequent, multifocal, or seen in couplets (two or more together), continuous monitoring should be provided and a physician notified. Usually, digitalis or propranolol are
the drugs of choice if treatment is deemed necessary.

Atrial Tachycardia

First, a test of your short-term memory. Do you remember the *minimum* and *maximum* inherent rates of SA
node discharge? Well, time's up . . . !

Age	Rate
0–1 month	100–180
1 year	80–180
5 years	70–150
10 years	60–125

In *atrial tachycardia*, the heart rate is usually in excess of 180 beats per minute, considerably *faster* than the inherent firing rate of the SA node (aren't you glad we reviewed those rate limits!). You will recall from Section 2, atrial tachycardia may be precipitated by (1) a single atrial ectopic site (P.A.C.) firing repeatedly, or (2) may result secondary to an anomalous circuitry within the atria, allowing an initiating ectopic stimulus (P.A.C.) to repeatedly re-enter and activate the atria in a circus-like fashion. (If you need a quick review of re-entry pathology, refer back to page 61.

This rhythm strip demonstrates a newborn sinus rhythm. The rhythm slows slightly after beat 4. Beat 6 initiates a burst of atrial tachycardia at a rate of approximately 200 per minute! Since there are definite P waves, we know the rhythm is atrial in orgin!

Atrial tachycardia has the following identifying features:

➤ Rate—greater than 220 beats/minute in infants less than 1 year; greater than 180 beats/minute in children.

➤ Rhythm—extremely regular.

➤ P wave—obvious before each QRS; if not obvious, but other features are met, the term supraventricular is utilized in lieu of atrial tachycardia.

➤ P-R may be prolonged owing to tissue refractoriness (the tissue must have sufficient recovery time if the next impulse is to conduct normally).

➤ QRS—usually of normal duration.

The onset of atrial tachycardia may be gradual, but more often is abrupt, as seen above. When the onset and conclusion is abrupt, the rhythm is called *paroxysmal atrial tachycardia*—P.A.T. to *close* friends.

As *stimulating* as it may be to feel like you have a machine gun firing in your chest, long bouts of atrial tachycardia cause decreased cardiac output which may progress to congestive heart failure!

Both dobees and don't bees are subject to bouts of atrial tachycardia. Atrial tachycardia, or P.A.T., is found in healthy children (roughly 50 percent of the cases), children with congenital heart disease, children with Wolff-Parkinson-White Syndrome (see page 78 for discussion), and in the presence of hypovolemia, hypoxia, hyperthermia, electrolyte imbalances, tamponade and a number of other conditions.

Remember the toilet example on page 61? You will recall that a rapid heart rate reduces cardiac output. (If you flush your toilet 180 times per minute . . . it's all coming back to you . . . I knew the toilet would do it!) So, treatment consists of correcting the underlying pathology (or cause), *slowing the heart rate* and *restoring the sinus*

Kidstuff 407

pacemaker. Adenosine (0.1 mg/kg) administered intravenously is the drug therapy of choice. It acts by slowing conduction through the AV node. Cardioversion may be the first line of treatment for children with evidence of cardiovascular compromise. The typical setting is 0.5 to 1.0 joules/kg body weight.

Older children with short bursts of atrial tachycardia may respond well to measures that increase vagal tone (carotid sinus massage, gagging, application of cold or ice water to the face, Valsalva maneuver, etc.). Infants, however, may not respond well to these tactics owing to the immaturity of the nervous system. Following restoration of a sinus rhythm, these children may be placed on digoxin for six months to prevent further recurrence.

Very *tachy* stuff, huh?

Well, sometimes an ectopic atrial impulse simply interrupts the underlying, normal rhythm.

Paroxysmal Supraventricular Tachycardia (P.S.V.T.)

P.S.V.T. is the most common dysrhythmia of clinical significance encountered in pediatrics. One finds a hyperexcitable ectopic focus within the atria or junctional tissue discharging rapidly or, encounters a re-entry phenomenon. (If you need a "re-entry refresher," please review page 63!) Basically, P.S.V.T. is a descriptive category. In other words, when a definitive distinction cannot be made between atrial tachycardia and junctional tachycardia, the rhythm is termed *supraventricular tachycardia.* If the rhythm is *paroxysmal* in nature, it is labeled *P.S.V.T.* Oftentimes, supraventricular tachycardia has a sudden onset. And often, owing to the rapid rate, one cannot determine where in the cardiac cycle P waves are occurring (before, during, or after the QRS). Look at a strip of P.S.V.T.

This rhythm strip demonstrates a supraventricular tachycardia at a rate near 300 beats per minute! It is impossible to determine whether the "bump" between QRSs is a P wave, a T wave, or both. In cases like this, the term supraventricular tachycardia is *most* appropriate! The term implies that the pacemaker is above the level of the ventricles. If the rhythm were ventricular in origin, the QRS would appear widened. (A widened QRS may occasionally be observed with a supraventricular rhythm, as well. This occurs when the AV conduction pathway has had insufficient time to recover between rapid fire stimulations, thus slowing ventricular depolarization. Slowed ventricular activation causes the QRS to widen.)

P.S.V.T. has the following identifying features.

➤ Ventricular rate—250–300 in infants; 160–200 in children.

➤ P waves—difficult to distinguish owing to the rapid rate.

➤ QRS—usually normal in duration (the initiating pacemaker is somewhere above the ventricles).

P.S.V.T. is *most often seen* in infants one to three months of age, but there are some *little ones* who like to begin life in the *fast lane* by demonstrating P.S.V.T. in utero. (Definitely type A personality babies!)

P.S.V.T. may also be associated with:

➤ congenital heart disease

➤ infections

➤ following cardiac surgery

➤ adolescents—fatigue, stress, caffeine, tobacco

➤ tension pneumothorax

➤ hypovolemia

➤ hypoxemia

➤ hyperthermia

➤ thromboembolism

➤ no known reason—*unfortunately*, the greatest percentage!

The problem with P.S.V.T. is one we have already encountered *numerous* times—as demonstrated with the toilet flushing on page 61. The rapid ventricular rate causes decreased ventricular filling and thus, decreased cardiac output.

The treatment for P.S.V.T. depends on the severity of the episode. Sometimes the rhythm will spontaneously convert. If of a brief duration, vagal stimulation (such as carotid massage, gagging, application of cold or ice water to the face, or ice water in the stomach) may convert the P.S.V.T. to a sinus rhythm. When associated with cardiac compromise, more definitive treatment is required! Adenosine is the typical drug therapy of choice. If the situation is more acute, cardioversion may be used. *(0.5 to 1.0 joules per kg. of body weight)*

Remember, patients receiving digitalis require a downward adjustment of the cardioversion current setting. Infants who have recurrent bouts of P.S.V.T. may be maintained on digitalis therapy for six months.

Atrial Flutter

Remember the "Jaws" movies? Well, for those of you who are too young, or who have better taste in movies, sharks have a *sawtooth* type fin that protrudes above the water. Atrial flutter resembles a *convention of all Pacific coast great white sharks*—multiple sawtooth waves (sawteeth) with QRSs interspersed.

A Convention of Great White Sharks

Do not color sharks . . . →   ← Water (Pacific Ocean)
they are white   Color this blue

P.S. We must humor the author . . .

Atrial flutter arises from an excitable ectopic site within the atria or occurs secondary to an anomalous atrial re-entry circuit. The atrial flutter rate is *usually* 240–360 beats per minute! However, not all of those impulses are passed through the AV junction. Commonly, one sees a 2:1, 3:1, or 4:1 conduction i.e., one QRS per four sawtooth waves). The sawtooth waves are "F" or flutter waves.

Atrial flutter has the following characteristics:

➤ Atrial rate 240–360 . . . therefore, the ventricular rate is usually $\frac{1}{2}$, $\frac{1}{3}$, or $\frac{1}{4}$, of 240–360.

➤ Atrial rhythm—regular.

➤ P waves—rather than P waves, there are continuous "F" waves.

➤ QRS is of normal duration; R-R interval may be regular or irregular depending upon the degree of physiologic block in the AV junction.

➤ Atrial and ventricular activity are related because the interval between a conducted flutter wave and its QRS is always constant.

Note: Flutter waves may cause distortion of the QRS, ST segment and T wave, owing to their continuous nature.

Atrial flutter is seen *rarely* in children, but may be associated with.

➤ chronic, severe rheumatic fever

➤ sick sinus syndrome

➤ hypoxia

➤ hypoglycemia

➤ following intra-atrial surgery

The following strip demonstrates a 2:1 atrial flutter . . . sometimes it's difficult to identify flutter waves. Try looking at the strip upside down to better view the flutter waves!

The atrial rhythm is regular at a rate of 300 per minute. Note the "SHARK" waves!

The object of treatment is to reduce the rapid ventricular rate and restore the normal sinus mechanism. (A rapid ventricular rate reduces cardiac output owing to the reduced ventricular fill time.) Adenosine is the first drug of choice. It serves to increase AV block, thus slowing the ventricular rate. In more serious situations (when the rapid rate is poorly tolerated), cardioversion may be the initial treatment of choice.

Atrial Fibrillation

In *atrial fibrillation* there are no waves, just bizarre, irregular, rapid deflections called "f" waves which distort the baseline. (The baseline *undulates* . . . remember?) The atrial activity has no rhythmic pattern. See for yourself!

Note the varying R-R interval of atrial fibrillation.

You will notice that there is no coordinated effort in the atria. To quote "the" author, "some parts of the atria are in a state of excitation and some are in a state of refraction."

The specifics of atrial fibrillation include the following characteristics.

➤ Atrial rate—400–600 per minute (but who's counting—who could count that!).

➤ Rhythm—irregularly irregular (everything is irregular).

➤ P waves—none present; instead, irregular f waves.

➤ QRS duration normal, but the R-R interval varies continuously.

➤ Ventricular rate—usually rapid in uncontrolled atrial flutter.

In children, one may see atrial fibrillation associated with

➤ electrolyte imbalance

➤ hypoglycemia

➤ hyperthyroidism

➤ intra-atrial surgery

➤ structural heart defects

As with the adult, treatment is aimed at *reducing the rapid ventricular rate* and restoring sinus rhythm. When the ventricular rate is rapid, there is a reduced cardiac output owing to the decreased ventricular fill time. Similar to other rapid atrial dysrhythmias, adenosine or cardioversion may be the first line of treatment, depending upon the child's tolerance of the dysrhythmia!

Wandering Atrial Pacemaker (W.A.P.)

The name says it all . . . the atrial pacemaker wanders! There is a gradual shifting between the SA node and other ectopic atrial foci to be the "big cheese" (site of impulse formation). A wandering atrial pacemaker may result when there is a slight slowing of the SA node impulse formation or when various sites within the atria have similar impulse formation rates.

Notice the changing appearance of the P waves, the slight variation in the
P-R interval and the variable heart rate.

The following are criteria which assist in identifying W.A.P.

➤ Rate—within normal limits.

➤ Rhythm—slightly irregular.

➤ P wave—constantly changing, may be SA, atrial, or junctional in origin (if the pacemaker wanders out of the atria), or may not be visible. P-P interval irregular.

➤ P-R interval—varies continuously (though the variation is seldom marked).

➤ QRSs—are related to all P waves; QRS duration within normal limits.

Usually W.A.P. is a benign dysrhythmia and frequently is seen in *otherwise* healthy children. However, it may also be associated with the following conditions:

➤ acute rheumatic fever

➤ increased vagal tone (i.e., increased intracranial pressure, hypertension, etc.)

➤ drugs—digitalis, propranolol

No treatment is required when a wandering atrial pacemaker is found in a healthy child. When associated with other clinical conditions, it is the underlying clinical problem that may require treatment.

Practice Exercise 3

A. The aims of treatment for any rapid atrial dysrhythmia (i.e., P.A.T.) are:

1. _____

2. _____

B. What are the identifying characteristics of a premature atrial contraction?

1. _____

2. _____

3. _____

C. Analyze this strip:

_____

_____

_____

D. Describe the identifying features of a wandering atrial pacemaker.

_____

_____

_____

E. Describe the treatment for paroxysmal supraventricular tachycardia?

_____

_____

✔ For **Feedback 3**, refer to page 434.

Input Section 15.4: Junctional Dysrhythmias and Rhythms

A little *junctional escape rhythm lore*—

The heart has many potential pacemakers: the SA node, the atria, the AV junctional tissues, and the ventricles. Only the dominant or fastest pacemaker will normally control the heart rate. If the sinus pacemaker fails to fire, *or* if the impulse fails to be conducted, *or* if the sinus node discharges impulses so slowly that the heart rate becomes inadequate, a lower, more distal pacemaker will assume the role of pacemaker. Whew!

Junctional Escape Rhythm

If a rhythm originates in the AV junctional tissue, it is known as a *junctional escape rhythm* or an *idiojunctional rhythm*.

This strip demonstrates a junctional escape rhythm in a five year old female. The heart rate is approximately 64 per minute. Notice that there are no visible P waves occurring before or after the QRS. In this example, the atria and ventricles are being activated at approximately the same time . . . thus, the P wave is hiding within the QRS. (If you need a refresher on *hiding* P waves, turn back to page 94.)

The specifics of junctional escape rhythms:

➤ Ventricular rate—usually 50–90 in infants and 50–70 in children, though rates may vary.

➤ Rhythm—regular . . . (escape rhythms are almost always regular).

➤ P—may be observed before or after the QRS . . . or may be hiding within the QRS. If visible, P waves will be inverted in leads II, III, and aVF. (If you need a refresher, refer back to page 91.)

➤ QRS—duration normal.

How could this happen, you ask??? **A junctional escape rhythm may be associated with the following conditions.**

➤ children who have an otherwise normal heart

➤ sick sinus syndrome

➤ increased vagal tone

➤ following atrial surgery and/or any open heart surgery

If the ventricular rate is adequate, treatment is usually not necessary. Remember, however, not only does the slower heart rate compromise the child, so does the loss of *atrial kick*. Therefore, if the child is hemodynamically compromised, epinephrine, atropine or pacing (in exaggerated cases) may be necessary.

Junctional Escape Beats

A *junctional escape beat* is an impulse arising from the junctional tissue due to a brief interruption of the sinus pacemaker. Junctional escape beats will come later than anticipated normal beats (better late than never!). As before, the P wave of the junctional escape beat will occur before or after the QRS . . . or be buried in the QRS. In leads II, III, and aVF the P wave will be inverted. Additionally, the P-R interval of the junctional escape beat will be shorter than the lower limits of normal.

The following tracing demonstrates a slowing of the sinus pacemaker which allows two junctional escape beats to come through. Remember . . . escape beats will always come later in the cardiac cycle than anticipated normal beats.

Single, infrequent junctional escape beats have no real significance. If the SA node persistently fires slowly or if the sinus impulse fails to conduct, a sustained AV junctional rhythm may be observed as demonstrated on page 412. Remember, escape beats or escape rhythms are *never* a primary phenomenon . . . they are *always* secondary to another event. They occur because of failure or disruption of the sinus apparatus. So, you would never want to eradicate escape beats or escape rhythms. It's the proverbial "you don't bite the hand that feeds you."

Premature Junctional Contractions (P.J.C.s)

Like P.A.C.s, *premature junctional beats* arise from an excitable focus. The P.J.C. arises within the AV junction, outside the normal conduction system, interrupting the underlying rhythm. The premature beats cause the rhythm to appear irregular. You will recall that a P.J.C. may have a P wave before or after the QRS . . . or the P wave may be "hiding" within the QRS. If visible, the P waves will be inverted in leads II, III, and aVF. Additionally, if a P wave comes before the QRS, the P-R interval will be less than the lower limits of normal. That's a mouthful! The location of the P wave varies depending upon the timing of antegrade and retrograde conduction. If you need a review of antegrade v.s. retrograde conduction, check out page 91! Typically, the QRS of the premature beat is within normal limits.

Single, infrequent P.J.C.s in otherwise healthy children have no clinical significance. They may also be associated with

➤ surgery near the AV junction

➤ hypoxic conditions

➤ hypoglycemia

Look closely at the above strip! Beat 2 is a P.J.C. that interrupts the otherwise normal rhythm. In this instance, the P wave of the P.J.C. is "hiding" in the QRS.

Usually P.J.C.s require no treatment, though it is important to note their presence and frequency. If the patient shows signs of diminished cardiac output, treatment may be started with adenosine (0.1 mg/kg).

Junctional Tachycardia

In *junctional tachycardia*, a hyperirritable ectopic focus within the AV junction assumes control of the rhythm owing to its rapid rate of discharge . . . usually 160–200 discharges per minute. Junctional tachycardia may result after surgery near the AV node, or be associated with digitalis toxicity or myocarditis. You will remember that the patient with junctional tachycardia experiences a reduced cardiac output from both the rapid ventricular rate and the loss of atrial kick. Atrial activation must be synchronized with ventricular activation to maximize cardiac output!

Let's look at an example of junctional tachycardia.

You will notice in this strip, retrograde P waves follow the QRSs indicating that ventricular activation precedes atrial activation. This is a junctional tachycardia with a rate of approximately 200 per minute.

Junctional tachycardia will have the following characteristics.

➤ Rate—160–220.

➤ Rhythm—regular (usually).

➤ P waves—may not be visible (buried in the QRS), or are inverted occurring before or after the QRS. **Often because it is difficult to establish definitive P waves, these rhythms are called supraventricular tachycardias.**

➤ P-R interval—if an inverted P wave occurs before the QRS, the P-R will be shorter than the lower limits of normal.

➤ QRS is usually of normal duration.

Treatment is aimed at decreasing the rapid ventricular heart rate and restoring the sinus pacemaker. Usually adenosine is the first line of drug intervention. If rapid treatment is required due to a deteriorating clinical condition, synchronized cardioversion is the treatment of choice *(0.5 to 1.0 joules per kg. of body weight).*

Anticipating that your energy may be on the downslope, practice exercise 4 will be relatively short!

Practice Exercise 4

A. What is the difference between a junctional tachycardia and an atrial tachycardia? _____

_____

_____

_____

B. What is happening in this strip, and why?

_____

_____

_____

_____

✔ For **Feedback 4**, refer to page 435.

Input Section 15.5: Ventricular Dysrhythmias

Well, you're still with us, and I believe the worst—meaning the most confusing—may be behind us!

Premature Ventricular Contractions (P.V.C.s)

P.V.C.s are extra beats arising in an excitable focus or site somewhere in either ventricle (outside the normal conduction system). There is no failure of the normal rhythm, merely additional beats arising from an irritable site or focus.

Rhythms displaying P.V.C.s typically have the following features.

➤ Rate—within normal limits for age group.

➤ Rhythm—underlying rhythm usually regular, interrupted by premature beats.

➤ P waves—no P wave visible prior to the abnormal QRS; may be a P wave following the abnormal QRS. Do you remember why? For a thorough explanation, see page 109.

➤ QRS—the QRS of the P.V.C. is wide and *bizarre* in relation to the other QRS complexes. You will remember that the QRS is wide because the premature impulse originates and travels outside the normal conduction system. Thus, conduction is slow!

➤ T wave—the T wave of the P.V.C. usually appears directionally opposite to the T wave of the normal QRS. In addition, there may be a full compensatory pause following the P.V.C.!
Let's look at some pint-size P.V.C.s!

Bigeminy P.V.C.s

This strip is interesting! Notice the artifact that disrupts the baseline midstrip. Bigeminy P.V.C.s are the order of the day!

The following two rhythm strips demonstrate frequent P.V.C.s and short bursts of ventricular tachycardia. These strips were taken from a thirteen year old overdose victim!

One may observe P.V.C.s in children with

➤ normal hearts

➤ congenital heart disease

➤ drug intoxication (e.g., digitalis)

➤ electrolyte imbalance

➤ hypoxia

➤ hypoglycemia

In a healthy child, occasional P.V.C.s are relatively harmless. When *associated* with an underlying cardiac condition, P.V.C.s represent *ventricular irritability* and may be the forerunner of ventricular tachycardia or ventricular fibrillation. *Not a good way to go!!* Additionally, multiformed, coupled, and frequent P.V.C.s and P.V.C.s precipitated by activity are usually significant.

P.V.C.s are usually treated with amiodarone (5mg/kg IV over 30–60 minutes), procainamide (15 mg/kg IV over 30–60 minutes), or lidocaine. Lidocaine therapy involves an initial loading dose—usually 1 mg/kg body weight, followed by a continuous drip (20 μg/kg/minute). If the P.V.C.s are related to drug or chemical imbalance, the treatment should be directed at the cause. Likewise, P.V.C.s related to hypoxia may be eliminated with the stabilizing of blood gases!

Ventricular Tachycardia

The following strip demonstrates ventricular tachycardia with a rate of slightly greater than 200 beats per minute.

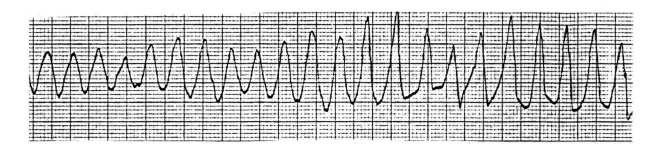

We will not dwell on *ventricular tachycardia* long, not because it isn't important, but because it is a *rare* finding in children.

Identifying features of ventricular tachycardia.

➤ Ventricular rate—slower than P.S.V.T., usually 120–180.

➤ Rhythm—basically regular.

➤ P waves—usually not visible. (If visible, they bear no relationship to QRSs.)

➤ Wide slurred QRSs.

You may find ventricular tachycardia associated with

➤ hypoxemia

➤ hypovolemia

➤ severe digitalis toxicity.

➤ myocarditis.

➤ severe electrolyte imbalance and metabolic disorders

➤ anesthesia.

➤ following cardiac surgery.

➤ hypothermia

➤ thromboembolism

Amiodarone is the drug treatment of choice, though procainamide or lidocaine may also be used.

If drug therapy is ineffective, synchronized cardioversion should be instituted. You will remember that the usual current setting for cardioversion is *0.5 to 1.0 joules per kg. of body weight.* In severely compromised situations, cardioversion may be the first line of intervention. Treatment will also be aimed at correcting the underlying disorder.

Ventricular Flutter

Ventricular flutter is most commonly a *transition rhythm* from ventricular tachycardia to ventricular fibrillation. In ventricular flutter, cardiac output is minimal owing to the rapid, feeble ventricular contractions!

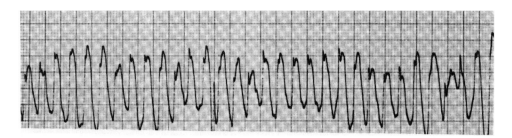

Ventricular flutter, rate 300 per minute.

Usually, the ventricular flutter rate is greater than 200 beats per minute. Ventricular flutter represents a *true* medical emergency. Immediate cardioversion is the treatment of choice if the rhythm persists. Owing to its transition nature, however, immediate defibrillation may be employed.

Ventricular Fibrillation

Well, you ask, *what could be worse than ventricular flutter?* The answer, *ventricular fibrillation! Ventricular fibrillation* represents chaotic, uncoordinated ventricular depolarization. There is *no* effective cardiac output. In effect, the fibrillating heart muscle quivers, but there is *no coordinated* ventricular activity. Death will occur in minutes without emergency intervention.

One usually observes P.V.C.s or some evidence of myocardial irritability prior to ventricular fibrillation.

Ventricular fibrillation may be associated with

➤ hypoxia.

➤ digitalis or quinidine intoxication.

➤ anesthesia.

➤ chest trauma.

➤ cardiac catheterization.

➤ hypothermia.

➤ drug overdose.

➤ severe electrolyte imbalance

➤ hypothermia

Coarse ventricular fibrillation

In ventricular fibrillation, one finds.

➤ Rate—no pulse.

➤ Rhythm—irregular, fluctuating baseline with no P, QRS, or T waves.

Ventricular fibrillation is a *medical emergency*. The treatment for ventricular fibrillation is electrical defibrillation (two joules per kg) followed by intravenous amiodarone or lidocaine. If a normal sinus rhythm resumes, usually prophylactic drug therapy is initiated and the underlying electrolyte factors corrected. **It should be noted that the use of AEDs is not recommended for children less than 8 years of age.**

Note: Ventricular fibrillation is a **rare** finding in children. More commonly, terminal rhythms are bradycardic in nature.

Practice Exercise 5

A. Why is the QRS of a P.V.C. *widened?* _____

_____

_____

_____

B. Ventricular fibrillation is a common/uncommon finding in children (circle one).

C. Draw a strip demonstrating ventricular fibrillation.

CONSTRUCTION ZONE

D. If electrical intervention is required for ventricular fibrillation one would use *synchronized cardioversion or defibrillation?* Why? _____

_____

_____

_____

✔ For **Feedback 5**, refer to page 435.

Input Section 15.6: Complex Dysrhythmias

Pulseless Electrical Activity (PEA)

Pulseless Electrical Activity (PEA) is also known as electrical-mechanical dissociation. Essentially, meaningful cardiac contractions are absent, though cardiac electrical activity (wave forms) is present on the monitor. Muscle contraction and perfusion does not follow electrical stimulation. The patient is pulseless, thus immediate CPR is required!

You will recall, in adults PEA is frequently the end result of cardiac insult caused by hypoxia and respiratory failure. **In children, the most common causes of PEA include**

➤ severe hypovolemia

➤ prolonged hypoxia

➤ severe acidosis

➤ electrolyte imbalance

➤ hypothermia

➤ pulmonary embolism

➤ tension pneumothorax

Treatment for PEA with visible ventricular tachycardia (VT) or ventricular fibrillation (VF) wave forms includes defibrillation (initially 2 J/kg). If ineffective, epinephrine is administered followed by repeat attempts to defibrillate. Antiarrhythmics, including amiodarone, may also be administered. Treatment for PEA associated with other visible rhythms or wave forms involves the administration of epinephrine in attempt to augment both the heart rate and myocardial contractility. Initial treatment (during the resuscitation procedure) must also focus on the identification and correction of the underlying causative condition(s).

There are four points to remember about PEA:

1. PEA is a descriptive classification rather than a distinct rhythm.

2. Pulselessness is a medical emergency requiring immediate CPR.

3. Visualization of a monitor rhythm does not assure patient well-being.

4. An underlying clinical condition(s) is responsible for PEA.

Inherited Long QT Syndrome (LQTS)

You will recall that the QT interval represents the total time for ventricular depolarization and repolarization. It encompasses the entirety of ventricular refractoriness (time when the ventricular myocardium is immune to further stimulation). On page 396, it was noted that in infants less than 6 months of age, the maximum QT interval is 0.45 seconds. In adolescents, the maximum QT interval is 0.425 seconds.

A prolongation of the QT interval (prolonged refractoriness) can be caused by drug effects or electrolyte imbalances. This type of QT prolongation is known as *acquired* long QT syndrome. It can also occur as an inherited disorder (*inherited or congenital long QT syndrome*). It is the inherited type that is commonly abbreviated LQTS. The inherited disorder is thought to relate to a mutation in genes that control sodium and potassium channels.

The presence of LQTS predisposes *the owner* to torsades de pointes (TdP) or polymorphic ventricular tachycardia which may lead to ventricular fibrillation and sudden death (refer to page 126 for a scholarly discussion of TdP! ☺) Though LQTS is believed to be relatively rare, children may present in the ER with syncopy, fainting or post cardiac arrest, and with no previous history of problems. Thought inconclusive, qualitative research has attempted to relate SIDS to LQTS.

In the presence of LQTS, dysrhythmias may be precipitated by the proarrhythmic effects of certain drugs (including certain bronchodilators and antibiotics), by adrenergic stimuli (like exercise or emotional upset) . . . or arrhythmias may occur with no known precipitating event or condition! Before puberty, the risk of cardiac events is greater in male than females. Post puberty, females have the higher risk.

Treatment typically consists of beta blockers (propranolol, nadolol, metoprolol), given for their adrenergic blocking properties, thus decreasing the risk of lethal cardiac dysrhythmias. Drugs such as amiodarone, flecainide, ibutilide, quinidine, sotalol are avoided due to their proarrhythmic effects. High risk children may have ICDs implanted (refer to page 245 for information on ICDs).

In summary, while a prolonged QT interval is not an absolute predictor of risk, one should be mindful of the association with lethal ventricular dysrhythmias. Since infant and juvenile QT intervals vary principally with age (rather than heart rate), the QTc interval (discussed on page 264, adult version) is *not* routinely calculated. Whew!! 😊

Now, on to complex practice!

Practice Exercise 6

A. Explain a PEA rhythm.

_____

_____

_____

_____

_____

B. Check (X) all of the true statements about QT intervals and LQTS.

   ❏ LQTS may predispose a child to polymorphic ventricular tachycardia.

   ❏ Pedi QT intervals vary principally with age.

   ❏ The QT interval represents the ventricular refractory period.

   ❏ LQTS is a genetic disorder.

✔ For **Feedback 6**, refer to page 435.

Input Section 15.7: Conduction Disturbances

Conduction disturbances are defined as *delays*, or worse still, sometimes *failure* of impulse conduction through the AV junction, through the bundle of His, down the bundle branches to the Purkinje fibers. There are three levels of heart block: first degree heart block; second degree heart block; and, third degree heart block. (Clever names.)

First Degree Heart Block

The only abnormality observed in *first degree heart block* is a prolonged P-R interval. Simple enough, huh!!

The above rhythm strip belongs to a five year old boy taking digitalis. Though it is somewhat difficult to measure here, the P-R measures approximately 0.18 seconds. A normal P-R interval for a five year old is 0.10–0.16 seconds. (If in doubt, check out the Pediatric P-R Interval chart on page 395.) So, for this little guy, we have a first degree AV block!

First degree AV block has the following identifying features.

➤ Rate—normal for age group

➤ Rhythm—usually regular

➤ P waves—normal in appearance and duration; P-R interval prolonged (remember, the duration of the normal P-R interval *varies with age*)

➤ QRS—normal duration

First degree heart **block may be associated with**

➤ increased vagal tone (e.g., increased intracranial pressure, hypertension, gastric dilatation)

➤ rheumatic fever

➤ atrial septal defect

➤ structural heart disease

➤ following myocardia surgery

➤ digitalis toxicity

First degree heart block usually does not require treatment. In infants, digitalis may be held if prolongation of the P-R interval is seen on the digitalis *predose* rhythm strip, or if, during the administration of digitalis, the P-R continues to increase in duration.

Well, that wasn't too complicated. Let's try second degree heart block. . . . ☺

Second Degree Heart Block
Mobitz Type I Second Degree Heart Block

In *Mobitz type I, Wenckebach*, there is a progressive prolongation of the P-R interval until a P wave is finally blocked (not conducted). In Wenckebach, as the P-R interval lengthens, the R-R interval shortens! Wenckebach may be observed in otherwise normal hearts or may be associated with underlying heart disease. You will remember that Wenckebach occurs because of progressive fatigue in the AV junction. (If you would like an in-depth review, turn back to page 150.)

The following are some of the *more frequent* causes of Wenckebach or Mobitz type I second degree heart block in children:

➤ increased vagal tone

➤ myocarditis

➤ structural congenital disease

➤ cardiac surgery near the AV junction

➤ digitalis toxicity

Let's have a look! Following is a strip of a four year old following recent atrial surgery.

Notice (above) that the P-R interval lengthens until a P wave is finally blocked or not conducted. Let's analyze the above strip!

1. The heart rate is within normal limits, which is common.

2. The rhythm is irregular. If you look closely, you will notice that the non-conducted P wave principally accounts for the irregularity.

3. The P-R interval progressively lengthens until the eighth P wave fails to conduct.

4. The duration of the QRSs are normal since there is no interference with ventricular activation.

Usually Wenckebach, or Mobitz type I, requires no treatment per se. Treatment is directed at the underlying cause.

Would you believe me if I told you I had a teddy bear named WENCKEBACH?

2:1 AV Conduction

Occasionally, a 2:1 (two P waves to one QRS) AV conduction pattern will be observed in children. Since *only* every other P wave is conducted, one cannot determine whether the P-R is constant or whether it becomes progressively longer (as in Wenckebach).

Generally, the causes of 2:1 conduction are the same as for Wenckebach. As a matter of fact, when a 2:1 conduction pattern has QRSs of normal duration, the rhythm is usually a manifestation of Wenckebach. In other words, if one watched a rhythm long enough, eventually two *consecutive* beats would be conducted . . . and one would note that the P-R of the second beat was longer than the first.

Study the following rhythm strip **carefully!**

The above rhythm strip belongs to a ten day old infant, two days post cardiac surgery to correct a structural anomaly. Notice that the ventricular rhythm is regular at a rate of 75 beats per minute. There are two distinct P waves for every QRS. HOWEVER, the morphology of the conducting P wave is different from the non-conducting P wave. The P-R interval of the conducted beats is constant. In a *textbook* 2:1 AV conduction pattern, one would expect all P waves to be uniform in appearance and to occur regularly (constant P–P interval) throughout the strip. Here, there is variation in the P–P interval. So . . . while this rhythm represents a 2:1 conduction pattern, it is atypical. (Likely, this rhythm is a multifocal atrial tachycardia with a bigeminal block pattern . . . or, an atrial tachycardia with bigeminal blocked P.A.C.s!)

This rhythm strip is included to emphasize the importance of analyzing all facets of a rhythm and to reinforce the value of an accurate description (rather than struggling with naming terminology)!

In a true 2:1 conduction pattern, *the P-R interval of the conducted beats will always be constant*. By contrast, in a third degree heart block, the interval between the P wave and the QRS will always *vary*, since there is no relationship between atrial and ventricular activity (see below, complete Heart Block).

Mobitz Type II Second Degree Heart Block

Mobitz type II is a *rare* finding in children. For that reason, we will not address the subject here. However, the *finer* identifying features of Mobitz type II (adult version), are discussed on page 152. Should Mobitz type II be observed in children, it is usually related to surgery on or near the bundle of His or the bifurcation of the bundle branches. Cardiac pacing may be considered.

Third Degree Heart Block (*AKA Complete Heart Block)

In *third degree heart block*, all atrial impulses are blocked from reaching and activating the ventricular system. None of the atrial impulses are conducted through to the ventricles to initiate ventricular depolarization. Though the sinus mechanism fires at a normal regular rate and activates the atria normally, none of the impulses reach the ventricular conduction system. Lower pacemakers sense the absence of sinus impulses, so . . . as a self-protection mechanism, a lower, more distal pacemaker assumes control of the heart (*self-preservation* you might say). The lower (escape) pacemaker may be initiated from either the junctional or ventricular tissue.

Circle the correct answer on the Pop Quiz found on the next page!

*AKA = *Also known as.*

Pop Quiz!

1. If an escape rhythm is initiated in the AV junction, the QRS complexes will usually be (widened or of normal duration).

2. If the escape rhythm is initiated in the ventricles, the resulting QRS complexes will be (widened or of normal duration).

If you answered *of normal duration* to question number 1, go to the head of the class! If you answered *widened*, go to page 412 for some quick review.

All right, down to facts. We have a regular sinus P wave representing atrial depolarization, but then going nowhere . . .

and a "survival" induced QRS, either junctional . . .

or ventricular . . .

When the atrial activity is combined with the escape mechanism, you will see evidence of the *two independent pacemakers*—the atrial pacemaker and the junctional, or ventricular, pacemaker. These two pacemakers are totally independent of one another. In other words, the electrical and mechanical activity is unrelated or dissociated (hence, the term *AV dissociation*).

In the above rhythm strip, you will notice that the atria and the ventricles function independently. The atrial activity occurs regularly at a rate of 83 per minute. The ventricular activity is regular, but slower at a rate of 44 per minute. Atrial activity is unrelated to ventricular activity . . . *how do I know*, you ask. Look at the P-R interval . . . it *always* varies. *This variation implies AV dissociation.* (AV dissociation is a descriptive term meaning that the atrial and ventricular activity occur independent of one another!) Often, the P waves are said to be *marching through the rhythm!*

Third degree heart block has the following identifying features.

➤ The atrial and ventricular activity occur in a regular pattern

➤ Atrial and ventricular rates are different, the atrial rate being faster than the ventricular rate (the atrial rate is usually normal for the age category).

➤ Atrial and ventricular activation are independent of one another . . . the P-R interval is *never* constant.

➤ The ventricular rate is slow and regular.

➤ The QRS may be narrow (junctional) or widened (ventricular).

Complete heart block may be associated with the following conditions

➤ congenital cardiac disease

➤ following cardiac surgery

➤ myocarditis

➤ digitalis toxicity

The aim of treatment is to restore hemodynamic equilibrium and an adequate ventricular rate. If ventricular activation is initiated by a junctional pacemaker, atropine may be the treatment of choice. Atropine inhibits vagal effect and, therefore, may speed up the junctional rate. Atropine *will not* eliminate the heart block . . . it may simply increase the rate of the junctional escape pacemaker! If the ventricles are activated by a ventricular pacemaker (widened QRS), epinephrine may be administered or external pacing may be initiated.

Occasionally, third degree heart block presents as a congenital anomaly, often associated with transposition of the great arteries. Though certain infants develop congestive heart failure, others adjust to the slow ventricular rate through compensatory mechanisms (such as chamber hypertrophy and increased stroke volume).

Bundle Branch Block

Our section on blocks would be incomplete if we did not discuss bundle branch blocks. You will remember that the conduction system consists of three fascicles. For a quick review of right and left bundle branch conduction defects, turn back to page 162.

Right Bundle Branch Block

Right bundle branch block is the most common form of ventricular conduction disturbance seen in children. Commonly, however, the right bundle branch is intact. The delayed right ventricular activation is often due to *congenital problems* that result in right ventricular volume overload (e.g., atrial septal defect). This volume overload and subsequent stretching of the right ventricle results in slower right ventricular activation!

In other cases, right bundle branch block patterns result secondary to right ventricular surgery, such as the repair of a ventricular septal defect or tetralogy of Fallot. In most instances, there is interruption of the Purkinje system rather than the right bundle branch. Just thought you might want to know that!

Unlike the adult patient, the rsR' or "M" pattern is a common finding in a *healthy juvenile EKG specimen*, though the QRS is within normal limits! If you have forgotten the normal pediatric QRS durations, you may want to review page 000. However, in a right bundle branch block, you can expect to see:

Right Bundle Branch Block Criteria

- rsR' in lead V_1
- QRS duration greater than the upper limits of normal for age
- wide, slurred S wave in lead I, V_5, and V_6

Take a look!

This is a sixteen year old female with right ventricular hypertrophy and a right bundle branch block. The heart rate is 62 per minute.

Left Bundle Branch Block

Left bundle branch block is extremely rare in children . . . in fact, so rare that we could not find a single example! We are told, however, that should *you* come across a *true* left bundle branch block, you can expect to see:

> - wide S waves in leads V_1 and V_2
> - QRS duration greater than the upper limits of normal for age
> - slurred and wide R waves in V_5 and V_6

So much for bundle branch blocks . . . right? Carry on!

Practice
Dead Ahead . . .

Practice Exercise 7

A. Describe the abnormality in this strip and the probable treatment. This is a five year old female with congestive failure.

B. Draw a picture of Mobitz type I (Wenckebach).

C. This rhythm strip demonstrates complete heart block. Describe the findings that support a complete heart block classification.

_____

_____

_____

_____

✔ For **Feedback 7**, refer to page 435.

Input Section 15.8: Drug and Electrolyte Induced Dysrhythmias

Potassium (K^+) norms vary in accordance with chemistry analyzers and clinical techniques. One should *always* verify accepted norm ranges in any pediatric setting!

Relative Serum Potassium Values	
Age	**Potassium Level Norms**
Premie	4.0–7.2 mEq. per liter
Full term	3.0–7.0 mEq. per liter
2 days–3 mos.	3.5–6.0 mEq. per liter
3 mos.–1 year	3.6–5.6 mEq. per liter
1–16 years	3.5–5.0 mEq. per liter

You will remember from earlier sections, potassium (K^+) ions play an important role in the repolarization activities of the myocardial cells. Since the T wave represents repolarization, look for changes in the EKG near the T wave.

Hypokalemia

Hypokalemia is the term used for potassium levels below the suggested low norm. On the EKG, hypokalemia may produce *depressed ST segments and prominent U waves.*

You will remember that the U wave is thought to represent late repolarization of the Purkinje fibers. Because of this add-on feature (the U wave), the QT interval appears prolonged. In reality, there is now a QU interval!

Whew!

Hypokalemia most commonly results from vomiting, diarrhea, or diuretic therapy. ***Hypokalemia causes electrical instability* and may produce any of the following dysrhythmias.**

➤ P.V.C.s

➤ atrial tachycardia or P.A.T.

➤ junctional tachycardia

➤ supraventricular tachycardia or P.S.V.T.

➤ ventricular tachycardia

➤ ventricular fibrillation

Unfortunately, U waves are *difficult* to spot . . . and we did not spot any! Usually, when an extreme hypokalemia is confirmed by lab values, one may be able to go back to a 12 lead EKG and discern U waves . . . though the U waves are never evident in all leads.

Happy Hunting!

Treatment for hypokalemia involves the administration of potassium supplement, oral or intravenous, depending upon the severity of the hypokalemia.

Hyperkalemia

Hyperkalemia is the term used for potassium levels that exceed the upper limits of the suggested norms (refer back to the table, p. 428).

In mild hyperkalemia, tall, peaked T waves may be observed.

As potassium levels increase significantly, the P-R interval prolongs and the QRS widens.

P-R Interval

In pronounced cases of hyperkalemia (K$^+$ levels *greater* than 9.0 mEq. per liter), the P wave may be absent and the widened QRSs may become diphasic . Look at this example!

Neonate showing EKG manifestations of hyperkalemia (10.9 mEq./L.)

Hyperkalemia may be associated with kidney damage or infusions of *excessive amounts of potassium replacements*. Hyperkalemia *depresses* the normal electrical activity of the myocardial cells. So, the child with hyperkalemia is at risk for *sinus bradycardia, first degree heart block, escape rhythms, ventricular fibrillation, etc.*

Treatment for severe hyperkalemia (*greater than 7.0 mEq. per liter*) is aimed at reducing the serum potassium levels. Drug treatment may include calcium gluconate (counteracts effects on the neuromuscular system), sodium bicarb (shifts serum K$^+$ into the cells), or concentrated glucose (increases cellular uptake of K$^+$). *These drug solutions do not remove K$^+$ from the body!* Rather, they shift serum K$^+$ into the cell. In addition, dialysis may be used. For mild cases of hyperkalemia, fluid or Kayexalate (orally or rectally) is administered.

This is mostly a review . . . right?!

Digitalis Toxicity

High serum levels of digitalis may provoke characteristic EKG pattern changes and dysrhythmias. We will look at specific dysrhythmias momentarily. *Please remember*, there are certain **predisposing factors** the child to digitalis toxicity, such as the following conditions.

➤ renal impairment

➤ elevated serum calcium (Ca^{++})

➤ acute hypoxia

➤ decreased serum potassium (K$^+$)

Digitalis toxicity usually involves disturbances in the formation and conduction of impulses. As you remember from page 377, digitalis in excessive amounts retards AV conduction, producing various forms of heart block—*sinus block, first degree AV block, second degree AV block, blocked P.A.C.s, paroxysmal atria tachycardia with block, escape beats*, etc. Additionally, one may find supraventricular tachyarrhythmias, premature atrial and junctional beats, and P.V.C.s (the multiformed or multifocal variety) associated with digitalis toxicity.

Following is a discontinuous rhythm strip associated with digitalis toxicity.

In the top strip, observe the junctional escape rhythm. In the second strip, the sinus pacemaker is evident for several beats, then gives way to the junctional escape rhythm. Finally, the sinus pacemaker resumes control. Remember . . . an escape rhythm will only be observed when there is failure or disruption of a higher pacemaker.

The most common EKG findings associated with *therapeutic* levels of digitalis are

➤ shortened QT interval

➤ slowed heart rate

➤ slight prolongation of the P-R interval

➤ changes in the ST segment

You should remember, a child "isn't only a heart"—a digitalis toxic child may have anorexia, nausea, vomiting, or diarrhea. Usually digitalis is held if the P-R interval is increasing, new dysrthymias are occurring, or the pulse is below 100 in infants or 70–80 in children.

Warning ▶ If a child is on digitalis, any new dysrthymia should be considered "suspect" for digitalis toxicity until ruled otherwise (by official "digitalis toxicity rulers" . . . otherwise known as physicians).

Practice Exercise 8

A. Abnormalities associated with potassium imbalance will be observed in the _____ segment of the EKG.

B. Construct an EKG complex demonstrating mild hyperkalemia.

C. Check (✔) the dysrhythmias that may be related to digitalis toxicity.

❒ sinus bradycardia   ❒ P.V.C.s   ❒ Wenckebach
❒ first degree heart block   ❒ P.A.C.s
❒ blocked P.A.C.s   ❒ junctional tachycardia

✔ For **Feedback 8**, refer to page 436.

Input Section 15.9: Kids' Artifact

Last, but not least, we need to acknowledge that children's monitors, like adults' monitors, occasionally display *artifact*. You may find it helpful to review Section 6 (beginning on page 000). *Artifact*, you will recall, is an electrical signal appearing on the monitor that originates from sources other than the heart! Sound familiar?

Owing to their high activity levels, children are prone to "creating" motion artifact. That means that special attention should be given to skin preparation. It is also helpful to secure the monitor cable and wires in a manner that reduces motion. (Tough job, right?)

Since Section 6 is comprehensive, we will not belabor the point.

Look at this rhythm strip (lead II) from a premie. Can you find the artifact? . . . And better yet, can you guess what is causing it?

Note the peculiar spiked waves occurring before complex 7 and before complex 20. These are hiccoughs! Neat, huh. Baby hiccoughs!

I thought about asking you to draw a baby hiccough . . . but, I reconsidered since this is the *last* input section!

. . . And, here's one more baby rhythm strip to ponder. This one belongs to an eleven month old *"little lamb."* See what you think!

Notice that the T waves of beats 1, 3, and 5 are distorted. Grounds for blocked P.A.C.s, right?! Well, *not* exactly, because there will *always be* pauses following P.A.C.s (conducted or blocked P.A.C.s). This is just one more example of baby artifact that may be confused with certain dysrhythmias!

There is no practice exercise associated with Input 9 . . . just be on the **lookout** for artifact!

A FINAL NOTE ♪

Pediatric dysrhythmias are generally classed as *stable* or *unstable*. Dysrhythmias are considered stable if the child remains asymptomatic, maintaining a healthy blood pressure, normal respiration and an unaltered mental status. Unstable dysrhythmias are associated with diminished cardiac output, decreased responsiveness, hypotension, and respiratory embarrassment or failure. **Generally, unstable pediatric dysrhythmias occur secondary to reduced cardiac contractility caused by extreme hypoxia and respiratory failure.**

NOW LEAVING

✔ Feedback 1

A. The heart rate, the duration of P-R, QRS, and QT intervals all vary with <u>age</u>!

   Circle the correct answer:

B. The heart rate increases / decreases with increasing age.

C. The P-R interval lengthens / shortens with increasing age.

D. The duration of the QRS is greater / lesser with increasing age.

E. The duration of the QT interval increases / decreases with increasing age.

F.

This is a normal cardiac complex with the exception that there is slight ST segment depression. Commonly, ST segment depression is associated with hypokalemia or digitalis administration.

✔ **Feedback 2**

GOOD WORK!

A. The easiest way to determine rhythm irregularity is to measure the P-P interval or the R-R interval.

B. This rhythm is a sinus tachycardia. For a normal six year old, a heart rate should be approximately 100 per minute. One would need to *investigate* and treat the underlying cause!

C. Sinus bradycardia in a child is defined as a heart rate of (less than 70) per minute. (Remembering heart rates is the most difficult part of this whole process!)

✔ **Feedback 3**

Hang in There

A. The aims of treatment for any rapid atrial dysrhythmia are:

   1. Reduce the rapid ventricular rate.

   2. Restore hemodynamic equilibrium—restore a sinus rhythm!

B. The identifying characteristics of a premature atrial contraction are:

   1. The beat is premature, interrupting the underlying rhythm.

   2. There is a P wave before the premature beat and characteristically, the premature P wave is of a different configuration.

   3. There is a pause following the premature beat, allowing the sinus pacemaker to reset itself.

C. This strip demonstrates an atrial flutter with a variable ventricular response. You will remember from page 00 that the ventricular response will be irregular if there is variable AV block. The identification of atrial flutter is confirmed by the rate and the regularity of the F (shark) waves. The atrial rhythm is regular at a rate of 300 per minute!

D. In a wandering atrial pacemaker, one finds:

   ➤ a normal rate

   ➤ a slightly irregular rhythm

   ➤ P waves that constantly change in appearance since the pacemaker wanders around in the atria

   ➤ a varying P-R interval

   ➤ the QRS duration usually within normal limits

E. The treatment for paroxysmal supraventricular tachycardia consists of using measures to slow the ventricular rate and restore the sinus pacemaker. Vagotonic maneuvers (carotid massage, gagging, ice water applied to the face) may *break* the rhythm. If these measures are ineffective, adenosine may be administered to increase AV block. In acute situations, cardioversion may be used. Cardioversion is usually applied using a current setting of 0.5 to 1.0 joules per kg. of body weight.

✔ Feedback 4

A little lamb

A. The difference between a junctional tachycardia and an atrial tachycardia is slight when it comes to heart rate! However, cardiac output will be more significantly reduced in a junctional tachycardia owing to the loss of atrial kick.

B. The underlying rhythm here is sinus rhythm at a rate of 75 per minute. (If this strip belongs to a newborn, it is a sinus bradycardia!) When the sinus pacemaker slows, a junctional escape pacemaker (safety mechanism) takes over for two beats. Then, back to sinus rhythm.

✔ Feedback 5

A. The QRS of a P.V.C. is wide and bizarre because the beat originates in the ventricular myocardium outside the normal conduction system. Because the impulse travels a retrograde (backward) pathway outside the normal conduction route, ventricular depolarization takes more time . . . therefore, the QRS is widened.

B. Ventricular fibrillation is a common / (uncommon) finding in children.

C. Your drawing of ventricular fibrillation should look something like this!

D. If electrical intervention is required for ventricular fibrillation, *defibrillation* is utilized because there is no effective cardiac activity. Synchronized cardioversion is only used when there is an effective underlying rhythm. (R waves are required to synchronize the patient's rhythm with the defibrillator unit). If you need a quick review, see page 000. The usual current setting for pediatric defibrillation is two joules per kg.

✔ Feedback 6

A. A PEA rhythm might be any rhythm. The electrical activity observed on the monitor is disassociated from the mechanical activity of contraction. Thus, the patient is pulseless. A PEA rhythm is a medical emergency requiring immediate CPR and other emergency interventions.

B. All of the statements about QT intervals and LQTS are true.

☒ LQTS may predispose a child to polymorphic ventricular tachycardia.

☒ Pedi QT intervals vary principally with age.

☒ The QT interval represents the ventricular refractory period.

☒ LQTS is a genetic disorder.

✔ Feedback 7

A. Since this is a rhythm strip from a five year old, the rhythm is a borderline sinus bradycardia. Normally the heart rate of a five year old would approach 100 per minute. In this example, the heart rate is approximately 94 per minute. Additionally, the P-R interval measures 0.18 seconds. The upper limits of normal for a five year old is 0.16 seconds. Thus, this is a borderline sinus bradycardia with a first degree AV block. Treatment probably is not warranted.

B. Hope your Wink E. Bach looks something like mine! Note the increasing P-R interval until finally, a P wave fails to conduct.

C. The ventricular rhythm is regular with a rate of 44 per minute. The QRS complexes are narrow, measuring 0.08 seconds. Atrial activity is regular occurring at a rate of 88 per minute. There is no relationship between atrial and ventricular activity (A-V dissociation). The narrow QRS indicates the escape pacemaker is of a junctional origin.

✔ Feedback 8

A. Abnormalities associated with potassium (K^+) imbalance will be observed in the <u>ST</u> segment of the EKG.

B. Hope you were in compliance with all construction codes! Your EKG complex should look *something like mine!*

C. *All* of the following dysrhythmias may be related to digitalis toxicity!

☑ sinus bradycardia	☑ P.A.C.s
☑ first degree heart block	☑ junctional tachycardia
☑ blocked P.A.C.s	☑ Wenckebach
☑ P.V.C.s	

★ STAR!

Notes

Notes

Test Your Skill

Objectives

Find a comfortable chair and complete this review exercise. And remember, it's okay to use the book to answer the questions . . . that's why the book is attached to the review exercise! ☺

When you have completed Section 16 you will be able to determine

1. areas of learning and accomplishment

2. content areas requiring further review or study

3. your readiness for Advanced Arrhythmia Interpretation Practice (Section 17)

Review Exercise

This is an exercise to tie all the loose ends together. Try to answer each question on your own. If you get stuck, **cheat!** (That's why the book is attached to the review exercise!)

1. Label the parts of the myocardial conduction system.

2. On EKG, the P wave represents _____.

The normal P-R interval measures _____ to

_____ small boxes wide, or _____

seconds. The QRS represents _____ and

should be *less* than _____ small squares or *less* than

_____ seconds. The _____ represents

recovery of the ventricles following depolarization.

3. Name three methods for calculating heart rate.

a.

b.

c.

4. The treatment for sinus tachycardia consists of _____

_____

_____.

5. The patient with atrial fibrillation has a/an _____ pulse.

The irregularity of the ventricular response is a result of _____

_____

_____.

6. In the normal heart, the AV junction is generally unable to conduct greater than _____ impulses per _____. The AV junction will _____ impulses greater than this rate. This is referred to as a _____ block.

7. "Saw-toothed" F waves are characteristic of _____. In this rhythm, there are actually two rates to calculate. The atrial or flutter rate may be between _____ per minute. Characteristically, the ventricular rate will vary between _____ beats per minute. Usually atrial flutter is a (regular/irregular) rhythm. What effect would digitalis have on atrial flutter? _____

_____

_____

_____.

If the heart rate (ventricular rate) is between _____ and _____ per minute, one should always *consider* atrial flutter.

8. What is an escape rhythm? When would one see an escape rhythm? What is the probable treatment?

_____

_____

_____

_____

_____

_____.

9. In order to qualify as a junctional beat, the P-R interval must be _____

_____.

10. Describe the criteria that must be met in order to identify a beat as a P.V.C. _____

_____

_____

_____

_____

_____.

11. P.V.C.s are harmful in patients with coronary disease; P.V.C.s indicate _____

_____, and may forewarn of _____.

12. Describe what is meant by "R on T" pattern when referring to P.V.C.s

_____

_____

_____

_____.

13. What are the identifying features of ventricular tachycardia—and how should it be treated?

_____

_____

_____

_____.

14. Describe myocardial activity and the EKG picture associated with ventricular fibrillation. What is the

appropriate treatment? _____

_____

_____

_____

_____.

And now, the fun part!

15. For each of the following rhythms, write one descriptive sentence that would help a new learner
    identify the rhythm. Then, draw a picture from what you have described!

    a. Mobitz type I (Wenckebach): _____

    _____

    _____

    _____.

    b. Mobitz type II: _____

    _____

    _____

c. Complete (third degree) heart block: _____

_____

_____

_____.

 Whew!

16. When looking at a 12 lead EKG, which chest lead is most helpful in identifying bundle branch blocks? _____.

17. Mild hyperkalemia may be suspected if _____

T waves appear on the EKG. Digitalis effect causes a _____

_____ of the ST segment.

18. With myocardial ischemia, the ST segment will appear _____.

ST elevation represents _____. The hallmark

finding on EKG indicative of a large scale myocardial infarction (tissue death) is the _____

wave in upright leads and the _____ wave in downwardly directed leads.

Describe the following EKG rhythm strips, including rate, regularity, etc. *If you feel comfortable*, apply a name. If you need help getting started, look back to page 00 for some tips on interpretation of abnormal rhythm patterns!

19.

_____.

_____

_____

20.

_____

_____

_____

_____

21.

_____

_____

_____

_____

22.

_____

_____

_____

_____

23.

_____

_____

_____

_____

24.

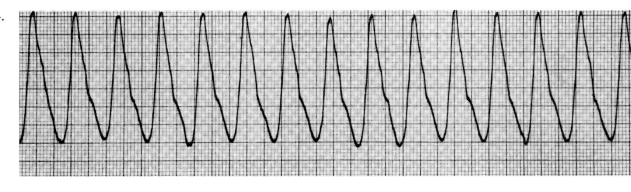

_____

_____

_____

_____

25.

_____

_____

_____

_____

_____

_____

ARE WE HAVING FUN YET ? 🙂

26.

_____
_____
_____
_____
_____

27.

_____
_____
_____

28.

_____
_____
_____
_____

29.

_____
_____
_____
_____

30.

_____
_____
_____
_____

31.

_____
_____
_____
_____
_____
_____
_____

32.

_____

_____

_____

_____

_____

33.

_____

_____

_____

_____

_____

34.

_____

_____

_____

_____

_____

35.

MCL₁

_____

_____

_____

_____

_____

36.

This is an example of motion artifact that masks the underlying rhythm. Describe actions that you would take to determine the significance of the rhythm disturbance. Then, describe methods for correcting the problem.

_____

_____

_____

_____

_____

_____

37. What are these two rhythms? Which dysrhythmia has the greater significance, and why?

A.

P-R = 0.14

QRS = 0.08

Heart Rate = 75

B.

P-R = 0.14

QRS = 0.08

Heart Rate = 75

_____

_____

_____

_____

_____

_____

_____

_____

40. This is a _____. The major distinctions between a pediatric and an adult

rhythm are:

a._____ rate

b. duration of the _____ interval

c. duration of the _____.

39. Reopro is classified as a _____ inhibitor.

40. List three reasons or three conditions warranting the insertion of a temporary pacemaker.

a. _____

b. _____

c. _____

41. Pacemaker non-capture means that _____

_____

_____

_____

_____

Draw a picture of ventricular non-capture.

42. Correctly match the following diagnostic abbreviations with the appropriate hemodynamic measurements.

CVP   left ventricular function

PCWP   myocardial contractile force

LVEDP   right heart preload

CO   left heart preload

43. Explain the differences between hospital defibrillators and AEDs (automatic external defibrillators).

_____

_____

_____

_____

_____

44. Pulseless Electrical Activity (PEA) commonly results from _____ and_____

_____. Check (X) those statements that are true.

☐ PEA is associated with monitor or EKG tracings.

☐ Defibrillation is the first emergency intervention.

☐ Secondary interventions include determining and treating the underlying cause.

☐ PEA is a true medical emergency.

45. When the major force of ventricular activation (depolarization) moves toward a positive ⊕ electrode, the resulting QRS will appear like which of the following? Circle the correct letter.

A.   B.   C.

46. Calculate the time elapsed for each of the following.

A. 5 big squares and 4 small squares _____ seconds

B. 6 small squares _____ seconds

C. 17 small squares _____ seconds

D. 15 big squares _____ seconds.

47. A demand-type pacemaker will generate a pacemaker impulse _____.

_____

_____

_____

48. Beta-blocker drugs produce which of the following effects? (Check all that apply.)

☐ increased heart rate

☐ decreased automaticity of the SA node

☐ an increase in the AV node refractory period

☐ decreased heart rate

49. Hypokalemia increases/decreases (circle one) electrical instability. Name three rhythms that might be associated with moderate to severe hypokalemia.

a. _____

b. _____

c. _____

50. Describe the following rhythm strip.

PHYSIO-CONTROL®

_____

_____

_____

_____

Great Performance!!

Remember, the major objective of this book was to assist you in describing EKG events . . . if you have learned some *jargon* and other facts along the way, that's a *bonus!* Just bear in mind that clinicians have a *great* tendency to disagree over terminology!

Answers for the review exercise begin on page 453.

Review Exercise Answers

The answers to questions 1 through 18 are strategically placed throughout the book . . . very clever, right? Since those questions have "concrete" answers, I will refer you to the appropriate page in the text. Then I will discuss the interpretations of the rhythm strips in detail!

1. Refer to page 16 to verify your answer.

2. Answers can be found on pages 17–22. If you had difficulty remembering any of these facts, you may want to reread Section I in its entirety.

3. Calculating heart rate (three methods) is discussed beginning on page 24.

4. The treatment of sinus tachycardia is discussed on page 53.

5. If you had difficulty with this question, refer to page 74.

6. Look back to the discussion on physiologic block, page 69.

7. Atrial flutter is discussed on pages 69 through 73. Reread the entire section if necessary.

8. Escape rhythms are reviewed on pages 90 and 132.

9. Double check your answers on page 92.

10. How did you do with this one? P.V.C.s are wide and bizarre in appearance interrupting the underlying rhythm; the QRS of the P.V.C. measures a minimum of 0.12 seconds; there is no P wave preceding the abnormal QRS. Review page 136 if you had difficulty!

11. Verify your answers on page 110.

12. This one was easy! If you experienced a memory lapse, see page 112.

13. Ventricular tachycardia is always difficult to "definitely" identify. You may want to reread page 120.

14. The chaotic, uncoordinated ventricular depolarization of ventricular fibrillation is discussed on pages 128–129.

My favorite part of this review exercise is question 15 a, b, and c! The best way to learn is to draw!

15a. Refer to page 150 for a textbook example and description of Wenckebach.

15b. Page 153 clearly depicts Mobitz type II.

15c. Complete heart block is discussed on page 159.

16. V_1 is the lead that most clearly identifies bundle branch block. See page 168.

17. Hyperkalemia and digitalis effects can be found on pages 266 and 377, respectively.

18. ST segment depression connotes myocardial ischemia. ST elevation represents current injury. And, the development of a pathologic Q wave in upright leads and the loss of R wave in negative leads represents myocardial necrosis. For a quick review see Section 11, pages 277–318.

Before we begin to discuss the various rhythm strips, I need to repeat myself. The important aspect of dys-rhythmia interpretation is accurately describing the electrical events. Do not compare how *I've written the interpretation* with how *you've written it*! Rather, make certain you have described what I have described! And remember, it is possible that you and I may see the same electrical events differently!

19. The rhythm appears regular. There is more atrial activity than ventricular activity. Atrial waves are "saw-toothed" in appearance and occur at a rate of 300 per minute. The QRSs are of normal duration and occur regularly at a rate of 75 per minute. Atrial waves (F waves) march through the rhythm. This is atrial flutter with 4:1 conduction (four flutter waves for every QRS). The fourth flutter wave is buried in the QRS—I know it is there however, because flutter waves are continuous, never stopping. If you need review, turn to page 69.

20. This one is easy! A normal sinus beat is followed by a P.V.C., then the whole cycle repeats. This is ventricular bigeminy. The heart rate should be determined by counting the patient's pulse for one full minute. It is helpful to count both apical and radial pulses because not all abnormal beats will be adequately perfused. The P-R interval of normally conducted beats is approximately 0.08 seconds. For review, see page 111.

21. The rhythm is irregular. There is a pause noted after the third beat. The underlying rhythm is a sinus rhythm with an approximate rate of 80 beats per minute—however, when a rhythm is irregular, it is important to count the rate over one full minute! The P-R interval is constant and measures 0.20 seconds; the QRS is constant and measures slightly less than 0.08 seconds. Looking closely at the pause, you will notice the preceding T wave is abnormally peaked. AH-HA! There must be a P wave sitting on top of the T wave! This is a P.A.C. that does not conduct. And as always, when a P.A.C. occurs, there is a pause allowing the sinus mechanism to reset itself. If you need review, turn to pages 59.

22. The rhythm is regular with a ventricular rate of slightly less than 60 per minute. The P-R is constant measuring approximately 0.16 seconds; the QRS is constant measuring approximately 0.08 seconds. There is slight scooping or depression of the ST segment. This is a sinus bradycardia with a slightly depressed ST segment. The ST depression may represent digitalis effect.

23. The rhythm is rapid and regular. The ventricular rate is approximately 120 per minute. The P-R is constant measuring 0.16 seconds; the QRS is constant measuring approximately 0.08 seconds. Giant, peaked, "tentlike" T waves are evident throughout. This is a sinus tachycardia with tall, peaked T waves (suggestive of hyperkalemia). If you need review, turn to page 266.

24. The rhythm is rapid and fairly regular with a ventricular rate of approximately 125 per minute. There is no obvious atrial activity; the QRSs are wide and bizarre. Though the rate is slower than a typical ventricular tachycardia and though there are no fusion or capture beats to confirm the "diagnosis," this is most likely ventricular tachycardia. This could, however, represent an accelerated idioventricular rhythm. For review, reread pages 120 and 132.

25. This is a poor quality rhythm strip, but a *great* thinking exercise! The rhythm is irregular. The atrial rate is regular occurring at a rate of approximately 68 per minute. The ventricular rate is slow and interrupted. The QRS is widened, measuring 0.14 seconds. Thus, a left a bundle branch block exists (check out lead V₁). The ominous finding in this strip is the 3.6 seconds of ventricular standstill! (This rhythm does *not* demonstrate A-V dissociation; a constant P-R interval is evident in all conducted beats). Intermittant ventricular standstill requires intervention. There is no assurance that ventricular conduction will continue. In ventricular standstill, *complete* bundle branch block exists (blockage of both the right and common left bundle branches).

26. You guessed it!!! Normal sinus rhythm. The ventricular rate is approximately 75 beats per minute. The P-R is constant measuring approximately 0.16 seconds; the QRS is constant measuring approximately 0.08 seconds. *I hope you don't need review!*

Whew!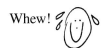

27. Here we have a regular, slow rhythm with a heart rate of 38 beats per minute. The QRS is within normal limits measuring 0.10 seconds. No P waves are visible prior to the QRS complexes. However, an inverted P wave follows each QRS. This is an idiojunctional or junctional escape rhythm. For review, see page 90.

28. The rhythm is irregular, so to determine the rate, I would need to count the pulse for one full minute. The P waves all appear uniform in appearance but the P-R interval gets progressively longer until a P wave fails to conduct. Then, the cycle repeats, though irregularly. This is good ol' Wenckebach (Mobitz type I second degree heart block). If you need review, turn to page 150.

29. The rhythm is regular with a ventricular rate of approximately 60 per minute. The P waves are uniform in appearance. The P-R is constant measuring almost 0.28 seconds. The QRS is narrow followed by significant ST elevation. So, this is a sinus rhythm with a first degree heart block and ST elevation. One would need to do a 12 lead EKG to determine in which leads the ST elevation is present. ST elevation is suggestive of current injury, and appears in the leads overlooking the area of injury. If you need a quick review, turn to pages 289.

30. The rhythm is regular and rapid with a ventricular rate of approximately 185 beats per minute. (I used the cheat guide on page 41.) It is difficult to identify any clear P waves, but the QRS is constant measuring 0.08 seconds. Therefore, I know the rhythm is not of ventricular origin. Since I am uncertain of P waves, I'm simply going to describe this strip as "supraventricular tachycardia, rate 185, QRS = 0.08 seconds."

31. The underlying rhythm here is sinus bradycardia with a rate of 50 per minute. The QRSs are wide and bizarre, *but* there is a P wave preceding each QRS. The P-R interval measures 0.16 seconds. The QRSs measure almost 0.20 seconds in duration! This is a bundle branch block. To know whether this is right or left bundle branch block, I would need to inspect lead V_1. So, in summary, this is a sinus bradycardia with bundle branch block! For review, see page 168. (Note: The delayed ventricular activation caused by the bundle branch block also distorts the ST segment.)

32. Everything about this rhythm is ***irregular!*** There is lots of atrial activity, but no definitive atrial wave forms. The QRS complexes are uniform in appearance, occur irregularly, and measure 0.08 seconds. This is our *old friend* atrial fibrillation. For a refresher, see page 74.

33. *OOOOOh!* Well, the underlying rhythm is a sinus rhythm with a rate of 70 per minute. The P-R interval is of normal duration though the P waves appear inverted. (For a better view of atrial activity, one would need to view lead II.) The R waves are absent and there is marked ST segment elevation suggestive of an acute anterior wall infarction! Beats 3 and 4 are P.V.C.s and beat 5 is a ventricular escape beat. A strip like this presents a *true* treatment dilemma! Refer back to page 280 for a review of R waves in lead V_1 and page 281 for review of left ventricular surfaces viewed by the various leads.

34. The beginning of this rhythm strip shows a supraventricular tachycardia at a rate of 166 per minute. I am calling it a supraventricular tachycardia because there is no clear evidence of P waves and the QRS duration is within normal limits. The rhythm then converts *spontaneously* to a sinus tachycardia with a rate of slightly greater than 100 per minute. The P-R interval of the sinus beats measures approximately 0.16 seconds. The QRS of the sinus beats measures approximately 0.08 seconds.

35. This MCL_1 strip demonstrates a sinus rhythm with *flipped* or inverted T waves, suggestive of myocardial ischemia. The P waves are biphasic in appearance and the P-R interval measures approximately 0.20 seconds. There is a 2.2 second pause between beats 3 and 4. This is a sinus pause since the *next anticipated event* during the pause is a P wave. The pause may relate to ischemic changes in the SA node. Clearly, a 12 lead EKG is in order. For a quick review, see page 284.

36. The significance of the disturbance can be determined by comparing the patient's pulse with the rhythm strip. When artifact is present, the pulse (rate and sequence) will assist one in locating QRS complexes. Motion artifact can often be eliminated or reduced by correct skin preparation and an ample quantity of gel on

the electrode patches. To prevent cable wire movement, the cable may be clipped to the patient's clothing. If motion artifact relates to respiration, reposition the lead away from the diaphragm. For review, see Section 6.

Note: Attaching the electrodes over bony areas will reduce motion artifact!

37. A *toughie!* Diagram A is a sinus rhythm with a blocked P.A.C. (notice that the unaccompanied P wave occurs *early* or prematurely in the cycle). There is a pause following the blocked P.A.C. The significance of P.A.C.s is the significance of the underlying disorder. Frequently, blocked P.A.C.s are observed in digitalis toxicity. Diagram B represents a Mobitz type II second degree AV block! In Mobitz type II, a P wave is suddenly blocked without warning. The blocked P wave is neither early nor late . . . it occurs *right on time*. Mobitz type II occurs because of intermittent bilateral bundle branch block and is almost always associated with *extensive* myocardial damage. Oftentimes, a pacemaker is prophylactically inserted when Mobitz type II is observed. ***Always determine if unaccompanied P Waves occur early, late, or right on time!*** For review, see pages 58 and 152.

38. This is a kid. The major distinctions between a pediatric and an adult rhythm are:
    a. heart rate
    b. duration of the P-R interval
    c. duration of the QRS

39. Reopro is classified as a GPIIb/IIIa inhibitor. If you need review of platelet inhibitors, turn to page 383.

40. A temporary pacemaker may be inserted to treat any of the following conditions:
    a. Mobitz type II second degree AV blocks associated with acute myocardial infarction
    b. drug-induced bradyarrhythmias
    c. third degree heart block
    d. symptomatic bradycardia

41. Pacemaker non-capture means that <u>a pacemaker generated impulse fails to produce the desired effect (atrial depolarization or ventricular depolarization)</u>. See page 217 for a quick review of noncapture!

VENTRICULAR
PACEMAKER SPIKE
↓

NON-CAPTURE—
THE STIMULUS DOES NOT
PRODUCE A QRS

42.
    CVP   Left ventricular function
    PCWP   Myocardial contractile force
    LVEDP   Right heart preload
    CO   Left heart preload

For a refresher, review section 13 beginning on page 333!

43. Hospital Defibrillator
    ➤ mobile
    ➤ used in hospitals
    ➤ capable of defibrillation, cardioversion, pacing
    ➤ requires manual programming by trained clinician
    ➤ requires clinician to interpret rhythm
    Refer to page 203 for a complete review.

Automatic External Defibrillator (AED)
    ➤ lightweight, portable
    ➤ used in the field and for rescue
    ➤ uses algorithms to "read" rhythm
    ➤automatically determines current setting

44. Pulseless Electrical Activity (PEA) commonly results from *hypoxia* and *respiratory failure* .The following statements are true.

  ☒ PEA is associated with monitor or EKG tracings

  ☐ Defibrillation is the first emergency intervention.

  ☒ Secondary interventions include determining and treating the underlying cause.

  ☒ PEA is a true medical emergency.

  For a review of PEA, refer to pages 130, 420.

45. When the major force of ventricular activation (depolarization) moves toward a positive ⊕ electrode, the resulting QRS will appear like diagram A.
    For a quick review, refer to page 4.

46. A. 5 big squares and 4 small squares <u>1.16</u> seconds
    B. 6 small squares <u>0.24</u> seconds
    C. 17 small squares <u>0.68</u> seconds
    D. 15 big squares <u>3.0</u> seconds.

47. A demand-type pacemaker will generate a pacemaker impulse on an as-needed basis, working in synchrony with the underlying rhythm.
    See page 214 for a quick refresher.

48. Beta-blocker drugs produce the following effects.

  ☐ increased heart rate

  ☒ decreased automaticity of the SA node

  ☒ an increase in the AV node refractory period

  ☒ decreased heart rate

  See page 374 for a review of beta-blocker drugs.

49. Hypokalemia increases electrical instability. Three rhythms that might be associated with moderate to severe hypokalemia include
    a. <u>atrial tachycardia</u>
    b. <u>junctional tachycardia</u>
    c. <u>ventricular tachycardia/ventricular fibrillation</u>
    Pages 263–265 provide an overview of hypokalemia.

50. This rhythm strip demonstrates an AV sequential pacemaker rhythm. Both atrial and ventricular activity are controlled by the two lead pacemaker. The atrial and ventricular rates are approximately 75 per minute.
    For a quick review of AV sequential pacemakers, refer to page 215.

NOTE FROM THE MANAGEMENT:
If an advanced practice section does not appeal to you, please find your "to be personalized" diploma following page 529!

Notes

The Final Analysis: Advanced Arrhythmia Interpretation Practice

Objectives

The purpose of this text has been to aid learners in gaining basic EKG interpretation competence. However, complicating rhythm strip interpretation is the fact that few

Textbook Cousins   Non-Textbook Cousins

"live" rhythms resemble their "textbook" cousins. Frequently, multiple anomalies can be found in one tracing. For example, ectopic activity may complicate conduction disturbances, or multifocused excitability may obliterate an underlying rhythm.

The analysis and interpretation of complex or "difficult" rhythms is aided by:

➤ knowledge of a patient's physical findings and overall sense of well being.

➤ review of the patient's underlying pathology, including current drug therapy and lab values (electrolytes, serum markers).

➤ observing the rhythm pattern over time (a six second strip is often too short to distinguish patterns)

➤ "tete to tete" consultation with a colleague

Blast Off

Remember: In all instances, the naming of rhythm anomalies is far less important than an accurate description of electrical events!

The following practice strips are included for their "less than textbook" quality. Use your best analysis skills and describe what you see! My analysis follows at the end of this section, beginning on page 510.

IMPORTANT NOTE: A ![cap] symbol precedes certain interpretations of mine. That symbol indicates the *debatable* nature of those complex rhythm presentations.

Advanced Practice Exercise

Review each strip carefully. Describe all that you see!

1.

_____

_____

_____

_____

_____

2.

_____

_____

_____

_____

_____

3.

_____
_____
_____
_____

4.

_____
_____
_____
_____

5.

_____
_____
_____
_____
_____

6.

_____

_____

_____

_____

_____

7.

_____

_____

_____

_____

8.

_____

_____

_____

_____

9.

10.

11.

12.

_____
_____
_____
_____

13.

_____
_____
_____
_____

14. A.

B.

_____
_____
_____
_____

15. A.

#1 #2 #3 #4 #5 #6 #7 #8 #9 #10 #11 #12 #13

B.

#1 #2 #3 #4 #5 #6 #7 #8 #9 #10 #11 #12

16.

17.

18.

19.

20.

21.

22.

23.

24.

_____

_____

_____

_____

25. A.

#1   #2   #3   #4   #5   #6   #7   #8   #9

B.

_____

_____

_____

_____

26.

_____

_____

_____

_____

27.

_____
_____
_____
_____

28.

_____
_____
_____
_____

29.

_____
_____
_____
_____

30.

_____
_____
_____
_____

31.

_____
_____
_____

32.

_____
_____
_____
_____

33.

_____
_____
_____
_____

34.

_____
_____
_____
_____
_____

35.

_____
_____
_____
_____
_____

36.

_____

_____

_____

_____

_____

37.

_____

_____

_____

_____

38.

_____

_____

_____

_____

39.

Note: the lower wave form is produced by a CVP monitor.

_____

_____

_____

_____

_____

40.

_____

_____

_____

_____

_____

41.

_____

_____

_____

_____

_____

42.

_____
_____
_____
_____
_____
_____

43.

_____
_____
_____
_____
_____
_____

44.

_____
_____
_____
_____
_____
_____

45.

_____

_____

_____

_____

_____

46.

_____

_____

_____

_____

_____

47.

_____

_____

_____

_____

_____

48.

_____
_____
_____
_____
_____
_____

49.

_____
_____
_____
_____
_____
_____

50.

_____
_____
_____
_____
_____
_____

51.

52.

53.

54.

55.

56.

57.

_____
_____
_____
_____
_____

58.

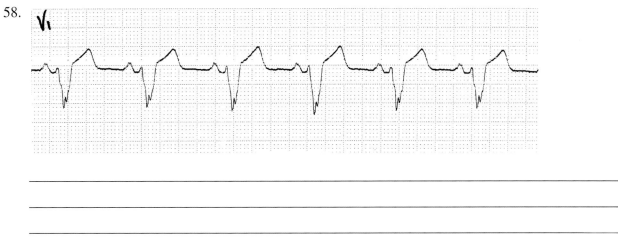

_____
_____
_____
_____
_____

59.

_____
_____
_____
_____

60.

61.

62.

63.

64.

65.

66.

_____

_____

_____

_____

_____

67.

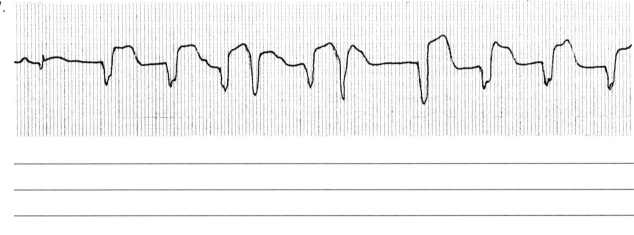

_____

_____

_____

_____

_____

68.

_____

_____

_____

_____

_____

69.

_____
_____
_____
_____

70.

_____
_____
_____
_____

71.

_____
_____
_____
_____

72.

_____

_____

_____

_____

73.

_____

_____

_____

_____

74.

_____

_____

_____

_____

75.

76.

77.

78.

79.

80.

CONTINUOUS STRIPS

81.

82.

83.

84.

85.

86.

87.

88.

89.

90.

91.

92.

93.

_____

_____

_____

_____

94.

_____

_____

_____

_____

95.

_____

_____

_____

_____

96.

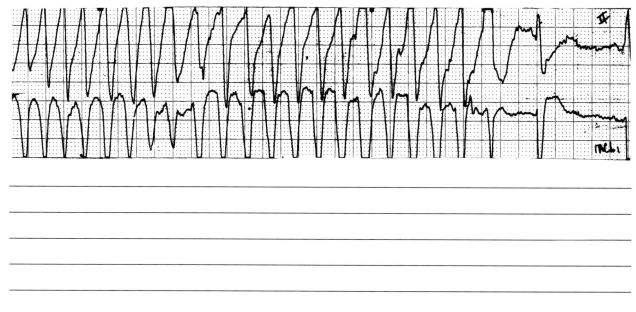

_____
_____
_____
_____
_____
_____

97.

_____
_____
_____
_____
_____
_____

98.

_____

_____

_____

_____

_____

99.

_____

_____

_____

_____

101.

495

102.

103.

105.

106.

107.

109.

110.

111.

112.

504

113.

114.

506

115.

116.

_____
_____
_____
_____

117.

_____
_____
_____
_____

118.

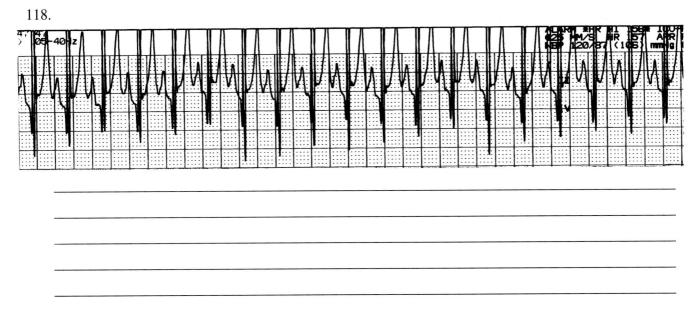

_____
_____
_____
_____

119. Continuous Strip

_____

_____

_____

_____

_____

_____

120.

_____

_____

_____

_____

_____

_____

Interpretations

No two individuals analyze rhythm strips in the same manner. Thus, I do not expect your verbage to match mine!! Be certain, however, that your descriptions contain the "fundamentals."

1. By eyeball analysis, this rhythm is irregular. Every QRS is preceded by a P wave. Certain P waves appear different in configuration. My tendency is to identify something familiar and work backwards. Beats #3 and #4 appear similar—slow sinus beats. Beats #3 and #4 have identical upright P waves and the P-R interval of those two beats measures 0.16 seconds. The QRS complexes measure slightly less than 0.12 seconds. The ST segments are significantly depressed and the T waves are inverted. Beat #5 occurs earlier than expected in the cycle, the P wave is of a different configuration, and the P-R interval is shorter in duration. This is a P.A.C. Following the P.A.C. is the normal anticipated pause allowing the sinus mechanism to reset itself. Beats #6 and #7 appear to be sinus beats. Now back to the beginning of the strip. Beat #1 is a sinus beat. (Note the constant P-R interval of beats #1, #3, #4, #6, and #7.) Beat #2 is a P.A.C., coming earlier than anticipated, and followed by a pause. Viola! The underlying rhythm is a sinus rhythm interrupted by P.A.C.s (beats #2 and #5). The ST depression and inverted T waves noted throughout are suggestive of ischemia. How did you do?

2. This rhythm is slow and irregular. Beats #1, #5, and #6 all look alike in that they have clearly identifiable P waves appearing before the QRSs. The P-R interval measures approximately 0.28 seconds—grounds for first degree AV block. The QRS complexes throughout measure a "hair less" than 0.12 seconds. Beats #5 and #6 represent the underlying rhythm, a pronounced sinus bradycardia (rate approximately 40) with first degree AV block. Measure the interval between beats #5 and #6 and compare that to the interval between beats #1 and #2. You will notice that beat #2 is inscribed later than expected. Beats #2 and #3 represent an escape rhythm generated from the AV junctional tissues (the QRSs are not preceded by a P wave and the QRS duration is within normal limits). Beat #4 may have a P wave, though the P-R interval is shorter than beats #5 and #6. (Limb leads would better display atrial activity.) Note the slight ST elevation throughout. In summary, the underlying rhythm is a *slow* sinus bradycardia with first degree AV block. There is a period of sinus arrest (a failure) and a resulting idiojunctional response. The sinus pacemaker resumes near the end of the strip. This patient was in the recovery phase of an acute M.I.

3. S L O W, irregular, ineffective ventricular rhythm. This is known as an agonal or dying heart rhythm. This rhythm strip followed an unsuccessful code arrest.

4. First, I have scanned the strip to determine that beats #1, #2, #3, #7, #8, and #9 appear similar. The P-R interval of those beats measures approximately 0.18 seconds. There is obvious artifact throughout the strip. Though somewhat difficult to measure precisely, the QRS appears to be 0.12 seconds in duration (normal duration is *less* than 0.12 seconds). The underlying rhythm is sinus rhythm (rate somewhere in the mid-sixties) with slightly delayed ventricular conduction. I would need to view lead V_1 for a better analysis and to distinguish right vs. left bundle branch block. Beats #4 and #5 are coupled P.V.C.s with the first P.V.C. falling near the vulnerable T wave of beat #3. Coupled P.V.C.s signify major ventricular irritability. Beat #6 is a "funny-looking beat" (FLB), but it is atrial in origin. In summary, this is a sinus rhythm with bundle branch block with coupled P.V.C.s.

5. The underlying rhythm is slightly irregular, probably secondary to a slight sinus arrhythmia (related to respiration). The approximate rate is 70 beats per minute. With the exception of beats #3 and #4, all P waves and QRS complexes appear identical. There is a "slight" first degree AV block present since the P-R interval measures approximately 0.21 seconds. Beat #3 is a P.V.C. though it does not interrupt the rhythm of the underlying pacemaker. This is an interpolated P.V.C. with the same significance of any other P.V.C. (you may wish to refer back to page 105 for review). Beat #4 is probably a sinus beat.

Interpolated P.V.C.s typically cause a prolongation of the P-R interval of the next beat. I suspect a P wave is hidden in the recovery phase of the interpolated P.V.C. In any event, this is a sinus rhythm with borderline first degree AV block interrupted by a P.V.C. (interpolated). Generalized ST scooping is present throughout. Note: Frequently a prolonged P-R interval and ST scooping is found with digitalis administration!

6. Here is a two lead view of a sinus rhythm. Note the ST depression in lead II and the ST elevation present in the V lead. You will also notice the absence of an R wave in the bottom strip. The ST elevation represents current injury; the loss of the R wave is evidence of infarct. The ST elevation seen in lead II is a reciprocal change. One would want to view a 12 lead EKG to identify the location and extent of damage.

7. This rhythm is slow and regular with a rate near 50 beats per minute. Identically appearing P waves precede each QRS. The P-R interval is constant and measures 0.18 seconds. The QRSs are uniform in appearance and measure 0.11 seconds. There is slight sagging of the ST segment. This is a sinus bradycardia with suspected ischemia.

8. Here we find an irregularly irregular rhythm. There are no clear P waves. The baseline appears to undulate. A lone P.V.C. breaks the ranks. This rhythm is atrial fibrillation with a P.V.C. One would need to count the rate for one full minute to accurately determine heart rate.

9. This strip presents another irregularly irregular rhythm with fairly marked ST depression. Though T waves are pronounced following the ST depression, there are no definitive P waves preceding the QRS complexes. QRS complexes measure within normal limits. For a better view of atrial activity, I would monitor on leads II, III, or aVF. This rhythm strip is fine atrial fibrillation with pronounced ST depression. If you think rhythm interpretation is tedious and frustrating, you are correct!

10. **Never panic!** Always make the monitor believe *you* are in control! My first eyeball analysis reveals that P waves come before every beat! Thus, I can relax. This is *not* a ventricular anything. I am going to begin my analysis at the beginning of the strip. The first five beats occur regularly with an approximate rate of 85 per minute. Though some notching exists, the P waves appear uniform and the constant P-R interval measures 0.20 seconds. (Notching of the P wave may represent atrial hypertrophy.) The QRS complexes measure 0.12 seconds in duration, grounds for bundle branch block. An analysis of the second half of the strip reveals an approximate rate of 85 beats per minute. The P-R interval measures 0.22 seconds. The QRS complexes measure 0.12 seconds in duration. The second half of the strip also reveals a bundle branch block. My best guess is that this rhythm represents alternating right and left bundle branch blocks—no doubt a function of severe myocardial ischemia/damage. Both the right and left bundle branch blocks produce ST-T wave distortion. To be certain, more information is warranted and a 12-lead EKG is in order!

11. Another strange rhythm strip! The underlying rhythm is regular (approximate rate 62) with a premature beat appearing midstream. A P wave presents before each QRS of the underlying rhythm. The P-R interval is prolonged, measuring 0.24 seconds. Thus, a first degree AV block is present. The QRS complexes of the underlying rhythm measure approximately 0.14 seconds, signifying bundle branch block. To determine right vs. left bundle branch block, one would need to view lead V_1. The underlying rhythm is a sinus rhythm with both first degree AV block and bundle branch block. The premature beat interrupting the rhythm has a QRS measuring 0.14 seconds. Is it ventricular or supraventricular in origin? I believe it is a P.A.C. with delayed ventricular conduction (prolonged QRS duration). There is a probable P wave resting on the downstroke of the previous T wave. I did not describe ST depression because, in the face of bundle branch block, repolarization occurs in a distorted manner.

12. The rhythm is regular with a rate of 125 beats per minute. P waves are present before each QRS and begin on the downstroke of the preceding T wave. The P-R interval is constant and measures slightly

less than 0.20 seconds. The QRS duration is constant and measures slightly greater than 0.08 seconds. This rhythm is a sinus tachycardia with marked ST depression.

13. Here is a nice, pretty, regular rhythm with an approximate rate of 58 beats per minute. The QRS duration is within normal limits and the T waves are peaked in appearance. No P waves are obvious prior to, or following, the QRS. This rhythm is a junctional (escape) rhythm. A potassium level may be in order since prominent peaked T waves are a primary feature of hyperkalemia. Also, hyperkalemia depresses normal electrical activity and may precipitate conduction disturbances such as junctional rhythms!

14. This is a tough one, so I thought two consecutive rhythm strips (A and B) might be helpful! I always look for something "known" when I begin analysis. The last three beats of the second strip (B) demonstrate a sinus rhythm with an approximate rate of 75 per minute. The P-R interval measures 0.18 seconds and the QRS is greater than the normal limits, measuring 0.14 seconds. So, the last three beats represent a sinus rhythm with bundle branch block. One would need to view lead V_1 to determine right vs. left bundle branch block. Now back to the beginning, Strip A. At first glance, the rhythm resembles a ventricular tachycardia. The rhythm is fairly regular, the QRSs are widened, and there are no clearly distinguishable P waves. However, in the middle of Strip A there appears to be two consecutive P waves. Presumably the second P wave conducts through to the ventricles (a sinus beat). The QRSs of the rapid rhythm are similar in appearance to those at the end of the second strip. If the rapid rhythm was ventricular in origin, the QRSs would be wide, but they would be configured *differently* from the sinus beats, secondary to retrograde or backward conduction. So, what is the rapid rhythm? I'm not certain either! It might be a "masked" atrial flutter given the two consecutive P waves (rate 300) in the middle of the top strip. Rather than risk confusion, I would simply describe this strip as a rapid rhythm (rate 150) of supraventricular origin. The rapid rhythm breaks spontaneously in the bottom strip. There is a pause, followed by a beat with an inverted P wave, then on to sinus rhythm. Treatment would be aimed at preventing a recurrence of the earlier rapid rhythm.

Whew!!

15. Another difficult strip for consideration! I hope having two consecutive rhythm strips helped. To be certain, this is a chaotic rhythm. In beginning my analysis, I look for beats similar in appearance! In the second strip (B), beats #2, #4, #5, #7, #8, #10, and #12 look reasonably similar, as do beats #1, #3, #9, and #11.

First, I'll consider beats #2, #4, #5, #7, #8, #10, and #12 (B). No clear (obvious) P waves precede these beats, but the baseline undulates. The QRS complexes are within normal limits, measuring 0.10 seconds and the R-R interval varies. Note the ST segment depression and biphasic T wave following those QRSs. The underlying rhythm here is atrial fibrillation with ST segment depression.

Now back to beats #1, #3, #9, and #11 in Strip B. One can easily be misled believing these are sinus beats with a bundle branch block configuration! However, there are *no* P waves preceding these prolonged QRS complexes (QRS measures 0.16 seconds)! Look back at the ST segment and T waves of beats #4, #5, and #7 of Strip B. What appears to be P waves preceding the widened QRSs are in fact the biphasic T waves of the previous beat. *Ugh!* So, these wide beats (#1, 3, 9, 11 in strip B) are most likely P.V.C.s. Beat #6 (Strip B) is also a P.V.C. but of a different configuration (signifying irritability of different ventricular focus).

Now back to Strip A. Beats #2, #4, #6, #7, #8, #10, and #12 are likely P.V.C.s! This rhythm is an atrial fibrillation with *extreme* ventricular irritability as is evidenced by frequent P.V.C.s, multifocused ventricular excitability, and consecutive P.V.C.s. Clearly, amiodarone therapy would be in order.

Press botton . . .

(electronic stripreaded activator)

. . . if you wish to continue!

16. This strip demonstrates a pacemaker generated ventricular rhythm. No doubt the pacemaker was inserted to correct failure or ineffectiveness of a higher pacemaker. Note the pacemaker spikes initiating each QRS. The ventricular pacemaker rate is approximately 75 per minute.

17. The underlying rhythm is a sinus rhythm with an estimated rate of 70 beats per minute. The P-R interval of the sinus beats measures 0.18 seconds and the QRS measures less than 0.12 seconds in duration. The rhythm is interrupted by unifocal P.V.C.s occurring in a bigeminal pattern. Note the artifact at the end of the rhythm strip.

18. This strip demonstrates a regular underlying rhythm, rate 88 beats per minute. The atrial activity is masked by a major artifact evident throughout the tracing. The QRSs of the underlying rhythm measure 0.12 seconds. Though distorted, there is evidence of significant ST depression. There is a probable run of P.V.C.s in the second half of the strip. As a first course of action, I would attempt to diminish the artifact (anti-artifact tips can be found on page 181). This rhythm is a sinus rhythm with bundle branch block interrupted by a short burst of ventricular tachycardia!

19. This strip seems simple compared to some of the previous examples! The rhythm is regular at an approximate rate of 66 beats per minute. The P-R interval is constant and measures 0.16 seconds. The QRS is abnormally wide, measuring almost 0.16 seconds. This is a sinus rhythm with a bundle branch block. One would need to review lead V_1 to accurately distinguish right from left bundle branch block.

20. The rhythm is regular with a rate of 136 beats per minute. When P waves cannot clearly be distinguished, I tend to use the term *supraventricular*. There may be P waves occurring on top of the T waves, but I am uncertain. Because the QRS is within normal limits (0.08 seconds), I know the rhythm cannot be of ventricular origin. Thus, we have a supraventricular tachycardia with a rate of 136 beats per minute. In all probability, this is a sinus tachycardia. P waves can be seen more distinctly when monitoring on leads II, III, or aVF. The ST segment sags throughout.

21. Ugh! The rhythm is regular, occurring at an approximate rate of 80 beats per minute. A widened P wave precedes each QRS (suggesting atrial hypertrophy) and the constant P-R interval measures 0.20 seconds. The QRS measures 0.11 seconds. Before naming this rhythm, I would want to view leads II, III or aVF to be assured that an atrial flutter is not hiding!

22. Here we have a sinus rhythm with a rate of 75 beats per minute. The rhythm is interrupted by a lone P.V.C. (note the retrograde P wave following the widened QRS). The P-R interval measures 0.20 seconds and the QRS of the sinus beats measures 0.20 seconds (major conduction delay). There is evidence of ST elevation; however, abnormal ventricular depolarization causes abnormal ventricular repolarization. One would need to view a 12-lead EKG for further analysis. This is a sinus rhythm with a bundle branch block and ST elevation interrupted by a P.V.C.

23. The rhythm is irregularly irregular with an undulating baseline. This is an atrial fibrillation. The QRS measures 0.08 seconds.

24. This rhythm strip demonstrates an undulating baseline with no evidence of effective ventricular activation. With no patient to observe, one would assume this is ventricular fibrillation and grounds for immediate resuscitation. However, the truth of the matter is that this patient lost his electrodes! In fact, the patient had a normal sinus rhythm once the leads were reattached!

25. Two continuous rhythm strips were presented to assist in rhythm interpretation. The first three beats in Strip A demonstrate a sinus rhythm with a rate of 75 beats per minute and marked ST elevation. The P-R interval measures 0.20 seconds and the QRS measures approximately 0.08 seconds. The P wave of beat #4 occurs on time, though the P wave is slightly more pronounced than in the previous three beats. The QRS of this beat is configured differently, but measures less than 0.12 seconds in duration. The pacemaker for this beat is located within the atria, but obviously travels a different pathway, resulting in a QRS with a different configuration. However, looking ahead to the next series of beats, I suspect that beat #4 is a fusion beat—partly formed by a sinus impulse and partly formed by an ectopic ventricular impulse. The remainder of Strip A demonstrates an accelerated ventricular rhythm, rate of 79 beats per minute. Some practitioners would call this a "slow ventricular tachycardia." Fortunately, near the end of Strip B, the sinus pacemaker again resumes pacemaker control! This type of rhythm presents somewhat of a treatment dilemma. Depending upon the underlying pathology, aggressive clinicians might elect to treat based on the premise that, if the faster ventricular rhythm is abolished, a slower sinus rhythm will prevail. Conservative clinicians may refrain from aggressive therapy if the patient tolerates the rhythm. The rationale behind conservative treatment is the concern that this may be a ventricular escape mechanism, and, if abolished, there may be no underlying sustaining rhythm. To me, the strongest clue supporting an ectopic vs. escape origin is beat #4, the fusion beat. It is helpful to know that this patient had an acute inferior wall myocardial infarction in progress.   Whew!!

26. The underlying rhythm is sinus rhythm (see mid-strip) with a rate of 80 beats per minute. The P-R interval and QRS measure 0.16 seconds and 0.11 seconds, respectively. Note the ST segment depression suggesting myocardial ischemia. The sinus rhythm is interrupted by bursts of ventricular tachycardia, rate approximately 160 per minute. You will note each "run" of ventricular tachycardia begins with a "funny-looking beat" that has a P wave, and a QRS less wide than those of the ventricular tachycardia. These funny-looking beats are fusion beats and strongly support a ventricular tachycardia classification. Clearly, there is pronounced ventricular irritability!

27. This strip is a killer! Note that the rhythm is irregular. Three slight pauses are evident in the tracing. At first glance, the atrial activity appears to be "a mess." QRS complexes measure approximately 0.14 seconds in duration, demonstrating delayed ventricular conduction (bundle branch block). To begin my analysis, I look at the last beat in the strip (#13) because it appears reasonably normal. I will use it as my guidepost as I examine other complexes. The trick is to determine what mechanism is causing the varying P waves and the irregular ventricular response. Beat #8 resembles beat #13, so I'll begin there. Beat #8 looks like a sinus beat with a P-R interval measuring 0.24 seconds. Beat #9 has no obvious P wave, but the T wave is exceptionally fat. There may be a P wave occurring on the downstroke of the T wave. If so, the P-R interval would be longer than the P-R interval of the preceding complex. The same thing goes for beat #10. There is no obvious P wave, but the T wave is distorted, and appears different. If a P wave is occurring on top of the T wave, this P-R interval would be even greater than in the previous beat. In beats #11 and #12, it is somewhat easier to measure the increasing P-R interval. Following beat #12, there is a pause. Then the cycle appears to begin again. The same pattern exists in beats #3 through #7, with a pause following beat #7. This is a second degree AV block—type I, Wenckebach, accompanied by a bundle branch block. (A conduction system filled with delays!) As is typical of Wenckebach, the P-R gets progressively longer and the R-R interval becomes increasingly

shorter until an atrial impulse fails to conduct. This conduction failure relates to refractoriness of the AV junction and is usually caused by ischemia! How are you doing? I'm stopping for dinner!

28. This rhythm is irregularly irregular and is interrupted by a P.V.C. This is a "fine" atrial fibrillation. The QRS measures 0.12 seconds. This ventricular conduction delay probably accounts for the early distortion (ST segment depression) of ventricular repolarization.

29. This is one of those "treat now and ask questions later" strips. This looks like a ventricular tachycardia at a rate of 166 per minute. See page 120 for a quick review.

30. This strip demonstrates a rapid rhythm with a rate of approximately 120 beats per minute. The QRS duration is 0.12 seconds. This *may* be a sinus tachycardia with a first degree AV block (P-R measures almost 0.24 seconds) and a bundle branch block. However, I am a suspicious character by nature. Any time I see a "sing-song" rapid, regular rhythm, it makes me suspect an atrial flutter. (Sometimes, turning the strip upside down assists me in detecting atrial flutter waves.) I would want to see a rhythm strip of leads II, III, or aVF where atrial activity is more pronounced. I have drawn dots on the strip where I suspect flutter waves. If I am correct, this is a 2:1 atrial flutter. If I am wrong, this is a sinus tachycardia as described above. Beyond looking at other leads, one might have the patient perform a Valsalva maneuver. The Valsalva maneuver momentarily increases the degree of AV block and may make flutter waves more obvious.

31. This rhythm is viewed from both a lead II and lead V_1 perspective. You will note the rhythm is slow with a rate of 42 per minute. The baseline reflects patient movement. Though somewhat indistinct, P waves are evident and the P-R interval is within normal limits. The QRS measures slightly less than 0.12 seconds. In lead II, there is pronounced ST depression. In lead V_1, ST elevation is present suggesting current injury. So, this is a sinus bradycardia with evidence of current injury in lead V_1. One would want to view a 12-lead EKG to determine an overall pattern and location of injury. The ST depression in lead II probably represents reciprocal change. Need review? Refer back to Section 11.

32. Here we have classic artifact. If you observe closely, you can walk regularly occurring QRSs through the strip. The first two complexes suggest that this is a sinus rhythm.

33. This is a borderline sinus bradycardia with tall peaked T waves. I would want to check out the serum potassium level!

34. This rhythm strip represents a borderline sinus tachycardia. The presence of P waves tells me the rhythm is atrial in origin. However, the notching of the P wave is suggestive of left atrial hypertrophy. The T waves are inverted, most commonly associated with a resolving myocardial infarction. I would want to inspect a 12-lead EKG.

35. Looking closely, you will note that no definitive P waves are evident. The baseline is chaotic and QRSs appear irregularly. This rhythm is atrial fibrillation interrupted by frequent P.V.C.s.

36. This rhythm strip is similar to the previous example with one exception. In this strip, the QRS of the underlying rhythm is widened, measuring greater than 0.12 seconds. This is atrial fibrillation with bundle branch block interrupted by a lone P.V.C. One would want to view a V_1 lead to distinguish right from left bundle branch block.

37. Here we have a sinus rhythm with evidence suggesting left atrial hypertrophy and hyperkalemia. Note the tall, tent-like T waves!

38. This is a sinus rhythm with a first degree heart block. The P-R internal measures 0.28 seconds.

39. They rhythm is irregular. At first glance this looks like Wenckebach where one would expect to see an increasing P-R interval until finally, a P wave does not conduct. However, upon closer inspection and measurement, one notes that the P waves vary in size and configuration and the P-R interval, while slightly variable, does not conform to Wenckebach standards. Likely, this rhythm represents a wandering atrial pacemaker interrupted by blocked P.A.C.s. Notice the variation in the T waves preceding the pauses. I think there is a P wave sitting on top of those T waves. The P.A.C.s may not be conducting owing to refractoriness of the previously conducted impulses.

    P.S.–the wave line at the bottom of the strip is a C.V.P. pressure tracing.

40. You are probably an expert by now! This is a sinus rhythm exhibiting slight ST elevation. One would want to inspect a 12-lead EKG to determine in which leads a current injury pattern might be evident.

41. Here baseline artifact makes rhythm detection difficult, at best! Because QRS complexes are relatively discernable, I can see that the rhythm regularity varies. A quick measurement of the R-R interval confirms this. I also note (see lead V_1) that when the rate slows, a pacemaker spike is visible. Measuring the R-R intervals, I note that when the rate drops below approximately 70, the pacemaker kicks in. Owing to the opposite directional inscription, I presume the final two complexes represent coupled P.V.C.s. Clearly, one would want to adjust electrodes and lead wires to diminish artifact.

42. This is a sinus rhythm with a bundle branch block. One would want to look at lead V_1 to distinguish right from left bundle branch block.

43. Here is a sinus rhythm with a first-degree AV heart block (P-R = 0.24 seconds) interrupted by a lone etopic beat (perhaps a premature junctional beat). Also note the slight ST elevation suggestive of injury.

44. This rhythm strip demonstrates a classic atrial fibrillation.

45. Never panic. Always make the monitor think you are in control! The first two complexes appear to be sinus beats (rate approximately 80). The QRS measures almost 0.20 seconds, grounds for bundle branch block. Following is a premature beat with a widened QRS and no obvious P wave. Because this premature beat is directionally inscribed in the same manner as the previous two sinus beats, I think this is a premature junctional beat. Its QRS is widened because of the existing bundle branch block. Complex 4 is also a sinus beat followed by a P.V.C. This is a P.V.C. for two reasons: First, the complex is directionally inscribed opposite to the sinus beats; second, a small retrograde P wave follows the complex. Then the patterns repeat. Interestingly, beat 7 is a premature junctional beat followed by a late (escape) junctional beat. For descriptive purposes, I would say that this is a sinus rhythm with bundle branch block (I would need to inspect V_1 to determine right or left) interrupted by both premature and escape junctional beats and a P.V.C. Often times, complex rhythm strips require a beat by beat analysis!

46. This is a sinus rhythm with evidence of slight ST depression. One would want to examine a 12-lead EKG to determine the significance of the ST depression.

47. Here we have a sinus rhythm with evidence of bundle branch block. The QRS measures approximately 0.14 seconds. One would need to view leads V_1 and V_6 to determine right from left bundle branch block.

48. This is a ventricular fibrillation! Hope you did not miss this one! It seemed timely to give you a break.

49. Again, this is a sinus rhythm with evidence suggestive of atrial hypertrophy. Also note the ST depression suggesting ischemia.

50. This is a rapid and irregularly irregular rhythm. Though baseline artifact makes precise interpretation difficult, this is most likely atrial fibrillation with one aberrantly conducted beat occurring early in the tracing.

51. Here we have sinus rhythm during deep slumber. Note the flipped T waves evident in the chest (V) lead. One would want to inspect a 12-lead EKG to gauge the significance of the T wave inversion.

52. This rhythm is fairly regular. Pacemaker spikes are evident throughout most of the rhythm strip producing a heart rate of 83 per minute. It would appear that the underlying rhythm, a sinus rhythm with bundle branch block, is occurring at a similar or competing rate with the pacemaker.

53. Here we have a regular sinus rhythm interrupted by a P.V.C. However, the P waves are pronounced and the QRSs are wide, measuring 0.16 seconds. So, this is a sinus rhythm with bundle branch block interrupted by a P.V.C. Note the expected pause following the P.V.C. allowing the sinus pacemaking mechanism to reset. The pronounced P waves suggest atrial hypertrophy.

54. This strip is irregularly irregular. The baseline appears to undulate. This is atrial fibrillation!

55. Yikes!! This is a *grab-the-Lidocaine-and-an-external-pacemaker-quickly rhythm*. This is a ventricular tachycardia (rate 187 per minute) that terminates spontaneously, giving way to a ventricular escape rhythm, rate 47 per minute. The object of treatment is to abolish the ventricular irritability and then support the underlying rhythm. This patient is gravely ill!

56. This is a two-lead view of sinus rhythm. Note the ST elevation present in the V lead. One would want to inspect a 12-lead EKG to determine other leads reflecting a current injury pattern.

57. Here is another interesting strip demonstrating the proper functioning of a pacemaker. The underlying rhythm is atrial fibrillation. When the rate of conduction slows, the ventricular pacemaker (rate 50) responds.

58. Here we have a sinus rhythm with evidence of a classic left bundle branch block. The QRS measures a touch less than 0.16 seconds.

59. This looks like a sinus bradycardia, rate approximately 50 per minute. However, upon closer inspection, one notes that a non-conducted P wave follows every T wave. One can *walk* the P waves through the strips, meaning that P waves occur regularly at a rate of approximately 100 per minute. The important question to answer is whether the atrial activity bears any relationship to ventricular activity. To determine that, I measure the P-R interval of the conducted beats. Because the P-R interval is constant, I know that this is a 2:1 AV conduction pattern. Because the QRSs are of normal duration, this is most likely a manifestation of Wenckebach, meaning that if one watched the rhythm long enough, two successive P waves might conduct. In that case, one would likely find that the P-R interval of the second conducted beat lengthened before the next non-conductive P wave. Whew!!

60. Ventricular tachycardia. Lidocaine, please. If the patient is losing consciousness, cardioversion is the first line of treatment.

61. This is a sinus rhythm with lots of motion artifact!

62. Here we have a sinus rhythm with pronounced first degree AV block. Note that the P-R interval measures 0.32 seconds. The appropriate question to ask is whether the patient is taking a digitalis preparation. If so, it is time to discontinue dosing the patient.

63. This is an atrial fibrillation interrupted by a P.V.C. Notice the QS pattern and ST elevation in lead V_1 and the reciprocal ST depression in lead II.

64. Some motion artifact complicates this rhythm strip. I presume this is an A-V sequential pacemaker. Having two leads to inspect is helpful given that all pacemaker spikes are not clearly evident in either lead. However, I would want to determine the type of implanted pacemaker and would want to verify two (dual) wires by chest x-ray. If this was a *runaway* or malfunctioning pacemaker, one would expect to see a variable P-R interval (interval between 2nd spike and QRS).

65. Here we have a sinus tachycardia (rate 107) with a first degree heart block. The P-R interval measures 0.28 seconds. The rhythm is interrupted by a premature beat of uncertain supraventricular origin. I know the premature beat is not a P.V.C. because the QRS duration is within normal limits.

66. This is a bit of a perplexing strip. Despite the fact that two leads are demonstrated, I would want to view a 12-lead EKG. Though at first glance the rhythm appears fairly regular, if one measures the R-R interval, rhythm irregularity is evident. The R-R interval always varies and there are no discernable P waves. Thus, the underlying rhythm is atrial fibrillation. Typically, one would expect QRSs within normal limits when associated with a reasonable heart rate. In this example, however, the QRS complexes are widened, measuring slightly greater than 0.12 seconds. Thus, a left bundle branch block (inspect lead V_1) exists, meaning that the conducted fibrillation waves travel in an antegrade (forward) fashion, but encounter delay secondary to a conduction disturbance in the left bundle branch.

POP QUIZ:

Q: What if the underlying rhythm was atrial fibrillation, but the widened QRSs were occurring regularly?

A: This would mean that all atrial fibrillation waves failed to conduct (usually related to a bilateral bundle branch block) and a lower, more distal pacemaker (ventricular escape) had assumed control of the rhythm!

---

67. Bummer. This one is tough! The very first complex is a sinus beat exhibiting a first degree block and ST elevation. After that, hold on to your hat. Because of the long pause following the initial sinus beat, it appears that an accelerated idioventricular pacemaker kicks in for three beats, and then is disrupted by a P.V.C. falling on the T wave of the preceding beat. That pattern occurs twice, then back to the probable idioventricular rhythm. The strip ends with a junctional escape beat. If the patient is relatively stable, I would want to observe a 12-lead EKG. It is possible that the patient has a bundle branch block confounding a junctional escape rhythm with interspersed P.V.C.s. Whatever be the case, the owner is in a compromised position. Most likely, treatment would consist of a transcutenous pacemaker followed by amiodarone.

68. This is a Wenckebach rhythm. Notice that the P-R interval increases prior to the non-conducted P wave. The non-conducted P wave is sitting on top of the T wave. Note the distortion of the T wave prior to the pause. As is characteristic of a Wenckebach rhythm, the R-R interval shortens.

69. This is a normal sinus rhythm with a right bundle branch block.

70. This rhythm is irregular and there is evidence of saw-toothed atrial activity. Though there is a bit of base-line artifact, one can *walk* the F waves through the strip (lead II). The flutter waves are occurring at a rate of 300 per minute. This is atrial flutter with variable A-V block. One would need to count the

complexes for one full minute to determine an accurate heart rate. Note that flutter waves are most obvious in leads II, III, and aVF.

71. This rhythm looks somewhat similar to the previous tracing in that saw-toothed waves are evident in the V lead. However, when one tries to *walk* those waves through the rhythm strip, they tend to fizzle out. In other words, try as I might, the saw-toothed waves are not quite regular. Often times this type of rhythm is referred to as atrial fib-flutter. Some would argue that it is a course atrial fibrillation. Since treatment is essentially the same, it does not really matter!

72. Here again is a sleeping pattern, reflecting deep respiration. The rhythm is a sinus rhythm with first degree block (P-R = 0.25 seconds) and a right bundle branch block. Respiratory artifact can be diminished by altering lead placement.

73. This is a sinus rhythm interrupted by P.A.C.s.

74. This is a two lead view of a borderline sinus tachycardia with a right bundle branch block. Do you remember that repolarization (ST and T wave) is anomalous secondary to bundle branch block? If not, refer to Section 5.7.

75. This is a sinus rhythm with first degree AV block. Note the ST elevation (current injury pattern) and the absence of an R wave (QS infarct pattern). One would want to inspect a 12-lead EKG to determine the location and scope of injury and infarct.

76. Clearly, one would want to see a longer rhythm strip in order to determine if three or more narrow complex beats occur consecutively. If so, one could determine the regularity or irregularity of those complexes. If regular, one could assume an underlying junctional rhythm (owing to the relatively slow rate and the absence of visible P waves). If irregular, one could assume that the underlying rhythm is atrial fibrillation. The bottom line is that one cannot determine the underlying rhythm from this short tracing. Thus, the best one can do is describe the rhythm as an undetermined rhythm interrupted by bigeminy P.V.C.s. The underlying rhythm demonstrates no clear P waves; atrial fibrillatory waves versus artifact exists. The QRS complexes of the base rhythm measure just slightly less than 0.12 seconds.

77. The rhythm is regular and the narrow QRS (<0.08 seconds) ventricular rate is approximately 65 beats per minute. The *eye catcher* here is the regular atrial waves occurring at a rate of 250 per minute $(6\overline{)1500} = 250)$. The critical question is whether the atrial activity is related to ventricular activity. A close measurement indicates that the 4th atrial wave (following each QRS) is equidistant to the next QRS, meaning that atrial activity is related to ventricular activity. Thus, this is a classic atrial flutter!

78. This rhythm is a classic left bundle branch block (LBBB) with a heart rate of approximately 80. The P-R interval measures 0.20 seconds.

79. Wish the gain had been turned up on this rhythm strip! The ventricular response is irregular necessitating that the rate be counted for one full minute. The QRS complexes measure within normal limits. There are an abundance of atrial deflections. The challenge is to determine the regularity or irregularity of those deflections and their relationship to ventricular activation. My first instinct is that this rhythm is an atrial flutter with varying degrees of physiologic block (which causes the irregular ventricular response). However, despite all my good instincts, precise measurement of the atrial deflections reveals some irregularity. In other words, the atrial waves will not walk precisely through this rhythm. Thus, the rhythm is probably a coarse atrial fibrillation. And, atrial fibrillation *always* has an irregular ventricular response.

80. Here is a partially pacemaker (demand-type) generated rhythm. Beats 1, 2 and 4 represent the patient's self-generated complexes, sinus beats with evidence of first degree AV block (P-R = 0.24 seconds). The heart rate of the first two beats is approximately 72 (1500 ÷ 21 small squares = 72). As the patient's heart rate slows below 68, the demand pacemaker assumes control (measure the distance between two

pacemaker generated complexes (1500 ÷ 22 small squares = 68). You will notice throughout the strip, various complexes are *joint creations* of the patient and the demand pacemaker (most obvious in beats 3 and 5, somewhat less obvious in beats 6, 8, 10, 11, 14, 15). This type of phenomenon is observed when the patient's actual heart rate is at or near the pacemaker set rate.

81. Here is a regular rhythm (heart rate approximately 84 per minute) with a widened QRS measuring greater than 0.20 seconds. The QRS morphology is bizarre, making precise QRS measurement difficult! There may be an inverted P wave (short P-R interval) occurring before the QRS. If so, this is a junctional rhythm with bundle branch block. More likely, however, there is no P wave occurring before the QRS. Thus, the rhythm is an accelerated idioventricular rhythm (ventricular escape rhythm).

82. The underlying rhythm (viewed from the last half of the rhythm strip) is a sinus rhythm (rate 88) with a bundle branch block (QRS measures 0.14 seconds). The P-R interval measures 0.16 seconds. Various ectopic beats interrupt the rhythm. The first beat originates in the AV junction as evidenced by the retrograde P wave following the QRS. Beat 2 is a sinus beat followed by a fusion beat. (The P wave before the fusion beat occurs on time and the P-R interval is short; thus, the beat is both formed by a normal antegrade impulse colliding with a P.V.C. traveling a retrograde path). Beat 5 is a FLB (funny looking beat). The P wave occurs on time and the P-R interval is consistent with the sinus beats. This beat is a normally conducted sinus beat (no bundle branch block). Notice the biphasic P waves throughout, a classic finding of bi-atrial hypertrophy.

83. This is an ominous rhythm in appearance with variation in QRS duration and morphology. The rhythm is irregular and the rate is slightly tachycardic. P waves are periodically visible; however, no clear pattern is visible (P waves cannot be walked through the rhythm). The most likely diagnostic option is an atrial fib/flutter in the presence of a bundle branch block with occasional differently inscribed (morphology) ventricular complexes. Obviously, various conduction abnormalities are present. Remember ST abnormalities are a characteristic of bundle branch block.

84. Here is another rhythm for debate! The non-controversial points of the rhythm are these: the rhythm is regular, the heart rate is approximately 84 beats per minute. The QRS is widened measuring approximately 0.13 seconds. This rhythm is likely one of two rhythms: (1) sinus rhythm with a mega first degree heart block (P-R interval measuring 0.40 seconds) and a bundle branch block or (2) a junctional rhythm (with a hidden P wave in the QRS) and a pronounced T wave, resulting in a prolonged QT interval of 0.44 seconds, in part owing to the widened QRS. (The normal female QT interval is 0.39; the normal male QT is 0.41). Clearly a 12 lead EKG and a clinical history (including pharmacologic agents) would be helpful. What do you think?

85. This rhythm is slow and irregular. A P wave precedes each QRS. The P-R is consistent, measuring 0.16 seconds, though the P wave morphology varies somewhat. The QRSs are within normal limits measuring 0.08 seconds. This a a pronounced slow sinus arrhythmia (the R-R interval of beats 1 & 2 is equal to the R-R interval of beats 3 & 4). This rhythm would likely be treated as a sinus bradycardia and may be related to toxic drug effects, electrolyte imbalances, or ischemia involving the sinus node.

86. Here we have an irregularly irregular rhythm, atrial fibrillation. Notice the fine atrial oscillations. Though one would need to view a longer rhythm strip to accurately determine the ventricular rate, this would appear to be a controlled rate atrial fibrillation.

87. The rhythm is regular at an approximate rate of 70 beats per minute. The P-R interval measures 0.16 seconds. The QRS is widened measuring slightly greater than 0.12 seconds. This is a sinus rhythm with a left bundle branch block (note the V pattern in lead MCL$_1$). The repolarization abnormalties occur secondary to the bundle branch block.

88. This rhythm is also an atrial fibrillation with coarse atrial fibrillatory waves. Notice the irregular irregularity. The "N" notations at the top of the rhythm strip are the computerized monitor notations, signaling that ventricular conduction (QRSs) are narrow, conducting normally (N).

89. As always, it is easier to identify the *known*, than work backwards to identify the unknown! The last five complexes represent a fine atrial fibrillation. (It is unlikely that the "bump" before beat 4 is a P wave). Returning to the beginning of the strip, the atrial fibrillation is interrupted by two unusual beats. The first of those, beat 2, is the "normal" QRS with aberrancy (same QRS configuration with a wider presentation). Beat 3 is an ectopic beat, probably of ventricular origin.

90. This is an interesting strip requiring some thoughtful analysis. Begin by noticing that the P waves vary (two different presentations) in configuration. As always, interpretation would be easier if a longer rhythm strip were available! The two different P wave configurations suggest that one is likely "normal" (sinus) and one is likely of ectopic origin. The positive (upright) P waves in complexes 1, 4, 6 and 9 identify sinus beats. The first sinus beat (beat 1) is followed by two ectopic atrial beats (beats 2, 3). A pause follows the third beat, allowing the sinus pacemaker to reset. Throughout the strip, the ectopic atrial pacemaker interrupts the normal rhythm. Very likely the ectopic pacemaker has a rate similar to the sinus rate; thus, the two pacemakers compete for control of the rhythm. The P-R interval of both presentations measures 0.16 seconds.

91. Here we need to turn up the gain to better visualize the baseline! The rhythm is virtually regular at a rate of 44 per minute. The QRS complexes measure 0.08 seconds. Assuming that the diminished gain is not obscuring upright P waves occurring before each QRS, this is a junctional rhythm with P waves hidden within the QRS complexes.

92. Here, a borderline sinus tachycardia (rate 100) presents with tall "tent-like" T waves, often suggestive of hyperkalemia. The corresponding V lead demonstrates flipped (inverted) T waves suggestive of ischemia. You will recall, in the initial hours of acute myocardial injury, the T waves will often appear tall and peaked owing to potassium leaking from ruptured myocardial cells. One would definitely want to observe a 12 lead EKG. The P-R interval is this strip measures 0.16 seconds.

93. Artifact always makes rhythm strip interpretation interesting! Despite the motion artifact, portions of this rhythm (complexes 4-7) occur regularly with distinguishable P waves. The P-R interval of those beats measures slightly less than 0.20 seconds. However, the QRS measures slightly greater than 0.12 seconds. thus the underlying rhythm here is a sinus rhythm (approximate rate 85) with a bundle branch block. It is helpful that the V lead is also included which identifies the block as a left bundle branch block. Complex 8 is a premature beat followed by a characteristic pause. The last two complexes are sinus beats with LBBB. Though somewhat obscured, the initial complex (beat 1) is probably a sinus beat followed by a premature beat and pause. It is difficult to identify the origin of the premature beats given both the artifact and the LBBB. However, given that the appearance of the premature beats is distinctly similar to the normal beats, my guess is that they are of atrial origin with the P wave masked by the preceding T wave! Whew!

94. <u>Important note.</u> Computerized monitors identify QRS configurations or patterns (V = wide), they do not identify the origin of the complex. Here we have a sinus rhythm (rate 62) with a right bundle branch block (RBBB). The P-R interval measures approximately 0.14 seconds.

95. The *eyecatcher* in this strip is the unexpected pause measuring slightly greater than 2.0 seconds. The underlying rhythm is irregular and artifact obstructs the ability to easily identify atrial activity. On *first pass*, this looks like an atrial fibrillation with a left bundle branch block . . . and a long pause possibly relating to drug therapy Vs. ischemia Vs. vagal stimulation Vs. blockage of both the right and left bundle branches (bilateral bundle branch block). However . . . a closer inspection reveals a constant R-R interval between beats 1-2, 3-4 and the final three beats in the strip. This R-R consistency leads me to believe the underlying rhythm may be a sinus rhythm with a left bundle branch block. In this scenario, beat 5 is a P.A.C. followed by a pause, resetting the sinus pacemaker. The long pause is a sinus pause which could relate to any of the previously named factors. Remember, there is no perfusion during the pause!

96. Hope you did not miss this one! This is a ventricular tachycardia (rate 250) that terminates spontaneously into a probable borderline sinus bradycardia with a left bundle branch block (LBBB). Evidence in support of ventricular tachycardia includes probable fusion beats (see MCL_1, beats 7 and 8).

97. Here we have an AV sequential pacemaker (rate 60) evident at both the beginning and end of the rhythm strip. Beat 3 and the second to the last beat appear to be jointly formed by the atrial pacer and the patient's own pacemaker. A *patient-generated* fairly regular, rapid (approximate rate 125) ectopic rhythm emerges beginning with beat 4, terminating at beat 10. The QRS is widened (0.12 seconds) in the ectopic sequence. Owing to baseline artifact, one cannot determine the presence or absence of P waves. Thus, this burst of ectopic activity could be of either a supraventricular origin (supraventricular tachycardia) with a bundle branch block or of ventricular origin.

98. This rhythm strip can be a fooler. At first glance, one thinks of a *classic* Wenckeback rhythm. However, close inspection reveals a varying P wave morphology (the P waves appear different) with only slight variation in the R-R interval (the R-R interval becomes only incrementally shorter). This is likely a wondering atrial pacemaker with "blocked" premature atrial beats. (Blocked beats are *assumed* because of the pause. In effect, the P waves are likely hiding in the preceding T wave). The assumed blocked beats do not conduct secondary to their prematurity.

99. This is a sinus bradycardia (rate 50) with a slight bradyarrhythmia likely associated with respiration. Peaked T waves are evident in Lead II. Lead MCL_1 demonstrates ST elevation suggestive of current injury. One would want to observe a 12 lead EKG to look for further evidence of injury/ischemia. The P-R interval (0.14) and QRS (0.08) are within normal limits.

100. Starting with the known, this is a relatively rapid, irregular rhythm with a left bundle branch block (lead V_1) pattern (QRS measures 0.12 seconds). Most obvious in the lead 2 rhythm strip, identifiable P waves are periodically visible (see beats 2, 5, 6, 12, 15), though the P morphology and the P-R interval changes slightly in the latter part of the rhythm strip. Presumably the rhythm is a sinus rhythm with left bundle branch block interrupted by short bursts of ectopic activity. The sinus mechanism, however is not dependable (notice the absence of P waves in the last 2 beats of the rhythm strip). Thus, there is some pathology involving the sinus mechanism (sick sinus, drug effects, ischemia, etc). Determining the origin of the ectopic bursts is a challenge. Options include a supraventricular versus a ventricular ectopic pacemaker. Ectopic beats of supraventricular origin would display a widened QRS owing to the bundle branch block (morphology consistent with sinus beats viewed from the same lead). Alternatively, an ectopic ventricular pacemaker arising in the right ventricle would produce a LBBB pattern in V. The clinical significance of the rhythm would drive therapy.

101. The first beat (obvious in leads I, II, III) is an ectopic beat of unknown origin. The remainder of the 12 leads reflect a sinus rhythm, rate approximately 78 per minute. The P-R interval measures 0.16 seconds. The QRS is widened, measuring 0.12 seconds, reflecting a bundle branch block. An inspection of the V leads reveals this is a left bundle branch block. The distortion of the ST segment is a characteristic of left bundle branch block.

102. Here we have evidence of an unhealthy patient! The rhythm is a sinus bradycardia (rate approximately 40) with first degree AV block (the P-R interval measures 0.28 seconds) and a bundle branch block (the QRS duration is 0.12 seconds). One would need to inspect a 12 lead EKG (the V leads) to determine right or left bundle branch block. Note: since this rhythm strip is from limb lead II, this is probably a left bundle branch block. A lone P.V.C is sandwiched (interpolated) between two normal beats. Owing to the slow rate, the P.V.C assists perfusion.

103. Here we have a 12 lead EKG overview of a sinus rhythm (heart rate 94). The P-R interval measures slightly less than 0.16 seconds; the QRS measures 0.10 seconds. Marked ST depression (ischemic pattern) is noted in leads I, aVL and V_1, V_2, V_3, and there is slight ST depression in leads V_{4-6}. Tall,

pronounced (hyperacute) T waves are evident in leads II, III and aVF. This EKG suggests current injury of the inferior myocardium with pronounced ischemia of the anterioseptal and lateral walls.

104. This EKG is a bit complicated, best identified by studying the lead II rhythm strip (bottom). Close observation of the P waves and measurement of the R-R intervals reveals that the pacemaker is wandering in the atria. Because the heart rate is rapid, this is a multifocal atrial tachycardia or, an atrial tachycardia with a wandering pacemaker. Commonly, wandering pacemakers are associated with pulmonary disease. Owing to the wandering pacemaker, the P-R interval varies slightly. The QRS measures 0.08 seconds.

105. This is a regular rhythm with a rate of 82 beats per minute. No atrial activity precedes the QRS. These leads do not assist the interpretation! The QRS is widened, though a precise measurement is difficult. It is unclear whether a retrograde P wave follows the QRS, though the last three beats in the top strip are highly suspect. Clearly, the patient has a conduction defect. This rhythm is either an accelerated junctional rhythm with a bundle branch block or an accelerated idioventricular rhythm.

106. This rhythm strip can fool you. On first glance, one might think this is a coarse atrial fibrillation owing to the irregularity and appearance of the baseline. However, close inspection identifies a regular rhythm pattern with premature beats, all confounded by artifact. The first three beats are sinus beats, followed by a P.A.C. (the P wave of the P.A.C. rests on the T wave of the preceding beat). The P.A.C. is followed by a pause, then two sinus beats occur followed by another P.A.C. That pattern exists until the end of the strip, where the last four beats are sinus beats. The heart rate is approximately 115 per minute. The P-R interval measures 0.12 seconds. The QRS is widened, measuring 0.12 seconds indicating a block in one of the bundle branches. Since lead MCL$_1$ is a proxy for lead V$_1$, this is a right bundle branch block. So, this is a sinus tachycardia with right bundle branch block interrupted by frequent P.A.C.s, sometimes occurring in a trigeminal pattern.

107. This one more rhythm strip demonstrating an atrial fibrillation. The QRS measures 0.08 seconds.

108. The underlying rhythm is a sinus rhythm, rate approximately 70 beats per minute. The P-R measures 0.14 seconds and the QRS duration is approximately 0.10 seconds. Looking first at the limb and augmented leads, one finds ST depression in leads I and aVL. Leads II, III and aVF demonstrate ST elevation (current injury) and prominent Q waves. This is an acute inferior Q wave infarct. The ST depression in leads I and aVL represents reciprocal charges. There is normal R wave progression across the precordial (V) leads.

109. Another challenging strip worthy of debate! The rhythm is rapid, averaging 150 beats per minute. There is slight irregularity of the rhythm and P waves are occasionally visible. The QRS duration varies between 0.18 and 0.21 seconds. My first impression was ventricular tachycardia, despite the slight rhythm irregularity. I presumed the more narrow QRS complexes (see beats 4 and 10, in particular) were fusion beats. However, a colleague consultation suggests that the irregularity of the rhythm favors a supraventricular origin. The widened QRS may relate to an underlying bundle branch block or a rate-related bundle branch block. As always, a clear description is more helpful than a name! Rhythm strip interpretation is an *imprecise* business!

110. The underlying rhythm is slow (slightly less than 40 beats per minute) and regular. The QRS measures 0.08 seconds. There are no P waves prior to the QRS, but an inverted P wave follows the QRS (most prominent in leads II, III and aVF). This is a junctional rhythm.

111. Here we have a rapid supraventricular tachycardia with a rate of 250 per minute. ST segment sagging (ischemia) is evident throughout, likely due to the rapid rate. The genesis of this rapid rate dysrhythmia may be a re-entry mechanism.

112. This is a borderline sinus tachycardia, rate 100 per minute, with a right bundle branch block. The P-R interval measures 0.16 seconds. The QRS is wide, measuring 0.13 seconds. You will recall that secondary ST changes accompany bundle branch blocks!

113. Here we have another coarse atrial fib with the QRS measuring slightly less than 0.12 seconds.

114. Leads II, III and aVF demonstrate marked ST elevation (current injury) and pathologic Q waves indicating acute inferior wall infarct. Recriprical ST segment depression is noted in leads I and aVL. Normal R wave progression is noted in the V leads though ST segment depression (ischemia) is observed in leads $V_2 - V_6$. The rhythm is a borderline sinus tachycardia (rate 100 per minute). The P-R interval measures 0.16 seconds. The QRS measures approximately 0.10 seconds.

115. Ugh! ST elevation is present in leads I and aVL (high lateral wall) and a pathologic Q wave is observed in lead I. Pathologic Q waves are also evident in leads II, III and aVF (interior wall). Unifocal P.V.C.s (most visible in the lead II rhythm strip) distort the precordial leads, though ST elevation (current injury) is evident throughout. Pathologic Q waves are evident in leads $V_4 - V_6$. Thus, this patient had current injury of the anterior, septal and lateral surfaces of the left ventricle and an age-undetermined Q wave infarct of the inferior wall.

116. This is a great rhythm strip! The baseline is erratic suggesting either atrial fibrillation or artifact.

No clear P waves are visible. The rhythm is regular at a rate of approximately 36 beats per minute. The QRS is widened, measuring 0.14 seconds. Atrial fibrillation is an irregularly, irregular rhythm. Complete heart block is the only condition that would allow a regular ventricular response in the presence of atrial fibrillation. Here we have an atrial fibrillation with complete heart block. The slow regular ventricular rhythm is produced by a ventricular escape pacemaker.

117. Brain break! Here we have a *classic* atrial flutter (4:1 conduction pattern). The atrial rate is 300 per minute.

118. The *bizarre* rhythm strip reflects two superimposed leads (lead II and V_1). The first corrective action would be to reduce the gain in attempt to independently view both leads.

119. Hope this continuous rhythm strip did not block you! The rhythm begins (first two beats) as a borderline sinus tachycardia (rate 100, P-R interval 0.20 seconds, QRS 0.10 seconds). Then the rate increases to 115 beats per minute and the QRS complexes change in morphology. Beat 3 demonstrates a clear P wave, occurring on time though the following QRS is premature in relation to the previous beat. No further distinct P waves can be identified in this second sequence rhythm pattern. The QRS is widened, measuring 0.14 seconds. In the middle of strip 2, the rhythm again reverts to sinus tachycardia (approximate rate 115) for four beats, then is interrupted by a presumed P.V.C. followed by a pause. Note that during the four sinus beats, the P wave morphology changes (inverted) and the P-R interval measures 0.18 seconds. A ventricular pacemaker (set rate of 75) appropriately kicks in following the pause for three paced beats. Then, the sinus rhythm (borderline sinus tachycardia) resumes at a rate of 100 beats per minute, again demonstrating upright P waves, and a P-R interval of 0.20 seconds. There are two uncertainties in this continuous tracing (1) the variation in P wave morphology and P-R duration (during the narrow complex rhythm) suggests alternate or competing atrial pacemakers (2) the etiology of the ectopic (wide complex) rhythm is probably ventricular, with the initial beat (beat 3) representing a fusion of the sinus pacemaker and a P.V.C.

120. Here is another somewhat challenging rhythm, subject to debate! The rhythm is irregular, occurring at an approximate rate of 150 per minute. There is slight variation in the QRS duration (0.12 and 0.10). Though artifact partially obscures distinct P waves, varied presentation P waves can be observed thoughout the rhythm strip. You will also note respiratory variation. Most likely, this is a multifocal

atrial tachycardia (MAT) with ventricular aberration occurring secondary to the rapid rate. This type of dysrhythmia is often associated with C.O.P.D. or respiratory failure.

SELF-RATING MEDAL AWARD FOR

OLYMPIC-LEVEL PERFORMANCE

GOLD   SILVER   BRONZE

(CHECK ONE. COLORING IS OPTIONAL)

Notes

INDEX

ACS, 279, 322, 326
AED, 203
AICD, 245
Ablation, 67
Acute myocardial infarction,
    see myocardial infarction
AV sequential pacemaker, 214, 215, 221
Absorption (drug), 367
Acetycholine, 370
Adenosine, 376
Afterload, 340
Amiodarone, 368, 369, 304, 380, 417
Amplitude, 24, 345
Anions, 262
Anteroseptal wall infarction,
    see myocardial infarction
Anti-artifact techniques, 181
Antiarrhythmic drugs, 372
Aortic stenosis, 356
Aortic valve, 335, 341
Apical (low lateral) wall infarction,
    see myocardial infarction
Athrectomy, 324
Artifact, 178, 432
    Baseline shifts, 183
    Motion, 182
    "Off the monitor", 190
    Pediatric, examples, 432
    Produced by electrical
        equipment, 189
    Sixty-cycle, 180
    Artifact identification, 193
Atrial depolarization, 18
Atrial fibrillation (adult), 73, 86, 240, 379
Atrial fibrillation (kids), 409
Atrial flutter (adult), 69, 85, 240, 379
Atrial flutter (kids), 408
Atrial flutter-fibrillation, 76
Atrial hypertrophy, 26, 393
    left, 24, 26, 335, 393
    right, 25, 27, 335, 393
Atrial kick, 74, 102, 133, 215
Atrial arrhythmia suppression, 240, 241

Atrial re-entry mechanisms, 63
Atrial tachycardia (adult), 61, 67, 84
Atrial tachycardia (kids), 405
Atrial tachycardia with block, 144
Atropine, 377
Auto capture, 238
AV block, adult, 141
    First degree, 147
    Mobitz type I (Wenckebach) second
        degree, 150
    Mobitz type II second degree, 152
    2:1 AV conduction, 154
    Third degree (complete), 157
AV block, pediatric, 421
    First degree, 422
    Mobitz type I (Wenckebach) second
        degree, 422
    Mobitz type II second
        degree, 424
    2:1 conduction, 423
    Third degree (complete), 424
AV dissociation, 157, 425

Baseline shifts, artifact, 183
Bazet's formula, 264, 273
Bedside monitoring, 9
Beta-blockers, 374
Bigeminy P.V.C.s, 111
Bi-ventricular pacing, 255
Blocked P.A.C.s, 59
Brady-tachy syndrome, sick sinus
    syndrome, 77, 403
Bundle branch block,
    adult, 162
Bundle branch block, kids, 426
Bundle of His, 16
Bypass re-entry mechanisms, 78

CABG, 324
Calcium, 268
Calcium channel blockers, 375
Calculating heart rate, 29, 216
Capture beats, 122

Cardiac catheterization, 323
Cardiac output, 339, 343, 356
Cardioversion, adult, 201
Cardioversion, kids, 418
Cardioversion (pacemaker), 248
Cations, 262
Cellular necrosis, *see* myocardial infarction
Central venous pressure, 343
Chronotropic incompetence, 229
Circulation, myocardial, 334
CK-MB, 313
Class I drugs, 373
Class II drugs, 374
Class III drugs, 375
Class IV drugs, 375
Compensatory pause, 110
Complete heart block, 157, 159, 424
Conduction system, 16
Contractility, 268, 340
Contraction, 262, 263, 268
Coronary angiography, 323
Coronary arteries, 288
Coupled P.V.C.s, 114
Coupling interval, 57, 108
Current injury, 289

Defibrillation, adult, 201, 202
Defibrillation, kids, 419
Defibrillation (pacemaker), 245, 247
Delta wave, 79
Demand ventricular pacemaker, 214
Depolarization, 2, 4, 18, 20
Diastole, 335
Dicrotic notch, 351
Digoxin, 376
    Dysrhythmias associated with
        toxicity, 377
    EKG effects, therapeutic ranges, 369
    Predisposing factors to toxicity, 377
    Symptoms of digitalis toxicity, 377
    Toxicity, adult, 377
    Toxicity, pediatric, 430
    Van Gogh, Vincent, 377

Dilantin, 378
Distribution (drug), 367
Dressler beats, 116, 118, 121
Drug classifications, 372
Drug eluting stents, 385
Drug Half-life, 368
Dysrhythmia interpretation, 35, 36

Early (premature) ventricular beats,
        109, 110, 136, 379
Echocardiogram, 323
EKG paper, 24
Electrical devices that produce artifact, 189
Electrical interference, 180
Electrode contact, 193
Electrograms, 235
Electrolytes, 262
Electrophysiology studies, 324
Endocardium, 288
Entrainment, 241
Enzymes, cardiac, *see* serum markers
Epicardium, 288
Epicardial pacing, 211
Excretion (drug), 368

F waves, 69, 418
f waves, 74, 418
Fib-flutter, 76
First degree AV block,
        AV block, 146, 147, 422
Fusion beats, 116, 118, 121

Generic drug names, 366
GPIIb/IIIa inhibitors, 383
Guide for determining heart rate, 41

Half-life, antiarrhythmic drugs, 368
Heart rate calculation, 29, 41
Heart rate, pediatric, 394
Hemodynamic monitoring, 334
His bundle electrograms, 145
Hypercalcemia, 269, 274
Hyperkalemia, adult, 266, 274
Hyperkalemia, kids, 429
Hypocalcemia, 269, 274
Hypokalemia, adult, 263, 274
Hypokalemia, kids, 429
Hystersis, 236

ICD, 245, 247, 251
Identifying artifact, 193
Idiojunctional rhythm, 90, 100, 412
Idioventricular rhythm, 132
Inderal, 374
Inferior wall myocardial infarction,
        see myocardial infarction
Inherent pacemaker rates
        Junctional, 132
        Sinus, 16, 132
        Ventricular, 132

Injury pattern, 289
Interpolated P.V.C.s, 114
Interpreting dysrhythmias, 35, 46
Ions, 262
Ischemia, myocardial, 283, 298

Junctional escape beats, kids, 413
Junctional escape beats, adult, 96, 105
Junctional escape rhythm, 90, 100, 412
Junctional tachycardia (adults), 100
Junctional tachycardia (kids), 414

LVEDP, 339, 355
Late (escape) ventricular beats, 131
Lateral wall myocardial infarction,
        myocardial infarction
Leads,
        Augmented leads (aVR, aVL, aVF),
                6, 9
        Bedside leads, 9
        12 lead EKG, 280
        Precordial or chest leads, 7, 8, 9
        Standard limb leads, 4, 5
Left atrial (LA) pressure, 352, 353
Left bundle branch block (LBBB),
        kids, 427
Left bundle branch block (LBBB),
        adult, 165, 166
Left ventricular end diastolic pressure
        (LVEDP), 355
Left ventricular surfaces, 9, 300
Lidocaine (xylocaine), 380
Lidocaine, pediatric dosage, 417
Long QT syndrome, 420

Magnesium, 272, 378
Metabolism (drug), 368
Metabolic syndrome, 325
Mitral valve, 335, 341
Mobitz type I, 146, 150, 423
Mobitz type II, 146, 424
Mode switch, 237
Motion artifact, 182
Multifocal atrial tachycardia (MAT), 62
Multifocal, multimorphic P.V.C.s, 112,
        113
Myocardial blood supply, 281
Myocardial infarction, 288
        Anteroseptal wall, 300
        Cellular necrosis, 288
        Current injury, 289, 303
        Electrical "window", 295
        Inferior wall, 300, 302
        Lateral wall, 300
        Loss of R wave, 295, 296
        Low lateral (apical) wall, 300
        Pathologic Q wave, 292
        Posterior, 310
        Resolution, 299
        Serum markers, 313

Treatment for acute myocardial
        infarction, 381
Myocardial muscle layers, 288
Myocardium, 288
Myoglobin, 313

NASPE pacemaker codes, 220
NSTEMI, 279, 322, 326, 327
Neointimal proliferation, 385
Neurotransmitter, 370
Nonsynchronized precordial shock, 201,
        202
Norepinephrine, 370

Overdrive pacing, 240, 241, 247

P wave, 18, 21, 27, 394
P.A.T. with block, 144
P-P interval, 48, 134
P-R interval, 17, 18, 28, 39, 147, 395
P-R limits (adults), 28
P-R limits (kids), 495
P-R segment, 18
Pacemaker capture, 217, 243
Pacemaker discriminators, 254
Pacemaker failure to sense, 219
Pacemaker generator, 210
Pacemaker identification codes, 230, 245,
        246
Pacemaker mediated tachycardia (PMT),
        242
Pacemaker programming, 220, 221
Pacemaker rhythm, 213, 214, 220
Pacemaker sensors, 231
Paper time, 24
Paroxysmal atrial tachycardia (P.A.T.),
        kids, 406
Paroxysmal atrial tachycardia (P.A.T.),
        adult, 61
Paroxysmal supraventricular tachycardia
        (P.S.V.T.), 407
Paroxysmal ventricular tachycardia, 123
Pause following premature beats, 58, 110
Pediatric dysrhythmias, 398
Pediatric heart rates, 394
Pericarditis, 290, 396
Permanent pacemaker, 211, 212
PCWP, 353, 354
Physiologic block, 69, 70
Platelet inhibitors, 383
Posterior wall myocardial infarction,
        see myocardial infarction
Potassium, 2, 263
Preload, 339
Premature atrial contractions (P.A.C.s),
        kids, 404
Premature atrial contractions (P.A.C.s),
        adult, 56, 83
Premature junctional beats, kids, 413
Premature junctional beats, adult, 98

Premature ventricular contractions (P.V.C.s), kids, 415
Premature ventricular contractions (P.V.C.s), adult, 109, 110, 136, 379
Pressure points (hemodynamic), 355
Proarrhythmic effect, 366, 379
Procainamide (Pronestyl), 380
Prolonged P-R interval, 147, 422
Pronestyl, 373
Propafenone (Rhythmol), 373
PTCA, 324
Pulmonary artery catheter, 343
Pulmonary artery pressure (PAP), 349
Pulmonary capillary wedge pressure (PCWP), 353, 355
Pulmonic valve, 335, 341
Pulseless electrical activity (PEA) Kids, 420
Pulseless electrical activity (PEA) Adult, 130, 381

Q wave, 19
Q wave, pathologic, *see* myocardial infarction
QRS complex, 19, 20, 39
QRS duration (adult), 28
QRS duration (kids), 396
QT intervals, adult, 22, 264, 272
QT intervals, kids, 396
QT prolongation, 305
Quinidine, 373
QTc, 264
QTd, 305

R wave, 20, 21, 28
R-R interval, 48
Rate dependent bundle branch block, 165
Rate modulation, 229
Re-entry phenomenon, 61, 63, 78, 124
Receptors, 370
Refractory period, 200
Reopro, 383
Repolarization, 2, 16, 22

Resolution of infarct, myocardial infarction, 299
Re-synchronization therapy, 257
Retrograde P waves associated with P.V.C.s, 109
Right atrial (RA) pressure, 346
Right bundle branch block (RBBB), kids, 426
Right bundle branch block (RBBB), adult, 163, 164
Right ventricle (RV) pressure, 348, 349
R on T Phenomenon, 111

S wave, 20
STEMI, 279, 296, 326, 327
Second degree AV block, 150
Serum calcium norms, 268
    Hypercalcemia, 274
    Hypocalcemia, 274
Serum markers, 313
Serum potassium (K+) norms, kids, 428
Serum potassium (K+) norms, adult, 263
Sick-sinus syndrome, 77, 403
Sinus arrest (pause), kids, 402
Sinus arrest (pause), adult, 142
Sinus arrhythmia (adult), 47, 81
Sinus arrhythmia (kids), 399
Sinus block, 142
Sinus bradycardia (adult), 50, 82
Sinus bradycardia (kids), 400
Sinus rhythm, 34, 46
Sinus tachycardia (adult), 53, 82
Sinus tachycardia (kids), 401
Sixty-cycle interference, 180
Skin preparation techniques, 193
Sodium Channel blockers, 373
Sotalol, 375, 380
Stents, 324, 385
ST segment, 22, 396
Standard EKG paper speed, 24
Starling's Law, 339
Streptokinase, 382
Supraventricular tachycardia, 66, 102
Swan-Ganz catheter, 343

Synchronized cardioversion, adult, 201
Synchronized cardioversion, kids, 418
Systole, 335

T wave, 22, 397
Temporary pacemaker, 210, 213, 221
Third degree AV block, AV block, 157, 424
Thrombolytic drugs, 382
Tocainide (Tonocard), 373
Torsades de pointes, 126
TPA (alteplase), 382
Transcutaneous electrical nerve stimulator (T.E.N.S.), artifact, 189
Transcutaneous pacing, 211
Transducer, 344
Tricuspid valve, 341, 352
Trifascicular conduction system, 142
Trigeminy P.V.C.s, 111
Troponin, 313
Trouble-shooting for artifact, 193

U waves, 22, 263
Unifocal, P.V.C.s, 113

Ventricular bigeminy, 111
Ventricular escape beats, 131
Ventricular escape rhythm, 131
Ventricular fibrillation (adult), 128
Ventricular fibrillation (kids), 418
Ventricular flutter, adult, 127, 138, 380
Ventricular flutter, kids, 418
Ventricular re-entry mechanisms, 124
Ventricular tachycardia, adult, 119, 120, 123, 137
Ventricular tachycardia, kids, 417
Verapamil, 376
Vulnerable period, 200

Wandering atrial pacemaker (W.A.P.), kids, 410
Wandering atrial pacemaker (W.A.P.), adult, 55
Wenckebach, *see* AV block
Wolff-Parkinson-White Syndrome, 78